Thyroid For Dummies, 2nd Edition

Maximizing Your Thyroid Health

For more information about these steps, see Chapter 22:

- Ask your doctor to screen you for thyroid disease at appropriate intervals; I recommend being screened every five years beginning at age 35.

- Check your thyroid function during times of major body changes, such as pregnancy.

- Make sure that you get enough iodine in your diet, especially if you're a vegetarian.

- If you've been taking thyroid-hormone replacement for several years to treat hypothyroidism (low thyroid function), ask your doctor if you can try stopping treatment to see if your thyroid can function without it.

- If you still experience symptoms of hypothyroidism while taking hormone-replacement pills, ask your doctor if you can try taking a pill that contains both types of thyroid hormone (T4 and T3).

- Be aware of medications that can interact with thyroid hormones. (For a complete discussion of drug interactions, see Chapter 10.)

- Protect your thyroid from radiation. Be sure that your doctor knows if your neck has been exposed to radiation in the past.

- Be aware of new discoveries in thyroid health and treatment. Appendix B features many Web sites that can help you.

Signs and Symptoms of Low Thyroid Function

Someone with *hypothyroidism* — a low-functioning thyroid — often experiences some of the following signs and symptoms. (Keep in mind that these symptoms alone can't diagnose thyroid disease, and thyroid disease may be present even if you don't experience all these symptoms. See Chapter 5 for detailed information about hypothyroidism.)

- Slow pulse

- Enlarged thyroid (unless it has been removed during prior thyroid treatment)

- Dry, cool skin that's puffy, pale, and yellowish

- Brittle nails and dry, brittle hair that falls out excessively

- Swelling, especially of the legs

- Hoarseness, slow speech, and a thickened tongue

- Slow reflexes

- Intolerance to cold

- Tiredness and a need to sleep excessively

- Constipation

- Increased menstrual flow

Thyroid For Dummies,® 2nd Edition

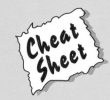
Cheat Sheet

Signs and Symptoms of Excessive Thyroid Function

Someone with *hyperthyroidism* — excessive thyroid function — may experience some or all of the following symptoms. (The same caution about symptoms of hypothyroidism applies here; these symptoms alone don't confirm a diagnosis. Only lab tests ordered by your doctor can confirm a diagnosis. See Chapter 6 for more information about hyperthyroidism.)

- ✔ Higher body temperature and intolerance to heat
- ✔ Weight loss
- ✔ Weakness
- ✔ Enlarged thyroid
- ✔ Warm, moist skin
- ✔ Rapid pulse
- ✔ Tremors of the fingers and tongue
- ✔ Increased reflexes
- ✔ Nervousness
- ✔ Difficulty sleeping
- ✔ Rapid mood changes
- ✔ Decreased menstrual flow
- ✔ More frequent bowel movements
- ✔ Changes to the eyes that make you appear as if you're staring

Medications to Watch Out For

Certain drugs can interact with your thyroid hormone to negatively affect your thyroid function. Chapter 10 goes into detail about this subject, but following are just a few commonly used medications that can impact your thyroid:

- ✔ Amiodarone
- ✔ Aspirin (more than 3,000 milligrams daily)
- ✔ Estrogen
- ✔ Iron tablets
- ✔ Iodine
- ✔ Lithium
- ✔ Propranolol
- ✔ Steroids

Wiley, the Wiley Publishing logo, For Dummies, the Dummies Man logo, the For Dummies Bestselling Book Series logo and all related trade dress are trademarks or registered trademarks of John Wiley & Sons, Inc. and/or its affiliates. All other trademarks are property of their respective owners.

For Dummies: Bestselling Book Series for Beginners

Thyroid

FOR

DUMMIES®

2ND EDITION

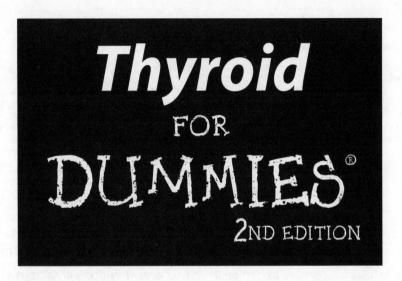

Thyroid
FOR
DUMMIES®
2ND EDITION

by Alan L. Rubin, MD

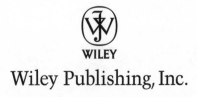

WILEY

Wiley Publishing, Inc.

Thyroid For Dummies®, 2nd Edition

Published by
Wiley Publishing, Inc.
111 River St.
Hoboken, NJ 07030-5774
www.wiley.com

About the Author

Alan L. Rubin, MD, is one of the nation's foremost experts on the thyroid gland in health and disease. He is a member of the Endocrine Society and has been in private practice specializing in thyroid disease and diabetes for over 28 years. Dr. Rubin was Assistant Clinical Professor of Medicine at UC Medical Center in San Francisco for 20 years. He has spoken about the thyroid to professional medical audiences and nonmedical audiences around the world. He is a consultant to many pharmaceutical companies and companies that make thyroid products.

Dr. Rubin has written extensively on the thyroid gland as well as diabetes mellitus. As a result, he has been on numerous radio and television programs talking about the cause, the prevention, and the treatment of conditions of the thyroid. He is also the best-selling author of *Diabetes For Dummies* and *Diabetes Cookbook For Dummies,* both now in second editions and translated into multiple languages including Chinese, Spanish, French, and Russian. His latest book is *High Blood Pressure For Dummies.*

Dedication

The second edition of this book is again dedicated to my wife, Enid. She smilingly let me do my work, sometimes into the wee hours of the morning, and missed many an opportunity to go out to dinner or a movie so that I could produce this book for you. If you have a fraction of the support in your life that she has given me, you are a lucky person, indeed.

Author's Acknowledgments

The great publisher and midwife, Kathy Nebenhaus, deserves enormous appreciation for helping me to deliver yet another bright-eyed baby. Her optimism and her enthusiasm actually made this book possible. Acquisitions editor Michael Lewis played a huge role in ironing out the inevitable problems that arise when book publishing and medicine meet.

My editor, Michael Baker, did a magnificent job turning my sometimes incomprehensible prose into words that you can understand. He also conducted a whole orchestra of other editors who contributed to the book, including Melissa Wiley. My thanks to Dr. Kathleen Bethin for the technical editing of the book.

Librarian Karen O'Grady at St. Francis Memorial Hospital was tremendously helpful in providing the articles and books upon which the information in this book is based.

My teachers are too numerous to mention, but one person deserves special attention. Dr. Francis Greenspan at the University of California Medical Center gave me the sound foundation in thyroid function and disease upon which this book is based.

Finally, there are my patients over the last 28 years, the people whose trials and tribulations caused me to seek the knowledge that you will find in this book. This book is written on the shoulders of thousands of men and women who made the discoveries, tried the medications, and held the committee meetings. Their accomplishments cannot possibly be given adequate acclaim. We owe them big time.

Publisher's Acknowledgments

We're proud of this book; please send us your comments through our Dummies online registration form located at www.dummies.com/register/.

Some of the people who helped bring this book to market include the following:

Acquisitions, Editorial, and Media Development

Project Editor: Mike Baker

(Previous Edition: Joan Friedman)

Acquisitions Editor: Michael Lewis

Copy Editor: Melissa Wiley

Editorial Program Coordinator: Hanna K. Scott

Technical Editor: Kathleen Bethin, MD

Editorial Manager: Christine Meloy Beck

Editorial Assistants: Erin Calligan, David Lutton

Cartoons: Rich Tennant
(www.the5thwave.com)

Composition Services

Project Coordinator: Adrienne Martinez

Layout and Graphics: Carl Byers, Andrea Dahl, Stephanie Jumper, Barbara Moore, Heather Ryan

Special Art: Kathryn Born

Proofreaders: Laura Albert, Leeann Harney, Jessica Kramer, Techbooks

Indexer: Techbooks

Publishing and Editorial for Consumer Dummies

    Diane Graves Steele, Vice President and Publisher, Consumer Dummies

    Joyce Pepple, Acquisitions Director, Consumer Dummies

    Kristin A. Cocks, Product Development Director, Consumer Dummies

    Michael Spring, Vice President and Publisher, Travel

    Kelly Regan, Editorial Director, Travel

Publishing for Technology Dummies

    Andy Cummings, Vice President and Publisher, Dummies Technology/General User

Composition Services

    Gerry Fahey, Vice President of Production Services

    Debbie Stailey, Director of Composition Services

Contents at a Glance

Table of Contents

Introduction

· ·

*W*hen the first edition of this book was published more than four years ago, I knew that knowledge of the thyroid and its diseases was minimal among the general public, but I had no idea of the burning desire of that same public to know more. Judging by the many thousands of copies that have been sold and the hundreds of e-mails that I have received, this book filled a huge gap. So many of you have written to thank me for helping you to understand what the thyroid does when it's working normally and how to tell when it isn't working normally.

The purpose of this second edition is to educate you about the newest developments since the previous edition and to fill in the areas that you tell me need more discussion and explanation. I thank you for your praise, your suggestions, and for allowing us specialists to study and understand you for the benefit of others.

As I entered the psychiatric medical unit at Bellevue Hospital the first day of my internship in 1966, I noticed a loud woman with penetrating eyes. I looked closely at her and saw that her neck was very enlarged. Because I was the new doctor on the unit, I picked up her chart and discovered that she had a case of Graves' disease, a form of excessive thyroid production. For the next few months, I became intimately involved with her problems. She taught me a great deal about thyroid disease and probably represents the explanation for my lifelong interest in this subject. I've taken care of many such patients over the years (though never again in a psychiatric unit), but she stands out in my memory like a first love.

For hundreds of years, people have understood that a connection exists between a strange-looking growth in the neck and certain diseases. Until about 60 years ago, confusion reigned because people with similar growths in their necks often had opposite conditions. One group would show excessive excitement, nervousness, and shakiness; the other would show depression, sleepiness, and general loss of interest. What the two groups had in common was that they consisted mostly of women.

Around 60 years ago, measuring the chemicals that were coming from those growths (enlarged thyroid glands) became possible, and suddenly the whole picture began to make sense. Since then, a vast amount has been learned about the thyroid, the chemicals (hormones) made in that gland, and the purpose of those hormones.

In this book, you benefit from the hard work of doctors and other scientists over the last few hundred years. You find that, with very rare exceptions, thyroid diseases, including thyroid cancer, are some of the most easily treated of all disorders (which is why many thyroid specialists say, "If I have to have a cancer, let it be thyroid cancer.")

After you read this book, I hope you're a lot less confused than the poor thyroid itself, which doesn't know where it is. I once heard the left side of a thyroid say to the right, "We must be in Capistrano. Here comes another swallow." If you've read any of my previous books, *Diabetes For Dummies, Diabetes Cookbook For Dummies,* and *High Blood Pressure For Dummies,* you know that I use humor to get my ideas across, a technique that characterizes the *For Dummies* series. I want to emphasize that I'm not trying to trivialize anyone's suffering by being comic. The work of Norman Cousins and others has shown that humor has healing properties. A positive attitude is far more conducive to a positive outcome than is a negative attitude.

About This Book

I don't expect you to read this book from cover to cover. Because the first few chapters are a general introduction to the thyroid, you may want to start in Part I, but if you prefer to go right to information about the thyroid condition that affects you, by all means do so. If you run across any terms that you don't understand, look for them in the glossary of terms in Appendix A.

I've written this book as a sort of medical biography of the Dummy family — Tami Dummy, Stacy Dummy, Linda Dummy, Ken Dummy, and other members of the clan whom you meet during your reading. These folks illustrate the fact that thyroid disease often runs in families. (Exceptions do exist to this fact, which I explain.) You meet members of the Dummy family, as well as some other fine fictional folks, at the beginning of each chapter that describes a thyroid disease so that you have a good picture of the condition I cover in that chapter.

One very big difference between thyroid disease and the other diseases that I wrote about in *Diabetes For Dummies* and *High Blood Pressure For Dummies* is that thyroid disease isn't a lifestyle disease. You can't cure any disease of the thyroid that I know of by changing your diet, exercising more, drinking less alcohol, or smoking fewer cigarettes. Although those changes are good for your health in general, you can't cure thyroid disease on your own. You need your doctor's help and sometimes the help of a specialist. What I hope you gain from this book is a good general knowledge of the thyroid gland and an understanding of the correct approach to thyroid disease. At the least, you should be able to ask much more informed questions and even decide for yourself how you want the doctor to approach your disease in some situations.

Many "facts" in the treatment of thyroid disease aren't so factual when you look at the medical research literature. For instance, one "fact" dictates that doctors always start with a low dose of thyroid hormone when treating an older person who has low thyroid function in order to avoid overstressing the older person's heart. But research doesn't support this rule. This book points out many such examples of incorrect "facts" that doctors often believe with no evidence to support them.

Conventions Used in This Book

To help you navigate this book, I use the following conventions:

- ✔ *Italic* text is used for emphasis and to highlight new words and terms that we define in the text.

- ✔ **Boldfaced** text is used to indicate keywords in bulleted lists or the action parts of numbered steps.

- ✔ `Monofont` is used for Web addresses. If you find that a specific address in this book has been changed, try scaling it back by going to the main site — the part of the address that ends in `.com`, `.org`, or `.edu`.

- ✔ Sidebars are shaded gray boxes that contain text that's interesting to know but not necessarily critical to your understanding of the chapter or topic.

And as much as I'd love to use all nonscientific terms in this book, if I did so, you and your doctor would be speaking two different languages. Therefore, I do use scientific terms, but I explain them in everyday English the first time you run across them. Plus, those difficult terms are defined in the glossary at the back of the book.

Three scientific terms come up over and over again in this book: *thyroxine, triiodothyronine,* and *thyroid-stimulating hormone* (also known as *thyrotropin*). I explain these terms in detail in Chapter 3. For these three words, I often use abbreviations: Thyroxine is T4, triiodothyronine is T3, and thyroid-stimulating hormone is TSH.

Assumptions

I make the assumption in this book that you or someone you care about has a thyroid condition that hasn't been treated or perhaps isn't being treated to your satisfaction. If this assumption doesn't apply to you, perhaps you suspect that you have a thyroid condition and want to determine whether you should see a doctor, or you can't get your doctor to run the necessary tests to determine whether a thyroid problem exists. Regardless of your individual situation, this book has valuable information for you.

I try to make no assumptions about what you know related to the thyroid. I don't introduce any new terms without explaining what they are. If you already know a lot about the thyroid and its functions, you can still find new information that adds to your knowledge.

How This Book Is Organized

The book is divided into five parts to help you find out all you want to know about the thyroid gland.

Part 1: Examining the Thyroid

Here is where you gain an understanding of the function of the thyroid and its location in your body. You're able to tell if the gland is working the way it should. In this part, you learn about the medical tests that help us determine if something is wrong with your thyroid. Your doctor orders these tests, but you need to understand their meaning and which ones are appropriate for the condition you have. This understanding helps you know the severity of your condition and when it's under control. A test that works in some situations isn't always valid in others. I try to let you know when exceptions occur. Be careful not to frighten your doctor with the extent of your knowledge.

Because you can't cure your thyroid disease without your doctor's help, and often without the help of a specialist, I tell you how to find a good specialist in this part. Although far too many patients with thyroid disease exist for each one to see one of the limited numbers of specialists, in some cases a specialist is essential, and you need to know how to fine a good one in your area.

Part II: Diagnosing and Treating Thyroid Conditions

This part explains each of the conditions that affect the thyroid and how they affect you. By the time you finish with this part of the book, I may be able to retire, because you will know just about everything I know about thyroid disease: how to identify it and how to treat it. External factors also influence your thyroid, particularly drugs you may take and irradiation that you may have had. I discuss these factors in this part of the book.

Many people who wrote to me asked if certain of their symptoms were found in one of the thyroid diseases I discuss. Many people who were already diagnosed with the disease asked me if a particular symptom was part of the disease process. I add a number of minor symptoms to the lists to be more inclusive. The question also arises as to whether the presence of certain symptoms after the disease has been cured means the disease is back. I clear up that issue as well.

Part III: Reviewing Special Considerations in Thyroid Health

Thyroid conditions can have a profound effect on your mental health. You understand what's happening in your brain along with the rest of your body when your thyroid gland is overactive or underactive. Unfortunately, such conditions impair your ability to think, so understanding this book may be more difficult for the person who hasn't received treatment for his or her thyroid condition, which gives me more reason to be as clear as possible. Let me know if I'm not completely successful in doing this.

Throughout the book are many mentions about the hereditary nature of many of the thyroid diseases. A chapter in this part explains how people inherit thyroid diseases. You can do little to alter your genes unless you know a way to choose your parents. In that case, you wouldn't be the same you anyway.

Three groups of people deserve special consideration in this book: pregnant women, children, and the elderly. Thyroid conditions take unusual directions in these groups, so the chapters in this part address their unique difficulties. The final chapter here offers suggestions for ways to improve your thyroid health — and your health in general — through diet, exercise, and lifestyle choices.

Part IV: The Part of Tens

Misinformation about the thyroid is rampant. In this part, I clear up some of that misinformation (though not all, because it accumulates faster than I can address it). I also show you how you can maximize your thyroid health. Thanks to all your questions, I have a new chapter in this part that answers the ten questions that recurred most often in your e-mails and seemed most important to clear up. Many things that seem so obvious to a person who has studied the thyroid and its diseases for thirty years may not be obvious for the person newly diagnosed with a thyroid disease. Keep those questions coming to me at thyroid@drrubin.com, and who knows — your question may appear in the next edition of this book.

Part V: Appendixes

In Appendix A, you find a glossary of medical terms that relate to the thyroid; you may want to bookmark the glossary so you can go back and forth with ease as you read other chapters. In Appendix B, I direct you to the best-of-the-best Web sites, where you can get dependable facts to fill in any blank spots that remain after you read this book. Remember that Web sites are in flux. Some begin, and some close. If you want to be aware of the latest and most reliable Web sites, check at my Web site, www.drrubin.com, every so often. At my Web site, you're able to click on a choice of one of three lists of "Related Websites" about diabetes, thyroid, and high blood pressure. They're the most up-to-date and reliable resources on these subjects. And when you're there, you may listen to my healthcasts (podcasts), several of which are about the thyroid gland.

Icons Used in This Book

Books in the *For Dummies* series feature icons in the margins, which direct you toward information that may be of particular interest or importance.

This icon means the information is essential. You want to be sure you understand it.

This icon points out important information that can save you time and energy.

This icon alerts you to situations in which you may need to dial up your doctor for some help.

This icon warns against potential problems you can encounter, such as the side effects of mixing medications.

This icon alerts you to information that, while informative, may provide a little more detail than you're looking for.

Where to Go from Here

Where you go from here depends on your needs. If you want to understand how the thyroid works, head to Part I. If you or someone you know has a thyroid condition, you may want to pay particular attention to Part II. For help in maintaining good thyroid health, turn to Part III. If you're pregnant or have a child or parent with a thyroid disorder, Part IV is your next stop. In any case, as my mother used to say when she gave me a present, use this book in good health.

If you've had an unusual or even a humorous thyroid experience you'd like to share, by all means, let me know about it by e-mailing me at `thyroid@drrubin.com`. Who knows — I may share it with the world in a future edition of this book.

Part I
Examining the Thyroid

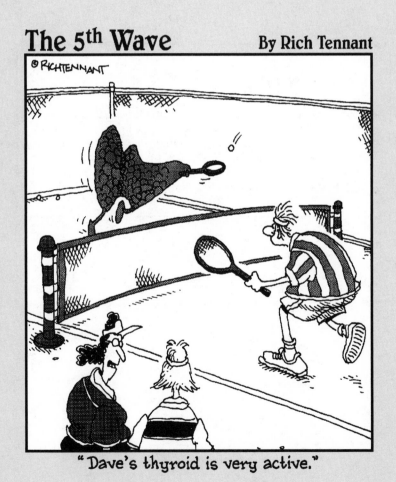

The 5th Wave   By Rich Tennant

"Dave's thyroid is very active."

In this part . . .

What exactly is the thyroid gland, and what does it do? In this part, you discover how important this little gland in your neck really is, what function it plays in your body, and how to determine if it is functioning properly. I also help you find a specialist who can help you fight thyroid disease.

Chapter 1

The Big Role of a Little Gland

*T*he thyroid is a little like Rodney Dangerfield: It doesn't get the respect it deserves. Anyone who watches those primetime TV news shows knows about the importance of other body parts — the heart and lungs sure get a lot of press time. But unless you come face to face with a thyroid problem, chances are that you don't hear much about what this little gland does and how important it is to your good health.

The fact that you're reading these words tells me that you've encountered a thyroid problem personally. (I suppose you could have just picked this book up off the shelf out of curiosity — or because you belong to the Dr. Rubin fan club — but I'm betting that a thyroid problem is the more likely impetus.) Maybe you've recently been diagnosed with a thyroid condition. Or maybe your husband, wife, mother, or friend is receiving treatment for a thyroid problem. You've probably found out at least a little about this mysterious gland. Now you're looking for answers to the questions that keep popping up in your mind:

✔ What causes this thyroid condition?

✔ What types of symptoms are related to this thyroid problem?

✔ How is this thyroid condition treated?

✔ What are the consequences of leaving it untreated?

✔ Does treatment end the problem forever?

✔ What can I (or my husband, wife, mother, or friend) do to help get back to optimal health?

I can't promise that this book will give you every possible answer to your questions. After all, doctors and researchers are constantly discovering new things about the thyroid — the information here is only as complete as our current knowledge. But if you're looking for concrete information about how the thyroid functions, what makes it malfunction, and what to do when a problem occurs, you're holding the right book.

Discovering the Extent of the Problem

Thyroid disease may be one of the most common diseases in the world. Research indicates that thyroid disease affects more than 200 million people worldwide. Table 1-1 shows the approximate incidence, or number of new cases a year, in 2004 of various types of thyroid disease in the United States, which has a population of more than 275 million.

Table 1-1	Incidence of Thyroid Disorders in the U.S.
Hypothyroidism (low thyroid function)	1.5 million
Hyperthyroidism (excessive thyroid function)	375,000
Thyroid cancer	37,500
Death due to thyroid cancer	2,250

The incidence of thyroid disease becomes even higher when you factor in careful autopsies done on people who didn't die of a thyroid condition. As many as 60 percent of these people show growths on the thyroid, and 17 percent have small areas of cancer that weren't detected during life.

These numbers are statistics, but thyroid disease affects individuals. Realizing that many people in the public eye have gone on to great accomplishments after receiving successful treatment for thyroid conditions may help you. Some of the people you may recognize include the following:

- Model Kim Alexis had hypothyroidism.
- Author Isaac Asimov had thyroid cancer.
- Golfers Pat Bradley and Ben Crenshaw both had hyperthyroidism.
- Former President George Bush, former first lady Barbara Bush, and even their dog Millie had hyperthyroidism.
- Runner Gail Devers had hyperthyroidism, while runner Carl Lewis had hypothyroidism.
- Supreme Court Chief Justice William Renquist had the very rare and most aggressive form of thyroid cancer.

✔ Roger Ebert, the movie critic, had thyroid cancer.

✔ Former second lady Tipper Gore received treatment for a thyroid growth, as did singer Rod Stewart.

I particularly enjoy the story of Isaac Asimov. He had thyroid cancer at age 52, and he died of unrelated causes at age 72. After his cancer surgery, he wrote about how he'd paid $1,500 for the surgery and then wrote an article about the experience, for which he received $2,000. Asimov said that he had the last laugh on the medical profession and was glad that he didn't finish medical school.

This list is far from exhaustive, but it should help drive home the point that if diagnosed and treated, thyroid conditions don't need to put a damper on your lifestyle, except in very rare cases.

Identifying an Unhappy Thyroid

Let's tackle some basics: Where is the thyroid, and how do you know when it needs some tender loving care? Chapter 2 gives you a detailed explanation of how to locate your thyroid, but for now, suffice it to say that it's just below your Adam's apple, at the front of your neck. If your thyroid becomes visible in your neck, if that area of your neck is tender, or if you have some trouble swallowing or breathing, consider visiting your doctor so that he or she can examine your thyroid. Any change in the size or shape of your thyroid can indicate that it's not functioning correctly or that you have growths on your thyroid, called *nodules,* which should be tested to rule out cancer (see Chapter 7). Soreness or tenderness in the area of your thyroid may indicate that you have an infection or inflammation, which I discuss in Chapter 11.

In addition to changes in the size and shape of the gland, some very common problems occur when your thyroid malfunctions. If your thyroid function is low, meaning that you aren't producing enough thyroid hormone, (you have *hypothyroidism*), you feel cold, tired, and maybe even a little depressed. I know that description doesn't sound very specific — those symptoms could indicate any number of other physical problems. But low thyroid function is so prevalent that asking your doctor to check it out is worth it if you experience such symptoms, especially if you're over age 35. Chapter 5 gives you the specifics about the causes and symptoms of hypothyroidism.

When your thyroid function is too high, meaning that you're producing too much thyroid hormone, (you have *hyperthyroidism*), you feel hyper and warm, and your heart races. You may have trouble sitting still, and your emotions may change very rapidly for no clear reason. These symptoms are a little more specific than those for low thyroid function, but again, they could easily result from some cause unrelated to your thyroid. The best way to determine whether a thyroid problem exists is to ask your doctor to check your thyroid function. Chapter 6 offers a detailed look at hyperthyroidism.

Recognizing Who's at Risk

A few key facts help doctors determine whether thyroid disease is a strong probability:

 ✔ Women experience thyroid problems much more frequently than men, as much as 10 to 15 times as often, depending on the condition.

 ✔ Thyroid conditions tend to run in families.

 ✔ Thyroid problems often arise after the age of 30.

These facts don't mean that a 20-year-old man with no family history of thyroid problems can't develop a thyroid condition. They simply mean that a 35-year-old woman whose mother was diagnosed with low thyroid function 20 years ago is at greater risk of having a thyroid problem than the young man. With this in mind, the young woman should be sure to tell her doctor about her family history. And she should definitely be tested periodically to make sure her thyroid function is normal.

About half (perhaps even more) of all the people with thyroid disorders are undiagnosed. The American Thyroid Association and other experts recommend that thyroid testing begin at age 35 and continue every five years thereafter. Women with family histories of thyroid disease may benefit from even more frequent testing.

Realizing the Importance of a Healthy Thyroid

Your thyroid gland influences almost every cell and organ in your body, because its general function is to control your metabolism. If your thyroid is functioning correctly, your metabolism should be normal. If your thyroid is working too hard (making too much hormone), your metabolism is too high. The result can be anything from an increased body temperature to an elevated heart rate. When your thyroid function drops below normal and you make too little hormone, so does your metabolism — you may gain weight, feel tired, and experience digestive problems.

Chapter 2 details how your thyroid affects various parts of your body, including your muscles, heart, lungs, stomach, intestines, skin, hair, nails, brain, bones, and sexual organs. (That's quite a list!)

Treating What Ails You

Depending on the specific thyroid problem, treatment options can range from taking a daily pill to having surgery to remove part or all of the thyroid. I discuss the details of treatment options and offer my opinions about which options are generally best throughout Part II of this book. But keep in mind that no matter what you read here (or anywhere else), you should always discuss your specific situation with your doctor. This book can help you have a more productive conversation with your doctor by explaining the pros and cons of each type of treatment and by suggesting questions to ask your doctor if a treatment doesn't seem to be working for you. It can't, however, act as a substitute for your doctor, because I don't know the ins and outs of your particular case.

However, following are the general approaches for treating the most common thyroid conditions:

- **Hypothyroidism:** In general, if you experience hypothyroidism (low thyroid function), your doctor prescribes a daily pill to replace the thyroid hormone that your body is lacking. Many people take this type of pill for the rest of their lives, but some people are able to stop taking it after a few years if lab tests prove that the condition has righted itself. See Chapter 5 for a detailed discussion of treating hypothyroidism.

- **Hyperthyroidism:** Three types of treatment options exist for someone with hyperthyroidism (an overactive thyroid). A patient with this condition may be placed on antithyroid drugs, may be receive a dose of radioactive iodine in a pill in order to destroy part of the thyroid tissue, or may undergo surgery to remove some or all of the thyroid gland. In the United States, most doctors recommend the radioactive iodine treatment for this condition, but I've seen antithyroid drugs work very well for many patients. Doctors generally perform surgery only when a patient can't have one of the other two treatments. Chapter 6 goes into the specifics about each treatment and explains why your doctor may suggest one treatment over the others, depending on your specific situation.

- **Thyroid cancer:** For patients with thyroid cancer, surgery is often required. Doctors may also use radioactive iodine to destroy any thyroid tissue that remains after the surgery. Chapter 8 discusses the treatment of various types of thyroid cancer.

- **Nodules:** Someone whose thyroid has *nodules* (bumps) may need surgery, may not need treatment at all, or may need a type of treatment that falls between those extremes, such as thyroid hormone replacement or radioactive iodine. See Chapters 7 and 9 for all the details about how your doctor may deal with thyroid bumps and lumps.

Sometimes the complications surrounding your thyroid condition are too much for the general physician to handle. At that point, you need a specialist. But how do you go about finding one that you know is competent? To answer this question, I've inserted Chapter 3 into this edition of the book. It tells you what to look for in a thyroid specialist and how to go about finding one. As much as I'd love to personally take care of all of you, considerations of time require that I send you to some other physicians. I give you directions in Chapter 3 to find the best qualified doctor to help you.

Once you have your specialist, he or she can help you to understand the various tests that doctors run to determine the severity of your thyroid condition and to follow the condition as it improves. These tests range from blood tests to various ways of visualizing the thyroid to biopsies. Chapter 4 provides a basic introduction to these tests and which tests your doctor should order and when. Some old-fashioned doctors are still ordering old-fashioned tests, and I explain these tests in Chapter 4 so you know their meaning. Don't hesitate to tell your doctor that you think a newer test is more appropriate. Refer the doctor to this book if he or she disagrees.

And as you can see from the preceding list of treatments, in the course of treatment for thyroid ailments, many people undergo surgery of the thyroid. I want you to understand what to expect if you have surgery, which is why I conclude the chapters on thyroid disease and its treatment with a chapter on surgery of the thyroid, Chapter 13. The most important aspect of such surgery is finding a highly competent surgeon, and I tell you how to do this.

Examining Additional Contributors to Thyroid Ailments

Many drugs have an effect on the thyroid, and Chapter 10 explains the most important of these effects: whether they're increasing thyroid function or blocking thyroid hormone production. The drugs that can impact your thyroid have all sorts of primary actions, but they also change thyroid function. If you're already on thyroid hormone, you need to understand that these drugs can change your dosage. You may need more or less thyroid hormone. Understanding what you need to do to maintain normal thyroid function while you take a drug for some other reason is important. Make sure you ask your doctor if a new medication interferes with your thyroid medicine.

Viruses and bacteria can also invade the thyroid. You may have a mild condition with a little pain in your neck or a severe illness with high fever, severe weakness, chills, and so much neck pain that you need a strong painkiller. Chapter 11 explains viral or bacterial forms of "thyroiditis," which are very different from other forms of thyroiditis, which I explain in Chapters 5 and 11.

Because thyroid hormones contain a lot of iodine, situations where too little iodine is in your body or too much iodine is in your body also change your thyroid function. Outside the industrialized nations, iodine deficiency causes major disease and even death for millions of people. Theoretically, death from iodine deficiency could be overcome without a great deal of difficulty, but the practical considerations of race and politics have made this very hard to do. In more industrialized nations, too much iodine is a greater problem, and Chapter 12 explains the consequences of both of these situations.

Realizing the Consequences of Delaying Treatment

Earlier in the chapter, I mention that at least half of all people with thyroid conditions are undiagnosed. Many people die of other causes without ever discovering their thyroid problem, which may lead you to wonder whether the diagnosis and treatment of thyroid problems is really necessary.

In some situations, a thyroid condition may be so benign that you don't even notice it. For example, many people with thyroid nodules never have any problems except for a little bump on the neck. In those cases, treatment may be unnecessary. Some patients have no symptoms at all, yet the laboratory tests of thyroid function indicate that they have low thyroid hormone production. Debate exists about whether such patients need treatment. I discuss this issue extensively in Chapter 5.

But for many other people, thyroid conditions are much more serious, having a significant impact on overall health and quality of life. The section "Realizing the Importance of a Healthy Thyroid," earlier in this chapter, gives you a sense of some of the consequences of delaying treatment. If you leave a low-functioning thyroid untreated, you could become so fatigued and depressed that you have trouble just doing your daily activities. With an overactive thyroid, you could experience heart trouble and extreme nervousness. A cancerous thyroid could be life threatening if untreated, depending on the type of cancer. And a thyroid with many nodules could become so enlarged or misshapen that it impacts your ability to swallow or breathe.

Unless your symptoms are already extreme, only lab tests can determine whether treatment for your thyroid condition is necessary. Given how important this little gland is to your health, both physical and mental, I can't imagine not asking your doctor to determine whether you need treatment.

Paying Attention to Special Groups and Considerations

I believe that everyone should have thyroid tests periodically, especially after age 30, to ensure that their thyroids are working as they should. But certain groups of people need to pay special attention to their thyroid function. Pregnant women, children, and the elderly have even more at stake than other folks when it comes to monitoring thyroid function. For this reason, I devote much of Part III of this book to these three groups of people, as well as to some other important considerations that you need to know about.

Doctors first discover that many patients have a thyroid condition when they have a breakdown in their mental health. They may be depressed, or they may be thought to be manic, unable to sit still and complaining that their heart is racing — situations where medication and other treatments can cure a disease that appears to be mental in origin if the thyroid is at fault. Chapter 15 shows you how your thyroid affects your mind and how your mind can return to health through treating the underlying thyroid condition. If I accomplish just one thing with this book, I hope I can raise your awareness of the mental consequences of thyroid disease, which can have such devastating effects if left undiagnosed and untreated.

A lot is new in our understanding of the thyroid in health and disease, which is the main reason that you're now reading the second edition of this book. I explore the most important of these advances in Chapter 16, so don't miss it. Nevertheless, science keeps finding even more valuable information, so be sure to go to my Web site at www.drrubin.com and click on "Thyroid" under the topic "Related Websites" to find the information that comes out even after this book is published, the stuff that will make it into the third edition.

Pregnancy can have a big impact on a woman's thyroid, whether she had a thyroid condition prior to the pregnancy or not. If she does have a known thyroid condition, her doctor monitors it closely during pregnancy, because her treatment may need altering. But if she doesn't have a thyroid condition, she and her doctor should watch carefully for signs and symptoms of thyroid problems, which the physiological changes she's experiencing can trigger.

Not only is a healthy thyroid crucial for the mother during pregnancy, but it's essential for the development of the fetus as well. For details about what to watch for during pregnancy and the types of problems a thyroid condition can create for mother and child, see Chapter 17. You also find information about the thyroid problems that can arise even after the pregnancy, which can be very devastating to the new mother.

Chapter 18 discusses the importance of thyroid screening after the baby is born. Screening is mandatory by law, because a healthy thyroid is necessary for proper mental and physical development. If you're a parent of an infant or young child, be sure to take a look at Chapter 18 so you understand what the screening is for, what risks children of parents with thyroid disease face, and how you and your doctor can reduce those risks.

The third group that should pay special attention to thyroid health is the elderly (for purposes of this discussion, people age 70 and over). The reason they're at such risk for thyroid disease is because the symptoms of a thyroid condition so often mirror symptoms of other ailments. If an elderly person is known to have a heart or blood pressure problem, a doctor may overlook a possible diagnosis of thyroid disease and attribute his or her symptoms to another condition. To confuse the issue even more, elderly people often experience symptoms that are *opposite* of what we expect to see with a certain thyroid condition. For example, an elderly person with a low-functioning thyroid may actually lose weight (instead of gaining weight, which would be expected), because he or she is depressed and loses interest in food. Chapter 19 helps you to understand how thyroid disease affects you if you're elderly or if you have an elderly relative.

Keeping the Rest of Your Body Healthy

So you or a loved one has received a diagnosis of a thyroid problem — what next? You start taking a prescription, or you undergo another type of treatment, and you wonder what else you should be doing to help yourself along toward better health. Did you do something that led to this problem in the first place? Can you make some change in your lifestyle that will lead to a cure?

I wish I could just tell you that if you ate more lima beans and got eight hours of sleep each night, your thyroid would return to perfect health. I could stop writing right now if that were the case. Unfortunately, the line between lifestyle choices and thyroid health isn't quite so straight. Your lifestyle definitely plays a role in your thyroid health, but lifestyle doesn't seem to cause thyroid conditions in the first place. If you receive a diagnosis of a hyperactive thyroid, for example, you most likely have the condition because you inherited a certain gene (or group of genes), as I discuss in Chapter 14. But if your life is full of stress, if you sleep only five hours a night, and if you drink lots of caffeine to get through the day, you definitely aren't doing your thyroid any favors. You may be aggravating the symptoms of your thyroid condition through your lifestyle choices. If you make some positive changes to your eating, sleeping, and exercise habits, your thyroid will definitely benefit.

In Chapter 20, I suggest ways that you can take a proactive role in upgrading your thyroid health by improving your diet, reducing your stress, exercising on a regular basis, and keeping a close eye on other aspects of your lifestyle.

Your thyroid gland doesn't exist in a vacuum. Your diet, the exercise you do, and your lifestyle in general all affect it. Although I've said that poor lifestyle choices don't cause thyroid disease, a healthy lifestyle will help to make any thyroid treatment work to its greatest extent, which is why I go into the basics of achieving a healthy lifestyle in Chapter 20. Chapter 20 informs you how the thyroid affects your weight. You may be surprised.

Finally, in the traditional Part of Tens, I offer ten or more things you need to know about myths surrounding the thyroid (Chapter 21) and about maximizing thyroid health (Chapter 22). You also find a new chapter that you've helped me to write in a way. In Chapter 23, I try to answer the major questions that you've asked me over the past few years since the first edition of the book was published. I hope you keep writing to me at thyroid@drrubin.com so I can continue to address your concerns about the thyroid gland. Many aspects of the thyroid that I take for granted may be unclear to you. I need you to let me know about them. If I can't put them into the next edition of this book, I can at least reply to your questions immediately through e-mail.

My goal is to help you preserve and defend your thyroid by knowing what to look for no matter what stage of life you're in. The more you know about the signs and symptoms of thyroid disease, the earlier you're able to alert your doctor that thyroid function tests may be a good idea.

Staying Informed

Doctors don't know everything. We do, however, tend to have an insatiable curiosity that drives us to always seek more information about the conditions we encounter. For this reason, new discoveries and treatment breakthroughs are popping up all the time. By the time this book is printed, doctors will have conducted hundreds of new studies that suggest or prove something new about thyroid diseases and their treatment.

I can't update this book every time I discover something new, but you can still stay on top of the latest discoveries thanks to the speed of the Internet. In Appendix B, I direct you to electronic resources that you can use to stay up to date on thyroid health. If you use only one of these resources, I hope that it's my own Web page, www.drrubin.com, which can link you to all the other sites I recommend, as I describe in the section "Paying Special Attention." And I promise a new edition of this book in a few years will gather together all the newest information so you can always be on the cutting edge of thyroid knowledge.

Chapter 2

How the Thyroid Works

The thyroid is a unique organ (or gland) that affects every part of your body by making hormones and sending them into your bloodstream, which carries them to every other cell and organ. (*Hormones* are substances made in one organ and carried by body fluids to another organ, where they produce an effect.) These hormones perform many different functions depending upon the particular organ your thyroid sends them to.

In this chapter, I show you how to locate your thyroid. If you're really perceptive and your thyroid is on the larger side, you may even be able to feel it. I describe the names of the various hormones that control your thyroid and that your thyroid produces. I show you what happens to your body when you produce thyroid hormones in excessive or insufficient amounts. And because your body contains many organs that perform various functions, I explain what thyroid hormones do in each organ to make that organ work more efficiently. This chapter also shows you how to recognize when the thyroid is abnormal in size and shape.

If you read this whole chapter, you'll know so much about thyroid function that you'll never suffer from *hamburger hyperthyroidism,* a real disease that results from eating cuts of meat that include the thyroid gland of the cow. When you finish this chapter, I expect that you'll have a much greater appreciation for your thyroid gland.

Picturing Your Thyroid

Have you ever seen one of those wonderful anatomy books where you can peel the layers away, starting from the skin and moving down, to see all the inner structures of the body? If you did that with the neck, as soon as you peeled away the skin, you'd find a bony, V-shaped notch created by the connection of the inside edges of the collar bones. The tissue that surrounds the front and sides of the *trachea* (windpipe) between the V and your Adam's apple is the *thyroid gland.* You can see the gland in Figure 2-1 with some of the more important surrounding structures.

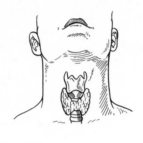

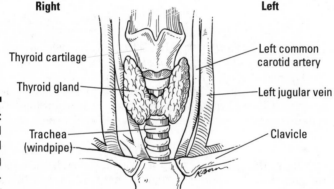

Right   **Left**

Thyroid cartilage — — Left common carotid artery

Thyroid gland — — Left jugular vein

Figure 2-1:
The thyroid
gland and
surrounding
anatomy.

Trachea — — Clavicle
(windpipe)

 If you want to find your thyroid (without peeling away your skin), place your index finger at the bony notch below your Adam's apple and push your finger toward the back of your neck. If you then swallow, you may feel something push up against your finger. You're feeling your thyroid gland!

In Figure 2-1, you see that the thyroid has the shape of a butterfly. The wings of the butterfly are called the *left* and *right lobes* of the thyroid. Connecting the lobes is the *isthmus,* a narrow strip of tissue between the two larger parts. Sometimes you can see a third thyroid lobe called the *pyramidal lobe,* another narrow strip of thyroid tissue rising up from the isthmus.

If you look at the thyroid under a microscope, you can see that it consists of rings of cells one cell deep with a clear center that contains the thyroid hormones. The rings are called *follicles* and are shown in Figure 2-2.

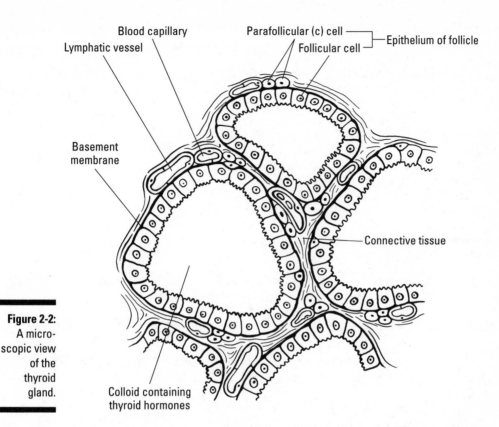

Lymphatic vessel

Blood capillary

Parafollicular (c) cell

Follicular cell

Epithelium of follicle

Basement membrane

Connective tissue

Figure 2-2:
A micro-
scopic view
of the
thyroid
gland.

Colloid containing
thyroid hormones

When the thyroid is normal in size, it weighs between 10 and 20 grams, or somewhere between one-fiftieth and one-twenty-fifth of a pound — not terribly large considering everything it does. Each lobe of the thyroid is only about the size of the last bone of your thumb underneath your nail. Even so, the thyroid is one of the largest hormone-producing glands in your body.

Examining the Production of Thyroid Hormones

The production of thyroid hormones actually begins in the brain, as shown in Figure 2-3. A structure called the *hypothalamus* (part of the brain that regulates many basic functions, such as body temperature) produces a hormone called *thyrotrophin-releasing hormone* (TRH). This hormone is carried a short distance in the brain to the pituitary gland, where it promotes the release of *thyroid-stimulating hormone* (TSH).

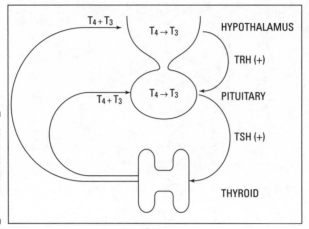

Figure 2-3:
Your brain
stimulates
thyroid
hormone
production.

TSH leaves the pituitary gland and travels in the bloodstream to the thyroid. When TSH reaches the thyroid, it prompts two reactions:

- ✔ It causes the release of existing thyroid hormone into the blood.
- ✔ It prompts the production of more thyroid hormones, which collect in the space inside the follicles (see the section "Picturing Your Thyroid" earlier in this chapter), awaiting future release.

Meeting the hormones

The two thyroid hormones are thyroxine (T4) and triiodothyronine (T3). T3 is the active form of thyroid hormone. T4 is considered a *prohormone,* a much weaker chemical that gains its potency only after it's converted to T3 by the thyroid or another organ of the body (wherever thyroid hormones do their work).

The thyroid gland normally releases about 13 times as much T4 as T3. However, your body as a whole produces only about three times as much T4 as T3. That T3 production gap is closed by organs such as the liver, kidneys, and muscles, which produce most (80 percent) of the T3 in your body through T4 conversion. The thyroid gland itself releases only 20 percent of the T3 it produces every day.

These production facts have profound importance for the treatment of thyroid hormone deficiencies. Most patients with *hypothyroidism* (low thyroid function) are deficient in T3 and T4, but during treatment, they receive only T4 (by ingesting daily doses of replacement thyroid hormone). Their bodies must get the T3 they need by converting the T4. Despite the conversion, some patients are still somewhat deficient in T3. I discuss this problem and possible solutions in Chapter 5.

Identifying the importance of iodine

Another substance that has a major effect on the production of thyroid hormones is iodine. When iodine is present in large amounts in the blood, it reduces the production of the hormones by blocking the stimulating effect of TSH. Doctors use this function, for example, when a patient is extremely hyperthyroid (see Chapter 6) to bring the patient under control rapidly. Iodine may also be used before surgery to remove large, overactive thyroid glands to quickly reduce the blood flow to the thyroid to reduce bleeding.

Interestingly, because much of the thyroid hormone *is* iodine, a lack of iodine also reduces the production of thyroid hormone. A large part of the world suffers from thyroid disease due to lack of iodine, which I discuss in Chapter 12.

Both thyroid hormones, T3 and T4, contain iodine (T4 contains four parts of iodine, which make up 65 percent of its weight; T3 has three parts of iodine, which make up 58 percent of its weight; see the sidebar "The birth of thyroid hormones" for more information), which means that the thyroid gland must trap iodine to make the hormones. Therefore, doctors can study the workings of the thyroid by substituting radioactive iodine for regular iodine. They can detect and measure radioactive iodine with a refined version of a Geiger counter (see Chapter 4) to perform a study called a *thyroid scan and uptake*.

Other organs, such as the breasts, the stomach, and the salivary glands, also trap iodine. However, no other organ in the human body besides the thyroid gland uses iodine for any important purpose. Thyroid hormones are the only significant chemicals that contain iodine in the human body.

The birth of thyroid hormones

Thyroid hormones are actually made in the follicular cells (see Figure 2-2). Enzymes in the cells add iodine to a compound called *tyrosine* to produce *monoiodotyrosine* (one iodine plus tyrosine) and *diiodotyrosine* (two iodines plus tyrosine). A monoiodotyrosine and a diiodotyrosine are combined to produce triiodotyrosine, or T3. Two diiodotyrosines are combined to produce thyroxine, or T4. These are combined together in a long chain called *thyroglobulin*, which is sent into the area of colloid in the center of the follicle. When thyroid hormones are needed in your body, thyroglobulin is broken down, and thyroid hormones flow into your bloodstream. The parafollicular cells, or C cells, another type of cell found in the thyroid, are important because they can form a tumor called medullary thyroid cancer (see Chapter 8).

Moving thyroid hormones around

After your thyroid releases T3 and T4, the hormones don't just travel loosely in the blood to their targets. Proteins in your bloodstream carry them.

Only *free* thyroid hormones can leave your blood and enter your cells. The rest are solidly bound to proteins, which means they're not available to perform the actions of thyroid hormone. Because 99.97 percent of thyroid hormone is attached to proteins, only 0.03 percent is free and active. When a doctor measures the *total* thyroid hormone in your blood, he or she measures bound hormone along with the unbound hormone. If the doctor knows only the total T4 amount in your blood, he or she needs to order a second test to determine the unbound T4 — the fraction of the total hormone free in your blood.

Knowing the distinction between free and bound hormones is important because many drugs and diseases alter the blood levels of *thyroxine-binding proteins* — one of the proteins that thyroid hormones bind to (see the following sidebar). If a drug like estrogen, for example, increases the amount of thyroxine-binding proteins in your body, your thyroid makes more thyroid hormone to bind to these proteins, keeping the unbound thyroid hormone constant and normal. Yet, the results of a total T4 blood test (see Chapter 4) will be elevated. Conversely, testosterone, the male hormone, causes a decrease in the thyroxine-binding proteins. If your testosterone level rises, your thyroid makes less thyroxine, and a measurement of total T4 shows a decrease (while the unbound T4 again remains normal). In both these situations, the measurement of total thyroxine will suggest that your thyroid function is not normal when, in fact, it is normal.

All aboard! Proteins carry your thyroid hormones

Exactly why proteins carry thyroid hormones isn't clear. Among the theories is that by having so much thyroid hormone bound to proteins and therefore inactive, large changes in the thyroid gland's output of thyroid hormones don't result in large changes in thyroid activity. Another theory is that the combination of the hormone and the protein produces a large molecule, which can't escape from the body through the urine, thus preserving iodine.

Three different proteins carry thyroid hormones. By far the most important is *thyroxine-binding globulin,* responsible for carrying 75 percent of the hormone in the blood. *Transthyretin,* which used to be called *thyroxine-binding prealbumin,* carries 20 percent of the thyroid hormones. *Thyroxine-binding albumin* carries the other 5 percent.

Regulating thyroid hormones with TSH

The released T3 and T4 circulate throughout your body, reaching, among other places, the pituitary gland. If the pituitary gland detects enough thyroid hormone, it continues to release the same amount of TSH. If your thyroid hormone levels drop for any reason, the pituitary releases more TSH to stimulate the thyroid to make and release more thyroid hormone, if it can. (If your TSH levels are elevated, it can also stimulate overall growth of your thyroid that can lead to an enlarged thyroid, called a *goiter.*) If your thyroid hormone levels are excessive, TSH release falls. (This is called the *negative feedback for TSH release.*)

In short, as thyroid hormone falls, TSH rises, and as thyroid hormone rises, TSH falls. Because T3, T4, and TSH can all be measured in the blood, it's simple to determine the state of your thyroid function (see Chapter 4).

TSH is also regulated by the release of thyrotrophin-releasing hormone (TRH) from the hypothalamus. Between TRH and thyroid hormones, the level of TSH in your blood remains very stable throughout life, and abnormal levels usually mean some disease is present.

Understanding the Function of Thyroid Hormones

Thyroid hormones are active in just about every cell and organ of your body. They perform general functions that increase the efficiency of each organ's specific functions, whatever they may be. The following sections tell you all about those functions of thyroid hormones and explain what too much or too little of the hormones would do to a healthy person.

Many bodily changes may be caused by other factors besides too little or too much thyroid hormone. For example, an infection can raise your body temperature, just as too much thyroid hormone can. Also, if you have a condition like menopause that tends to be associated with dry skin, this symptom may predominate even if you have hyperthyroidism that tends to cause moist skin. The information in this section shows you what classic symptoms of thyroid problems look like, but each case can have individual variations.

How thyroid hormone works

Thyroid hormone attaches to compounds called *receptors* in the membranes' surrounding cells and enters the cells with these receptors. Once inside the cells, the combination of hormone and receptor interacts with the DNA, the material that makes up the genetic code. The end result is the activity of thyroid hormone in that particular cell. This way of affecting your cells explains why it takes weeks to feel the effect of thyroid hormone. Changes in the DNA take a long time both to do and undo, so when you stop taking thyroid, it takes weeks before your body realizes that it is not getting thyroid any longer and you begin to feel low thyroid function. On the other hand, when you give antithyroid drugs that block the production of thyroid hormone, there is a large store of thyroid hormone in the follicles of the gland that must be used up before the concentration of thyroid hormone falls in the blood.

For example, in heart muscle, thyroid hormone and its receptor act to stimulate the formation of the proteins of muscle cells that increase contraction of heart muscle while suppressing the proteins of these same muscle cells that reduce contraction. The ratio of proteins changes in favor of more contraction, and the muscle cell contracts harder as it is exposed to more thyroid hormone.

Another example is that the combination of thyroid hormone and receptor stimulates metabolic activities in all cells throughout the body by increasing the activity of genes that produce enzymes, the proteins that are necessary for chemical reactions in the body. As these chemical reactions are revved up, much like increasing the fuel entering an engine, the body heats up, and this is translated into an increased body temperature. If thyroid hormone is reduced, metabolism declines, less heat is produced, and the body temperature falls.

General functions

In every cell, thyroid hormones cause that cell to make more *protein enzymes,* the chemicals that promote your *metabolism,* the sum total of all the chemical reactions going on in your body to form more tissue and to create energy. Think of your body as a machine. Adding extra thyroid hormone is like adding a richer fuel to it. The result is usually a revving up of the machine — like going from 2,000 revolutions per minute to 4,000 or more revolutions per minute, depending upon the amount of hormone added. Thus, when more thyroid hormone is present in your body, more chemical reactions are taking place.

Metabolism

The *basal metabolic rate* (BMR) is an overall measure of the amount of metabolism that's taking place in your body. Increased thyroid hormone may increase your BMR by as much as 60 to 100 percent. Any machine that increases its activity heats up; likewise, your body heats up with more thyroid hormone, and the result is a higher body temperature. At the other end of the spectrum, not enough thyroid hormone results in an abnormally low body temperature as your "machine" cools down.

As more metabolism takes place, your body burns more of your food intake for energy, so less is left to be stored. Your body detects the need for more energy and you get hungrier, but your faster metabolism usually more than offsets any increase in food intake. The net result is that you lose weight. However, if you take in too much extra food, you can actually gain weight. Check out Chapter 20 for more information on the relationship between your metabolism, your thyroid, diet, exercise, and weight loss.

Development

Normal development requires sufficient thyroid hormone. In one of the early thyroid experiments that showed this fact, researchers deprived tadpoles of thyroid hormone. The result was that they didn't develop into frogs. People deprived of thyroid hormone don't develop normally, either. In particular, the human brain fails to develop, and mental retardation is the result.

Muscle function

Your muscles need thyroid hormone for proper functioning, but too much isn't a good thing. An excess of thyroid hormone results in muscle wasting, as your body consumes muscle tissue for energy. As you lose muscle, you become weaker. If too much thyroid hormone is present, the nerves going to the muscles also show increased excitability, resulting in increased reflexes and tremor in the muscles.

Don't use thyroid hormone in an attempt to lose weight. Many diet programs, recognizing that increased thyroid hormone results in weight loss, use thyroid hormones. An overabundance of thyroid hormone results in muscle loss, so the weight that you lose isn't just fat, but also muscle, the so-called lean tissue of your body. You don't want to lose lean tissue.

Energy sources

In addition to the protein found in your muscles, thyroid hormone affects the other sources of energy in your body, namely *carbohydrates* and *fats*. Carbohydrates are the main sources of immediate energy in the body, so your body uses them up faster than normal when thyroid hormone levels rise, resulting in more heat production. Your body also uses up fat faster than normal. The result is a lowering of the different kinds of fat in your body, namely *cholesterol* and *triglycerides*. On the other hand, when thyroid hormone levels drop, the fats accumulate in your liver, and the level of cholesterol in your blood rises.

Because chemical reactions require vitamins, your need for vitamins increases when your body produces more thyroid hormone. Increased thyroid hormones cause a more rapid breakdown of the vitamins. Vitamins have little effect on the thyroid gland itself, except for those that contain iodine (often in the form of kelp or seaweed).

Avoid vitamins that contain iodine when you're being treated for hyperthyroidism or have a condition like multinodular goiter (see Chapter 9), where the iodine maybe used to make too much thyroid hormone.

Organ-specific functions

Every organ in your body requires thyroid hormone to function normally. When that hormone is lacking, the organs tend to do less of their usual functions. When too much thyroid hormone is present, the organs do more than they should. In this section, you find the most important changes brought on by abnormal amounts of thyroid hormone in your body. By no means is this discussion complete; that would require a large book by itself, and many of the changes that occur are too subtle to result in signs or symptoms that you can detect.

The heart and blood vessels

Your heart needs thyroid hormone for proper pumping. If an insufficient amount of thyroid hormone is present, the heart slows down and its pumping action decreases. If thyroid hormone is severely lacking, heart failure can result. Conversely, when thyroid hormone levels rise, your heart rate becomes too rapid. Your heart pumps out more blood at first, but if this increased pumping is allowed to go on for too long, the end result may be decreased heart strength because excessive thyroid hormone causes muscle wasting. (The heart is made of muscle.)

Depending upon the level of your physical activity, your normal resting heart rate should be between 60 and 80. (If you're in good physical condition, your heart rate should be around 60.) People with too much T4 often have a heart rate of 120 or faster.

Thyroid hormone also stimulates blood vessels to open up more, which increases blood flow in many organs of the body. One of the main objects of this increased blood flow is the thyroid gland itself. So much blood is flowing through the gland that you can actually feel the movement of the blood when you place a hand over your thyroid gland, and you can hear the whoosing sound of increased blood flow when you place a stethoscope over the gland.

The lungs

Thyroid hormone is necessary for proper formation of the lungs, because lung cells require thyroid hormone to grow properly. When animals are deprived of thyroid hormone during their development, their lung weight is decreased compared to animals that have enough thyroid hormone.

As you increase your metabolism, you need more oxygen for the chemical reactions in your body to take place. Oxygen comes into the body through your lungs. Your respiration rate, normally about 16 times per minute, speeds up to bring in more oxygen. However, even an increased respiration rate may fail to provide the body with enough oxygen if the muscular diaphragm and chest muscles are wasting from excess thyroid hormone.

The stomach, intestines, and liver

Thyroid hormone is required for the muscles of the stomach and intestines to push food along for digestion and excretion. When an insufficient amount of thyroid hormone is present, intestinal movement slows, as well as the absorption of food. The common complaint is constipation. On the other hand, too much thyroid hormone speeds up the bowels. Loose bowel movements, more frequent bowel movements, or diarrhea may be the result.

Thyroid hormone also permits normal development of the liver and the enzymes that the liver uses to break down many substances in the blood and to form sugar from other substances. Thyroid hormone is needed for the liver to form bile and handle cholesterol properly.

The skin, hair, and nails

Thyroid hormone is necessary to maintain your skin, hair and nails. Skin temperature is controlled by the flow of blood to the skin, which is maintained by your thyroid.

The increase in blood flow with increased thyroid hormone is especially prominent in your skin. The skin often feels warm, and perspiration may increase, so it also feels moist. When thyroid hormone levels fall, the skin often becomes dry and may scale, and it feels cold to the touch. The nails can't achieve their proper toughness without enough thyroid hormone and may break easily. The hair, likewise, is fragile, dry, and brittle, and excessive hair loss is a common complaint when an insufficient amount of thyroid hormone is present.

The brain and cerebral functioning

As the brain develops, it requires thyroid hormone to form its cells. Absence of thyroid hormone can lead to mental retardation. Even after birth, the brain is still developing and requires thyroid hormone to develop properly for up to three years. The right amount of thyroid hormone is necessary for normal mental function later in life.

Chapter 15 details the changes in mood that occur with too much or too little thyroid hormone. A person with excessive thyroid hormone may feel as if his or her brain is racing, which can result in extreme nervousness. The person may feel anxious without knowing why and become worried about minor things. In extreme cases, the result may be paranoia. Not enough thyroid hormone can lead to mental dullness and depression.

Sexual functioning and menstruation

Normal sexual development requires thyroid hormone, especially in women. Without it, sexual development is delayed, and the onset of menstrual function comes later. Proper development of the uterus requires thyroid hormone as well.

Thyroid hormone is also needed for normal sexual function. Both men and women lose interest in sex when an insufficient amount of thyroid hormone is present. They don't necessarily have increased interest in sex when thyroid hormone levels rise, because so many psychological and physical problems result from the increase.

The menstrual cycle depends on adequate thyroid hormone to proceed normally. Women with a lack of thyroid hormone may have trouble conceiving a baby. They tend to have increased menstrual flow and may become anemic (resulting from losing too much blood). Too much thyroid hormone often decreases the menstrual flow or causes missed periods.

The bones and teeth

Thyroid hormones help keep bone growth normal. When too little thyroid hormone is present in early life, your bones show delayed development and don't grow to their correct length. The result is a dwarf with short arms and legs and a larger trunk. If thyroid hormone is lacking after growth has stopped, your bones appear more dense than normal because of decreased bone turnover.

With an overabundance of thyroid hormone, due to taking too much thyroid hormone or inadequate treatment of hyperthyroidism, bone turnover and loss increases. The result may have the appearance of osteoporosis, the kind of bone loss that occurs in women after menopause. However, it rarely results in bone fractures if the increased thyroid hormone is controlled with treatment (because the bone loss stops).

Your teeth require thyroid hormone to erupt at the proper time and to grow to the proper size. When thyroid hormone is lacking, the roots of your teeth grow more slowly, your dental enamel is thinner, and you lose your "baby teeth" much later.

Chapter 3

Finding a Thyroid Doctor

. . . .

In This Chapter

▶ Asking the right questions

▶ Searching your insurance plan

▶ Checking with your doctor, friends and family

▶ Approaching major medical centers

▶ Looking at magazines

▶ Making use of the Internet

. . . .

*Y*ou may have a good idea that your thyroid gland is the cause of your medical problem but don't know much about it. You do know that you need the help of an expert, because your regular doctor doesn't know much about thyroid disease. How do you go about finding the specialist who can help you? As much as I'd like to schedule you for an appointment with me, my schedule is stretched to the breaking point. Instead, this chapter will provide you with everything you need to find a qualified thyroid doctor in your area. Plenty of qualified specialists are out there whom I would go to if I had a problem.

I do, however, make the time to answer general questions about thyroid disease, which I receive all the time by e-mail. You can write me at `thyroid@ drrubin.com`. But I have an unbreakable rule: I never answer specific questions about your case without the opportunity to ask you questions directly and examine you with my own hands. Any doctor who answers your specific questions without examining you personally breaks one of the basic rules of our profession.

In this chapter, I tell you the process that I use to find a good doctor, and you can apply this process not only to finding a thyroid doctor but a doctor for any special and unusual medical problem that you feel your general physician isn't adequately addressing. Although some of my recommendations don't apply exactly to physicians other than thyroid doctors, as you can see, most of them do.

You're fortunate, because your options for finding an excellent doctor are vast, especially if you possess the essential tool for conducting your search — a computer with an Internet connection. As this chapter shows you, you may find a doctor long before you need to search the Internet, but even if you do, you can still use the Internet to verify your doctor's qualifications. Qualifications may not be the first thing you research about your doctor, but as I explain below, they should definitely be the last.

Asking the Right Questions

You may think that I'm starting at the end by telling you the right questions to ask potential specialists before even signing on with them. First, you're probably thinking, I've got to find a doctor. But most of these questions can and should be answered — correctly — before you get to the doctor's office. A few of the following questions do require a face-to-face meeting with the doctor; so wait to ask those questions at your first appointment. But if your candidate fits in with the criteria I list here, feel pretty confident that you've found the right office. As you read through this material, you also get an introduction to the doctors who work with thyroid patients.

If the answer to either of the following first two questions is no, you probably don't want to go to that doctor.

Is the doctor board certified in endocrinology?

The medical profession is very careful to permit only the most qualified doctors to take care of complicated medical problems. The U.S. system of medical education ensures that doctors don't graduate before they are fully qualified to manage the problems they want to treat. Early in their education, medical students choose to pursue one path of medicine, surgery, pediatrics, or psychiatry. After that, they're observed by other doctors who already possess the qualifications they are trying to obtain. After young doctors have gone through the years of training thought necessary to achieve expertise in their specialty, they take an examination, called a "board" examination because one of the educational organizations accepted by all physicians — the American Board of Internal Medicine, the American Board of Surgery, the American Board of Pediatrics, or the American Board of Psychiatry — administers it.

If the doctor passes a board examination, he or she is said to be qualified to practice in the general specialty of internal medicine, surgery, pediatrics, or psychiatry the doctor has chosen. The doctor who wants to be able to call himself a subspecialist, isn't done yet. After enough years of training in that subspecialty, whether it is *endocrinology,* which mainly treats people with diabetes and thyroid disease (but covers diseases of many other glands that happen to occur less commonly), or *nephrology,* which treats people with kidney disease or *cardiology,* which treats diseases of the heart, the doctor must take and pass another examination. This examination emphasizes the skills that someone in that subspecialty must possess, and only when the doctor passes it can he call himself a board-certified subspecialist in that particular field, and he must have a certificate to prove it.

After he or she picks a subspecialty, the doctor can choose to take care of all the various components of that subspecialty or focus on one of them. For example, endocrinologists can further specialize in diabetes, thyroid disease, adrenal disease, parathyroid disease, and so forth or work in only one of them as a kind of "sub-subspecialist." There's no examination that a sub-subspecialist takes. Doctors who choose only one area, like thyroid disease, are often found at medical centers, while doctors who take care of all areas are often found in the community, but this isn't always the case.

Any doctor can call himself a specialist in anything and can even have some certificate that seems to confirm it, but you can check for yourself by searching for a doctor's name on the Web site of a particular specialty board. For the internal medicine specialties, you can go to www.abim.org and click on "Who is Certified." By filling in the name of the doctor, you can find out whether that doctor is certified and in what specialty and subspecialty. Your potential thyroid doctor should be board certified in the specialty of internal medicine and the subspecialty of endocrinology and metabolism.

Finding out if a doctor who is a surgeon is board certified isn't quite so easy. You have to call the American Board of Surgery at 215-568-4000 to verify the board status of the doctor you name. For written confirmation, you must provide a written request. You can write them at: The American Board of Surgery, 1617 John F. Kennedy Blvd., Suite 860, Philadelphia, PA 19103.

If the doctor is board certified, you know she possesses a very good knowledge of her specialty and has trained for enough years to be allowed to take the test. However, she may have taken the test 25 years ago and trained before that. The boards offer re-certification examinations, so if she has passed a re-certification examination in the last few years, that's an excellent sign of a doctor who wants to keep up to date. You can't pass these examinations without a strong knowledge of your subject.

Does the doctor belong to a specialty society?

To further medical education, the medical profession has organized itself into specialty societies that hold meetings at least annually and usually publish a monthly journal containing articles about their specialty. Your potential doctor should belong to one of these specialty societies and, hopefully, even attend meetings regularly.

How can you answer this question? You can go to the Web site of one of the societies and see if your potential doctor is listed as a member. The societies for thyroid disease and their corresponding Web sites are

- ✔ American Thyroid Association at www.thyroid.org
- ✔ American Association of Clinical Endocrinologists at www.aace.com
- ✔ American Association of Endocrine Surgeons at www.endocrine surgery.org
- ✔ Endocrine Society at www.endo-society.org
- ✔ Lawson Wilkins Pediatric Endocrine Society at www.lwpes.org

If you need a specialist, such as an eye doctor for thyroid eye disease, you can find a clickable list of doctors participating in specialty societies at the following Web site, maintained by the National Institutes of Health: www.nlm.nih.gov/medlineplus/directories.html.

To find out whether your potential doctor attends a specialty society's meetings, you have to ask the doctor. Unfortunately, knowing a doctor attends a meeting still doesn't tell you if he spends his time at the educational programs or the roulette table.

Where was the doctor trained?

If the answers to the previous two questions are yes, you don't need to ask where your doctor was trained. If the answer to either one of them is no, you probably don't want to go to this doctor. But if you still do for other reasons, like your mother-in-law swears by him, find out where he did his medical-school and post-graduate training.

The states license doctors. To receive a license, doctors must prove they are qualified to practice, but some medical schools aren't as good as others, particularly schools outside the United States on small islands. Plenty of great medical schools exist outside the United States. Just make sure your potential doctor went to one of them if she was not educated here.

Competent thyroid specialists should have done their post-graduate specialty training in a hospital that is known for its division of endocrinology with endocrine fellows. *Fellows* are doctors who have completed their general training in internal medicine and are now devoting their time to their subspecialty of endocrinology. Even some American hospitals fail this test.

Ask doctors' nurses or receptionists where doctors trained. Find out where the doctor did her fellowship in endocrinology. Any unwillingness to provide this information should lead you to seek a doctor elsewhere.

Has the doctor been disciplined for any infraction?

The licensing department of the state in which the doctor practices can tell you whether a doctor has been disciplined. States often make accessing doctors' infractions very easy by providing a Web site that lists pertinent information after you type in the doctor's name.

Be wary of doctors who have been disciplined. By the time the state licensing department disciplines a doctor, that doctor has already taken every possible route to avoid discipline. The fact that discipline took place anyway suggests that there's definite substance to the infraction. Examples of infractions include using illegal drugs or excessive amounts of alcohol, failure to answer licensing questions truthfully, sexual contact with patients, and a host of other possibilities.

Consulting Possible Sources

You may be limited to certain doctors in your insurance plan, you may have total trust in your personal physician, or you may feel that your family and friends are the best source for information about doctors. This section discusses how you use these various resources to find the best possible medical care.

Searching your insurance plan

All insurance plans, in order to be competitive, offer a number of doctors in each medical specialty and subspecialty. Your plan may mandate that you can go to only doctors who have a contract with your plan. Sometimes a plan pays almost all the cost of seeing a doctor within the plan and less for seeing a doctor outside the plan. If you don't want to end up with a big financial burden, find out your plan's stipulations before you go.

Most plans now offer a Web site where you can find the names of the specialists who belong to it and whether the specialists are accepting new patients. The fact that a health plan lists a doctor is reassuring because it shows the plan has done a certain amount of checking on a doctor's credentials. But you still need to ask the hard questions I discuss in the preceding section, "Asking the Right Questions." If you have a choice of several specialists, then the questions I give you can separate them out so you choose the one who looks the best.

Checking with your doctor

If you trust your general doctor, he or she may be the best source for finding a specialist. Your doctor usually knows the other physicians in the community, refers patients to many of them, and has an idea of the quality of the work that other doctors do. You can always ask your doctor that old standby question, "Would you send your mother to this physician?" Of course, you don't know if your doctor particularly cares for his mother. But I don't recommend following up with "Do you love your mother?"

Even if your doctor recommends the specialist, still use the information I provide in the "Asking the Right Questions" section of this chapter to evaluate the specialist. You have to weigh the value of a specialist who, for example, fails the tests of board certification and membership in a specialty society but holds the respect of your primary doctor.

Some insurance plans actually require that you have authorization from your primary physician before you can see a specialist, and then only one that is within your plan. If you don't get this authorization, you have to pay out of your own pocket.

No doctor has the right to tell you not to see another doctor, in any specialty. If you feel you need different advice, are not satisfied with the advice you are getting, or just want to talk to someone else, feel free to do so.

Turning to family and friends

Second to your doctor's advice, you may find the advice of family and friends helpful. Because thyroid disease is often hereditary (found in multiple members of the same family, who have many similar genes), chances are that your mother, sister, or aunt has seen a thyroid specialist at one time or another and can happily offer you a recommendation. (Thyroid disease is much more common among women than men.) And because thyroid disease is so common, as I discuss in Chapter 2, one or another of your friends has likely seen a thyroid specialist. You can first judge the quality of their health before listening to their advice. Then you have to decide how much respect you have for their opinion.

Don't fail to use the key criteria I discuss in the first sections of this chapter for doctors your family and friends recommend as well. Your aunt or college roommate probably has a good idea of how much time the doctor spends with her patients and whether she listens to them. But unless your aunt has read this book or a similar resource, she doesn't know how to judge the doctor's knowledge of endocrinology.

Finding the perfect physician is hard. You may have to make compromises, but if you do, for the sake of your health, give up a little of the art of medicine in favor of the science of medicine. A doctor who doesn't keep you waiting but gives you the wrong advice isn't for you. A full waiting room is also a poor reason for choosing a doctor. I wrote this book because the general knowledge of thyroid disease is very sparse. Most people don't even know the thyroid exists, much less how knowledgeable their specialist happens to be.

Approaching major medical centers

You can't go far wrong if you seek a specialist in a major medical center. Places like the Mayo Clinic and the Cleveland Clinic or university centers like New York University or the University of California–San Francisco Medical Center are bound to have experts on your condition. The benefits of seeing a specialist in a major medical center are numerous:

- ✔ **Specialization:** Major medical centers usually have a division of endocrinology. Within their endocrinology division, they have subdivisions devoted to thyroid disease, diabetes, pituitary disease, and all the other sub-subspecialties that make up endocrinology, leaving little doubt of the quality of the physicians working in such medical centers.

- ✔ **Credentials:** Medical centers do all the research on doctors for you by checking their references and following their skills carefully before promoting them to the position of assistant professor or professor. Your task is to find the right doctor within a center's massive structure.

- ✔ **Experience:** In addition, doctors at major medical centers have seen multiple examples of complicated medical cases and have much more experience than doctors in private practice. This depth of experience is particularly significant if your condition is especially complicated.

- ✔ **Shared knowledge:** Major medical centers usually have multiple specialists in each division. Your task is to select from among the many specialists. Your own doctor may know the reputation of one or another of them, or you can take a chance. If your problem is complicated, the chances are good that you get to meet all members of the group at one time or another and benefit from the accumulated knowledge of the whole group.

Make sure that your professor is a clinical professor, not a research professor. In medical institutions, the production of research papers, which may have little to do with intact human beings, often earns people promotions. Make sure that your potential doctor regularly sees patients and doesn't spend all of his or her time in a laboratory.

Major medical centers need new patients constantly, just like any doctor who isn't retiring. So they make it relatively easy for you to get a handle on who's who within the organization. Most centers have a book that lists all their sub-divisions and the names of the doctors within them. You can find a copy of a center's book of doctors in its medical library. Often, medical centers send copies to local doctors so doctors know how to refer their patients. Most major medical centers also have a large representation on the Internet, where you can find their list of doctors and the specialist that you need.

Looking at magazines

Many publications take it upon themselves to rate doctors. The good ones rate doctors by their level of knowledge and the efficiency of their office. When you run across a publication that rates doctors, don't simply take it at face value. Read the small print and ascertain how the ratings were put together. Make sure that you can answer "yes" to the following questions:

- ✔ Does the publication ask doctors in the community for the names of the best specialists in their opinion?
- ✔ Does the publication send out questionnaires to its subscribers, asking them to rate their doctors like they rate their car repair shops?
- ✔ Does the publication check with nurses to see which doctors they feel are most qualified?

Consumer Checkbook, an offshoot of *Consumer Reports Magazine,* which has been providing highly reliable information for the consumer for over 50 years, publishes one of the best examples of a trustworthy rating of doctors. *Consumer Checkbook* asked about 260,000 physicians to name the physicians they would send their loved ones to for care. The result was 20,000 doctors around the country. At the present time, *Consumer Checkbook* publishes local versions of the magazine for seven areas around the country: Boston, Chicago, Delaware Valley, Puget Sound, San Francisco/Oakland/San Jose, Twin Cities, and Washington, DC. *Consumer Checkbook* has also posted the results for those areas in past issues of its national magazine. However, to help you locate the best doctors as well as the best hospitals, it publishes the national guides *Consumers' Guide to Top Doctors* and *Consumers' Guide to Hospitals.*

Your local city magazine may also have a guide to the best doctors in your area. For example, my local magazine, *San Francisco Magazine,* in its January 2005 issue published "520 Best Doctors, Top Bay Area Physicians." Similar to *Consumer Checkbook,* the magazine featured the opinions of other doctors in the community. Check back issues of your local publication or call the office of the magazine to find out if it has published such a guide.

Making use of the Internet

If you want a list of the doctors who are specialists in thyroid disease in your area, you can use the following Web resources to find a specialist. Start at my Web site, www.drrubin.com, and click on "Thyroid" under "Related Web sites" on the left side of the page. You then come to a list of the best resources on the Web for thyroid disease, including links to the following societies for thyroid disease.

American Thyroid Association

Start by clicking on the address for the American Thyroid Association (www.thyroid.org). If you click on "Public and Patients," you come to a page where you can click on "Find a Specialist," which takes you to a map of the United States. Now click on your state, select a state from the drop-down list, or select another country from the non-U.S. residents list. After you click on a state, you see a list of thyroid specialists from that state.

The listing of specialists on the American Thyroid Association Web site isn't an endorsement by the American Thyroid Association, which the association makes clear on the page with the map on it. The specialists on the listing are simply members of this organization who have agreed to take new patients. Their membership in this organization suggests that they are knowledgeable in this field but doesn't prove it.

American Association of Clinical Endocrinologists

Go back to the list of thyroid addresses on my Web site and click on the American Association of Clinical Endocrinologists link (www.aace.com). On the first page, find "Services" on the left side. By clicking on it you can choose "Find an Endocrinologist." On the page that pops up, choose the U.S. or your country of residence. By choosing the U.S., you bring up a box where you fill in your city, state, zip, distance you are willing to travel, and the particular specialty you are seeking a doctor in. Choose "Search," and up pops the names of the members of this organization in your chosen specialty who are practicing in your area and want to be listed. Again, the list isn't an endorsement.

Endocrine Society

Return to the list of thyroid addresses on my Web site and click on the address for the Endocrine Society (www.endo-society.org). On the page that comes up, click on "Information for Patients," found at the top under "The Hormone Foundation." On the top, left-hand side of the next page, click the "Find an Endocrinologist" link. Type in your zip code, the distance from that zip code you are willing to travel, and the specialty you are seeking a doctor in, and a list of lots of names appears. The same caveat applies: The list isn't an endorsement, simply a list of members of the Endocrine Society who are willing to see new patients.

American Association of Endocrine Surgeons

The lists for the previously discussed societies contain the names of highly qualified thyroid surgeons. But if you want to go to the site that contains surgeons in their own society, find the American Association of Endocrine Surgeons (`www.edocrinesurgery.org`) on my thyroid addresses page. On the association's home page, choose the "Members" link on the left-hand side of the page. Then choose "Membership List" on the top of the next page that appears. To access the list, you need to have Adobe Acrobat installed on your computer, which you can download free of charge. Doctors' names appear under their resident state and city. If you page down to California, for example, you find a large number of names that I know include some of the best thyroid surgeons in the country.

National Institutes of Health

The National Institutes of Health maintains a list of all the specialty societies for doctors that can help you find a specialist in any field that may have to do with thyroid disease. For example, you may need an eye doctor if you have the eye disease associated with hyperthyroidism (see Chapter 6) or a skin doctor if you have the skin disease also associated with this condition. Check out the "Does the doctor belong to a specialty society?" section earlier in the chapter for the Web site.

Questions for and Observations about the Doctor on First Meeting

Asking your potential doctor the following questions gives you a chance to find out if the doctor practices the art as well as the science of medicine. You receive little benefit from the most highly trained doctor if you can't communicate with her. Some key questions to ask the doctor are:

- ✔ Will you call or e-mail me or permit me to call you about test results within a few days, or do I have to wait until our next appointment? (Appointments may be months apart, while test abnormalities sit in the doctor's file until you show up again.)
- ✔ May I e-mail you with questions and expect to hear from you soon after?

Some key questions to ask yourself as you observe your potential doctor, his staff, and surroundings are as follows:

- ✔ Does the doctor look at you when she talks to and examines you?
- ✔ Does the doctor listen to you and respond to your questions?
- ✔ Do you feel you are getting enough time or being rushed?

✔ Are the doctor's staff members helpful and happy? Their positive attitude suggests they feel good about working for this caregiver.

✔ Does the doctor's office appear clean and well maintained?

✔ Do other patients in the waiting room seem to be happy to be in this office?

A white lab jacket doesn't confer godliness or special knowledge. Some of the best physicians (I humbly include myself in this category, at least with respect to my clothes) never wear white coats.

Reviewing Special Considerations When Choosing a Thyroid or Eye Surgeon

Surgery of the thyroid gland is fairly complicated. Despite the fact that the thyroid is so close to the surface of the skin, it is intimately associated with many nerves, blood vessels, other glands, the trachea, and esophagus. You want a surgeon who has a lot of experience with thyroid surgery. The consequence of making an error may be permanent hoarseness, loss of function of the parathyroid glands, which control calcium, and even more severe damage.

Try to find out how many thyroid surgeries the doctor does annually. If the number is less than ten, you probably want to find another surgeon. If it is between ten and fifty, this is a surgeon who can do most thyroid operations in which the gland is located in the neck and the operation involves removal of part or all of a thyroid that has not been operated upon previously. When the thyroid is under the breastbone, is being operated upon for a second time, or is involved with rapidly spreading cancer, you need a highly trained surgeon who does at least fifty operations on the thyroid per year. You probably have to go to a medical center, as described earlier in this chapter, to find one. Check out Chapter 13 for more information on surgeons and thyroid surgery.

Most of the time, a regular ophthalmologist can handle 95 percent of the eye problems that thyroid patients, especially those with hyperthyroidism, experience (see Chapter 6). For the other 5 percent or less, an eye surgeon who has done surgery on the bony orbit of the eye is essential. The biggest complication may be blindness if the surgery isn't done right and sometimes may still result even though it is. You can find such a super specialist only at medical centers. Preserving your vision is definitely worth a trip to such a center. If you are in that exceedingly rare group of patients that requires such surgery, make sure the surgeon has successfully done this operation in the past and what his or her success rate is.

Chapter 4

Testing Your Thyroid

*T*hese days, we take for granted our ability to precisely measure thyroid function. Yet only 60 years ago measurements were so primitive that we depended more on a patient's physical and emotional state than the lab tests to make a diagnosis. Past limitations were unfortunate because the patients with obvious signs and symptoms of thyroid disease are just the tip of a huge iceberg of those folks facing thyroid abnormalities.

Today, the tests that measure thyroid function are getting more and more sensitive. Tests now enable doctors to identify many people with *subclinical* thyroid disease (thyroid disease in which symptoms aren't yet apparent to the patient or the doctor), which may be slowly damaging the patient and will become clinical sooner or later. Thyroid tests' increasing sensitivity is especially useful with our aging population, whose symptoms of aging are so similar to the symptoms of mild hypothyroidism. Although you can't order the tests I describe in this chapter for yourself, the information I provide can increase your understanding of what various tests involve and what their results mean. The information in this chapter can help you have better discussions with your doctor about your diagnosis.

Checking Thyroid-Hormone Levels with Older Tests

Many doctors practicing today learned about thyroid disease when only older tests were available to measure the amount of thyroid hormone in our blood, and some doctors still use the older tests. Inn case your doctor orders such tests or you have copies of old test results you want to understand, in this section I explain how some of the older blood tests work (although the sooner they're dropped from the list of tests that labs do, the better for patients). The *total thyroxine* and *resin T3 uptake* tests, as I discuss in the following sections, should be used in combination to determine your *free thyroxine index*. (For information on more accurate tests, skip ahead to the "Checking Your Levels with the Best Tests" section.)

Total thyroxine

Thyroxine (T4) is considered a *prohormone,* a weaker thyroid hormone that gains its potency only after it's converted to T3, the other thyroid hormone (see Chapter 2). The *total thyroxine test* (sometimes called the *T4 immunoassay*) measures all the T4 thyroid hormone in a given quantity of blood. (Total thyroxin is often abbreviated as TT4.) But most of the hormone measured in a total thyroxin test is bound to protein, so it doesn't get into cells where it does its job (see Chapter 2). By itself, the total thyroxine test doesn't tell you how much thyroid is available to get into the cells. To give a more accurate picture of your available thyroid hormone function, your doctor should combine the total thyroxine test with a test that measures what percent of the total thyroxine is bound and what percent is free.

The TT4 test can also be deceiving because many drugs and clinical states raise the level of TT4 in your blood (because they raise the amount of thyroxine-binding protein in your system) yet don't impact your amount of free thyroxine.

Some of the drugs that can raise the level of TT4 in your blood include

- ✔ Estrogenic hormones taken for hormone replacement or birth control
- ✔ *Amiodarone,* a drug used for the heart
- ✔ Amphetamines
- ✔ Methadone

Some clinical states that can raise TT4 levels include

- ✔ High estrogen states, such as pregnancy
- ✔ Acute illness, such as AIDS or hepatitis
- ✔ Acute psychiatric problems

Conversely, some drugs and physical conditions tend to lower the results of a TT4 test (because they depress the amount of thyroxine-binding protein) while not impacting the amount of free thyroxine.

The drugs that can lower TT4 levels include

- ✔ *Androgens,* male hormones taken to build muscle
- ✔ *Steroids,* usually given to reduce inflammation
- ✔ *Nicotinic acid,* given to lower harmful blood fats
- ✔ Aspirin in high doses (more than 3,000 milligrams daily)

Physical conditions that can lower TT4 levels include

- ✔ Severe chronic illness, such as kidney failure or liver failure
- ✔ Starvation

A normal range of TT4 is 5 to 11 micrograms per deciliter of blood.

Different laboratories may use different techniques to perform the same test, resulting in slightly different normal values. Even when different labs use the same technique, slight variations in the normal values may occur from lab to lab because values originate from each lab's own group of people without thyroid disease.

If your doctor chooses to use the total thyroxine test to monitor your thyroid function, he or she must make certain you aren't taking any of the drugs or experiencing any of the physical conditions I list in the preceding section. In addition, your doctor must also order the next test, the resin T3 uptake, to get a complete picture of your condition.

The total T4 test is actually a better measure than the free T4 test that I describe below in one important situation — pregnancy. Because of the method almost all labs use to measure free T4, the free T4 test gives an incorrect level when a woman is pregnant. During pregnancy, the total T4 is used instead, and should be one and a half times the normal total T4 when the woman isn't pregnant. The TSH may not give a correct reading until the end of pregnancy, so the total T4 is the measurement of choice. (See Chapter 17 for more information on the thyroid during pregnancy.)

Resin T3 uptake

The *resin T3 uptake* measures how many sites on thyroxine-binding proteins are available for T3 hormone (active thyroid hormone) to bind to. Lots of sites are available when the TT4 is low (and therefore takes up very few of the sites) or the binding protein levels are very high.

The usual result of a resin T3 uptake is 25 to 35 percent, depending on the lab. Here's the explanation for results that vary from this range:

✔ **Higher results:** Anything that reduces the binding sites leaves very few binding sites for any more thyroid hormone to bind to. If T3 is added to a sample of that blood, little T3 will be bound, leaving a lot of measurable free T3. The resin T3 uptake will be high.

✔ **Lower results:** Anything that raises the binding sites also leaves a lot of binding sites available for added T3. The amount of free T3 measured is low, giving a decreased resin T3 uptake.

Free thyroxine index

As I indicate in the previous sections, your doctor must use the total thyroxine (TT4) test and the resin T3 uptake together to be valuable. In the "Total thyroxine" section, I note several drugs and physical conditions that can alter the results of the TT4 test (and that also alter the resin T3 uptake results). The impact of such drugs and physical conditions always affects the TT4 and resin T3 uptake results in opposite directions: If the TT4 is depressed, then the resin T3 uptake is high; if the TT4 is elevated, then the resin T3 uptake is low.

Take, for example, the effect of estrogen pills. As I note in the "Total thyroxine" section earlier in the chapter, estrogen pills tend to raise the amount of thyroid-binding protein, resulting in many more binding sites for thyroid hormone. Free thyroid hormone is taken up from the blood, so the total thyroxine, which measures all the thyroid hormone in the blood, is higher. If radioactive T3 is added to the same blood, so many binding sites for the T3 still remain that little T3 is left in the free state, and the resin T3 uptake is low.

Likewise, as I note in "Total thyroxine," pregnancy raises the number of thyroid-binding proteins. If the doctor only measures the total thyroxine, the measurement is high, and the doctor thinks the patient has hyperthyroidism (see Chapter 6). The patient receives treatment, inappropriately, for hyperthyroidism with antithyroid drugs and possibly becomes hypothyroid, which isn't good for the mother or the baby. However, if the doctor measures resin T3 uptake as well, the doctor finds the product of total thyroxine and resin T3 uptake to be normal.

Conversely, androgens lower the amount of thyroid-binding protein. T4 releases from binding sites to become free T4. As soon as your body detects an excess of free T4, it reduces the release of T4 from the thyroid so the level of free T4 remains normal. The total measured T4 is lower than normal, because far fewer binding sites containing T4 exist. If radioactive T3 is added to this blood, it has fewer binding sites to attach to, and most of it remains free. All this free T3 attaches to the resin, giving you an elevated resin T3 uptake. Again, when you multiply the low total T4 by the high resin T3 uptake, the product is normal. And when you take steroids for an inflammatory condition like arthritis, for example, they reduce the number of thyroid-binding proteins. If your doctor measures only total T4, it is low and the doctor may incorrectly prescribe thyroid hormone, making the patient hyperthyroid. By measuring the resin T3 uptake, the doctor can find the correct state of normal thyroid function by multiplying the low total T4 and the high resin T3 uptake.

To determine a useful test result, doctors multiply the TT4 level by the resin T3 uptake. The result, the *free thyroxine index,* is an indicator of thyroid function and usually falls between 1.25 and 3.85. A free thyroxine index below 1.25 indicates low thyroid function, and a result above 3.85 indicates increased thyroid function.

Even if you're taking one of the drugs or experiencing one of the physical conditions I list in the "Total thyroxine" section, your free thyroxine index should be within the normal range if your thyroid is functioning normally.

Checking Your Levels with the Best Tests

Numerous blood tests can measure thyroid function, but the most accurate and sensitive tests for determining thyroid function are the *free thyroxine* (FT4) and the *thyroid-stimulating hormone* (TSH) tests, both of which I describe in this section. (Free thyroxine is the tiny portion of thyroid hormone in the blood that's free to get into cells; see Chapter 2.) The vast majority of people who take FT4 and TSH tests receive accurate diagnoses. If your doctor is screening you for thyroid function and wants to order just one test, that test should be the TSH test because of its accuracy and the fact that it's a simple blood test.

Free thyroxine (FT4)

The *free thyroxine* (FT4) *test* is the best way to measure the amount of free thyroid hormone in your blood. The FT4 test measures the 0.03 percent of T4 that's not bound to protein — the T4 that's free to interact with your cells (see Chapter 2). All the factors that can change the amount of total thyroxine in your system, such as the drugs and physical conditions I list in the "Total thyroxine" section earlier in the chapter, don't affect the amount of FT4 in your blood. Depending on the test method your particular laboratory uses, the usual FT4 level is around 1 to 3 ng/dl (that's nanograms per deciliter).

The level of FT4 in your blood is high if you have hyperthyroidism and low if you have hypothyroidism. (As I explain in more detail in Chapter 6, in rare cases a patient with hyperthyroidism has too much T3 rather than too much T4 in her blood, and her FT4 test can come back normal or even low.)

Free triiodothyronine (FT3)

The free triiodothyronine (FT3) test measures the free T3 hormone in the blood. The FT3 test is rarely necessary, except when a patient is hyperthyroid yet has a normal FT4 test result. The usual level of FT3 is 0.25 to 0.65 ng/dl (nanograms per deciliter). A hyperthyroid patient has a high FT3 result. A hypothyroid patient has a low FT3 result.

Thyroid-binding proteins affect T3 in a similar way to T4. As thyroid-binding proteins rise, the proteins absorb more T3, and the thyroid gland makes more T3 to take its place. As thyroid-binding proteins fall, the proteins absorb less T3, and the thyroid reduces its production of T3. The total T3 doesn't give an accurate measurement of active T3, and a measurement of resin T3 uptake must accompany it to accurately measure thyroid function.

The FT4 isn't a perfect test, because certain conditions make the FT4 level appear abnormal when the patient actually has normal thyroid function. Fortunately, your doctor can easily recognize these conditions, which include the following:

✔ Patients with severe chronic illness (not thyroid disease) may have slight decreases in FT4.

✔ People producing or eating large amounts of T3 have decreased FT4.

✔ The rare patient with resistance to T4 has high levels of FT4 yet isn't hyperthyroid, possibly due to a hereditary condition.

✔ Patients on heparin to prevent blood clotting may have slight increases in FT4.

✔ Patients with an acute illness may briefly have elevated FT4 as binding proteins suddenly fall.

Sometimes the FT4 test may be the only useful way of knowing if thyroid function is normal. When a hyperthyroid patient receives treatment, the FT4 result falls. But the TSH level, the other highly sensitive test that I describe as the best screening test for abnormalities of thyroid function, may remain low for months and finally return to normal. Your doctor can't and shouldn't use the TSH test to determine thyroid function in hyperthyroidism that is under treatment. Similarly, many patients have a low TSH and a normal FT4 score. If the TSH is the only test a doctor looks at, the doctor incorrectly labels the patient hyperthyroid. Patients with a low TSH and normal FT4 score actually have pre-hyperthyroidism (euthyroid Graves' disease) and don't need treatment as long as their free T4 remains normal.

Thyroid-stimulating hormone (TSH)

The *thyroid-stimulating hormone* (TSH) test is the most sensitive test of thyroid function in most circumstances. The TSH rises when the T4 level in the blood falls, and the TSH falls when the T4 rises (see Chapter 2). The chemical tests that measure TSH are the most accurate assays currently being done, so the TSH test is an excellent test to measure thyroid function. If you have hyperthyroidism, your TSH level is low (because the high level of T4 in your blood is suppressing TSH production). If you have hypothyroidism, your TSH level is high (because your body is trying to stimulate the production of more T4). As always, depending on the particular laboratory doing the test, the TSH is usually 0.5 to 5 mU/ml (that's microunits per milliliter).

Many experts, myself included, don't agree with the standard normal range of TSH and believe it should be narrower because of the many people who aren't thought to have thyroid disease yet have elevated levels of thyroid autoantibodies (see section below on thyroid autoantibodies). We believe that such patients have chronic thyroiditis with subclinical hypothyroidism. The patients have a normal free T4 but an elevated TSH. So we feel that the upper part of the "normal" range is actually abnormal for patients with chronic thyroiditis. The normal range in adults, after taking patients with chronic thyroiditis with subclinical hypothyroidism into account, is probably 0.5 to 2.5 mU/ml (microunits per milliliter).

A low TSH doesn't necessarily mean you have hyperthyroidism. Some of the many conditions and factors that can decrease your TSH include

- ✔ Excessive treatment with T3 or T4 hormone

- ✔ Thyroid nodules that make excessive T3 or T4 (see Chapter 7)

- ✔ The first trimester of pregnancy (A woman's body produces a hormone called *chorionic gonadotrophin* during the first trimester, which has TSH-like properties and stimulates the production of T4, thereby suppressing TSH.)

- ✔ The cancer *choriocarcinoma* or molar pregnancy, both of which are associated with the production of large amounts of the hormone chorionic gonadotrophin

- ✔ A pituitary tumor that destroys TSH-producing cells

- ✔ Euthyroid Grave's disease, where hyperthyroidism is present in the thyroid but the thyroid isn't making excessive levels of T4 (see Chapter 6)

- ✔ Acute depression

Several conditions can cause an increase in your TSH level, even if your thyroid isn't underactive. The following conditions require consideration when your doctor discovers a high TSH:

✔ A pituitary tumor involving the cells that make TSH

✔ Recovery from a severe illness

✔ Insufficient dietary iodine

✔ Resistance to the action of T4

✔ Failure of the adrenal gland to make adrenal hormone

✔ Psychiatric illness

Many of the conditions I list in this section are temporary, meaning that a patient's TSH level will return to normal if she just waits. Other conditions, such as a pituitary tumor, require action (such as the removal of the tumor) to restore the TSH to its normal level.

Sometimes a condition that suppresses production of TSH, such as hyperthyroidism, produces a low TSH level for some time even after you've returned to a normal metabolic state with treatment. If your FT4 is normal but your TSH remains low, your doctor can't use the TSH as a reliable guide to thyroid function and has to rely on the FT4 instead.

After your doctor establishes a diagnosis for a thyroid problem, you may have repeated TSH tests during the course of your treatment to monitor your progress. If you're receiving treatment for hyperthyroidism, however, repeated TSH tests may not be the most effective way to monitor progress, because your TSH may not recover for a long time after your metabolism returns to normal.

Taking Nonhormonal Blood Tests

Having thyroid disease doesn't necessarily mean that your thyroid is functioning too much or too little. For example, a patient who has thyroid inflammation or thyroid cancer could have normal levels of FT4 and TSH. In this situation, blood tests other than the ones I describe in the preceding sections may be helpful in making the correct diagnosis. In this section, I help you understand when nonhormonal blood tests are necessary and how you interpret their results.

Thyroid autoantibodies

Many thyroid conditions, which I explain in detail in later chapters, are called *autoimmune diseases* because they appear to result from the body rejecting its own tissue. If you look at diseased thyroid tissue under a microscope, it contains many of the same cells you'd find if a foreign invader were present in the body, such as if an organ were transplanted from one person to another. An *antigen* is the tissue, cell, or chemical that the body is trying to reject. An *antibody* is the chemical (usually a protein) that the body manufactures to reject an antigen. An *autoantibody* is an antibody directed against yourself, or your own tissue.

Many autoantibodies play a role in autoimmune thyroid disease, but the two principal ones are *antithyroglobulin autoantibodies* and *thyroid peroxidase autoantibodies* (sometimes referred to by their older name, *antimicrosomal autoantibodies*). Doctors find thyroid peroxidase autoantibodies more often than antithyroglobulin autoantibodies. (Bet you can't say that three times fast.)

If your doctor wants to confirm a diagnosis of autoimmune thyroid disease, he or she orders tests of your antithyroglobulin autoantibodies and thyroid peroxidase autoantibodies. If either test returns at a level of over 100 international units per milliliter, the test confirms the diagnosis.

Antithyroglobulin and thyroid peroxidase autoantibodies are found at the highest levels in patients with a condition called *Hashimoto's thyroiditis* (which I explain in Chapter 5), but they are also found in patients with Graves' disease, a form of hyperthyroidism (see Chapter 6). Autoantibodies are found at lower levels in up to 10 percent of normal people (the percentage increases with age). As noted above, some thyroid specialists believe that people with low levels of autoantibodies actually have subclinical (non-symptomatic) thyroid disease — if this is true, the population with thyroid disease is far greater than previously thought.

If autoantibodies aren't present in abnormal amounts, a doctor can't make a diagnosis of Hashimoto's thyroiditis.

Although I discuss each autoimmune thyroid disease in its own chapter, these diseases are actually different clinical presentations of the same underlying condition. The evidence for this is based upon the following facts:

- ✔ The thyroid tissue appears the same in the different autoimmune diseases.

- ✔ Autoimmune thyroid disease runs in families.

- ✔ One person may pass through Graves' disease, Hashimoto's disease, and hypothyroidism at different times.

- ✔ The same types of autoantibodies are present in all three groups.

Finding autoantibodies may be a clue that thyroid disease will occur in the future. Relatives of people with autoimmune thyroid disease often have autoantibodies, and many of them develop thyroid disease at some point in life.

Some autoantibodies stimulate the thyroid, while others suppress the thyroid by blocking the activity of thyroid-stimulating hormone. At any given time, the condition of a patient with an autoimmune thyroid disease depends on which group of antibodies is present at the highest levels. If more suppression than stimulation is occurring, the patient will have low thyroid function. If more stimulation than suppression is occurring, hyperthyroidism will result. The patient may start with high function, go back to normal, and end up with low thyroid function. Treatment sometimes does nothing more than speed up this natural process of going from high thyroid function to normal thyroid function to low thyroid function.

In up to 25 percent of patients, an autoimmune thyroid disease goes away after a time. A higher concentration of autoantibodies doesn't mean that a patient is sicker than someone who has a lower concentration. A higher concentration of autoantibodies may simply mean that the illness is less likely to go away. However, the rate of miscarriages is greater in women who have high levels of thyroid peroxidase autoantibodies compared with low or no autoantibodies.

One other autoantibody may be especially important in patients who have hyperthyroidism — *thyroid-stimulating immunoglobulin* (TSI). TSI acts like TSH in stimulating the thyroid to make and release more hormones. Its importance lies in that it can pass through the placenta from the hyperthyroid mother to her growing baby. The baby may then become hyperthyroid as well, but when the connection between the mother and her fetus is broken at birth, the baby's hyperthyroidism goes away. The risk of the baby becoming hyperthyroid during the pregnancy is greatest for the babies of mothers with the most severe hyperthyroidism. And a hyperthyroid baby doesn't develop normally in its mother's body.

Serum thyroglobulin

Thyroglobulin is the form in which thyroid hormones are packaged and stored within the thyroid follicle (see Chapter 2). Thyroglobulin is present in the blood of normal individuals, but its levels are much higher when thyroid damage exists (for example, with cancer of the thyroid or inflammation of the thyroid). A normal level of thyroglobulin is between 3 and 42 nanograms per milliliter.

Doctors won't test the level of thyroglobulin in your blood for the purpose of making a diagnosis of thyroid disease, because several different conditions cause thyroglobulin elevations. Rather, a thyroglobulin test follows the course of a patient already diagnosed with a thyroid condition — especially a thyroid cancer patient, who shows an increase in thyroglobulin if the cancer grows and spreads. Immediately after surgery for thyroid cancer, the thyroglobulin level is very low, but if the cancer remains present and spreads, the thyroglobulin increases.

Determining the Size, Shape, and Content of Your Thyroid

As I mention earlier in their respective sections, free thyroxine (FT4) and thyroid-stimulating hormone (TSH) levels are normal in patients who have thyroid conditions in which hormone activity is normal. Therefore, other types of tests may be necessary to gather information about the size, shape, and content of the thyroid gland. Even when a doctor has already diagnosed an abnormal thyroid activity, one or more of the following studies may help to differentiate the causes. Each test is easy and painless and provides information that a doctor can obtain no other way.

Radioactive iodine uptake and scan

The thyroid concentrates iodine from the blood in order to make thyroid hormones (see Chapter 2), a fact used for decades to perform a study of the dynamic activity of the thyroid. The procedure is performed in the hospital in the nuclear medicine laboratory. If a patient takes radioactive iodine (in the form of a capsule the patient swallows), a device like a Geiger counter can be passed over the thyroid to count the radioactivity. This count is done 6 and 24 hours after the radioactive iodine is swallowed to measure the speed with which the thyroid takes up the iodine.

A normal thyroid appears like a butterfly (see Chapter 2) at the lower end of the neck. The counts of radioactivity are uniform throughout. On paper, the counts register as dots. If the gland is normal, dots in every part of the gland are uniform, and the picture on paper shows the shape and two-dimensional size of the gland.

When one thyroid nodule is overactive, most of the radioactive iodine concentrates in that nodule, giving it a darker appearance on paper. The overactivity suppresses production of TSH so the rest of the thyroid isn't stimulated to take up iodine. Because of its appearance, the dark spot of overactivity on the thyroid is called a *hot nodule.* The rest of the gland is suppressed and appears lighter and is therefore said to be "cold." A *cold nodule* is a nodule that doesn't concentrate as much iodine as the rest of the gland. Thyroid cancers are generally "cold," because cancerous parts of the thyroid don't produce thyroid hormone in the usual way. However, most cold nodules aren't cancer.

Theories explaining autoantibody production

Exactly why the body forms antibodies against its own tissue isn't known, but several theories exist. Ordinarily, certain cells in the body prevent production of antibodies against parts of your own body. People who form thyroid autoantibodies may be deficient in protective cells at some point early in life. Another possibility is that a foreign invader (like a virus) with antigens similar to antigens in thyroid tissue attacks the body at some point. In making antibodies to fight the foreign antigens, the body makes antibodies that fight its own tissue as well.

In addition to showing the size and shape of the gland, a radioactive scan and uptake measures how active the thyroid is. When the thyroid is overactive, it takes up more iodine than normal. When it's underactive, it takes up less than normal. The maximum uptake of radioactivity usually occurs about 24 hours after swallowing the iodine. At this point, a normal thyroid has taken up between 5 and 25 percent of the administered dose of iodine. An overactive thyroid takes up 35 percent or more. Uptake between 25 and 35 percent is borderline.

Figure 4-1 shows the appearance of a normal thyroid scan and a scan that indicates hyperthyroidism. The second scan is much darker and shows a larger thyroid gland, which is consistent with the increased uptake and growth of the thyroid in hyperthyroidism.

Figure 4-1:
A normal thyroid and a hyperactive thyroid as shown in a radioactive iodine scan.

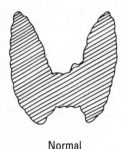 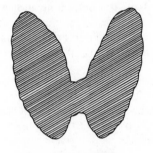

Normal   Hyperthyroid

A few situations prevent obtaining a thyroid scan and uptake. If a patient takes in large amounts of iodine, the iodine then both blocks iodine uptake by the thyroid and dilutes the administered dose. If you take thyroid replacement hormone, the hormone blocks thyroid activity and reduces the uptake of radioactive iodine. Diseases such as silent thyroiditis (see Chapter 11), where the iodine leaves the thyroid rapidly, also prevent a proper study.

In the past, doctors generally did the radioactive iodine scan and uptake to make a diagnosis of an overactive thyroid. Doctors don't do these tests as much anymore, because the blood levels of T4 and TSH are usually definitive along with the physical examination. Doctors use the scan and uptake more often for a thyroid that's abnormal in shape to establish whether multiple nodules are present (see Chapter 9) and to determine whether a nodule is overactive. The thyroid scan also assists in the management of thyroid cancer (see Chapter 8). It helps to determine if any thyroid tissue is left after the thyroid is removed by surgery and later to find new growths of cancer that have developed in the neck or elsewhere in the body.

Thyroid ultrasound

The *thyroid ultrasound,* also known as an *echogram* or *sonogram,* is a study that uses sound to measure the size, shape, and consistency of thyroid tissue. An ultrasound study uses no radiation. To get a thyroid ultrasound, you go to the testing facility and lie on your back on a table with your neck hyperextended. A gel is placed on your neck to assist in the transmission of the sound. A device called a *transducer* passes over the area of the thyroid, sending out high-pitched sound waves that tissue reflects back and a micro-phone collects. Tissue that contains water gives the best reflections, while solid tissue like bone gives poor reflections.

A thyroid ultrasound can measure the size of the thyroid or nodules very pre-cisely. It can be used to follow treatment for an enlarged thyroid or nodule to see whether it's shrinking. It can tell the difference between a cyst filled with fluid (which is almost never a cancer) and a solid nodule that may be a cancer. Ultrasound is much better than a physical examination in detecting thyroid cancer spread into the neck. Therefore, your physician should find any possi-ble site of cancer in the neck before thyroid cancer surgery so the surgeon can remove it.

This test is often used after a radioactive iodine scan detects an area that's cold. But is it cold because it contains no thyroid tissue, which is how a cyst appears, or is it cold because it contains cancerous thyroid tissue that's solid? The ultrasound can differentiate a cyst from a solid mass but can't tell you whether the mass is cancer. (Most of the time, the mass isn't cancer.)

Figure 4-2 shows a normal ultrasound study of the thyroid and one in which a prominent nodule is solid.

Deciphering ultrasound

A beam of sound from an ultrasound device consists of high-frequency sound waves. The frequency is far higher than anything the human ear can hear. Such a beam can be focused and directed just like a beam of light. When the beam strikes tissue, the tissue reflects a certain amount of sound back — the amount depends on how dense the tissue is. Air hardly reflects back any of the sound beam at all, while tissue, which consists of many layers and contains water, sends plenty of sound back. Different tis-sues absorb the sound differently, reflecting the sound to a different extent. A cancer appears differently on an ultrasound than normal thyroid tissue or a cyst filled with fluid. When the reflec-tion returns, the sound energy is converted to light energy and electrical energy. The electri-cal energy can be displayed on a cathode ray tube or made into a permanent record by expos-ing a film to the light energy.

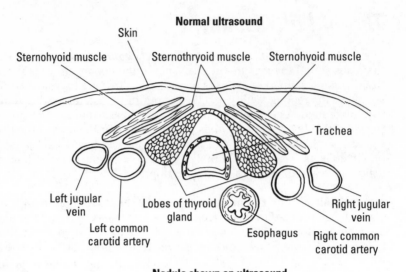

Normal ultrasound

Skin

Sternohyoid muscle   Sternothryoid muscle   Sternohyoid muscle

Trachea

Left jugular
vein

Lobes of thyroid
gland

Right jugular
vein

Left common
carotid artery

Esophagus

Right common
carotid artery

Nodule shown on ultrasound

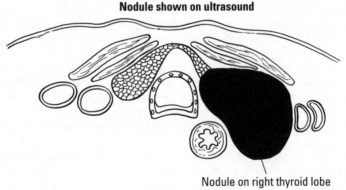

Figure 4-2:
A normal
ultrasound
study (top)
and an
ultrasound
that shows
a solid
nodule
(bottom).

Nodule on right thyroid lobe

Fine needle aspiration biopsy (FNAB)

When a doctor has a question about the type of tissue making up a growth on the thyroid, the *fine needle aspiration biopsy* (FNAB) may be the definitive test. It's just about painless and free of complications. It is done in your doctor's office with no anesthesia. After cleaning the area with alcohol, a small needle is introduced into the growth and, pulling back on the plunger to create a vacuum, removes tiny bits of tissue. The needle is moved to a few different places. You don't usually have to stay to be observed, because complications from the FNAB are so rare.

Ultrasound of the thyroid can guide the needle into the questionable thyroid tissue. You can see both the end of the needle and the tissue at the same time to make sure that you're getting the specimen you want and not some normal tissue next to it.

The tissue is sprayed on a fixative, stained, and examined for signs of cancer. Most of the time, FNAB can rule cancer out or in. Occasionally, the tissue won't provide a clear diagnosis, and your doctor does a core needle biopsy or removes the lobe (side) of the thyroid that contains the lump.

FNAB has saved thousands of patients from surgery and is often the first test performed to check for cancer, skipping the thyroid scan and the ultrasound. The Willie Sutton theory is the basis for using an FNAB first to check for thyroid cancer. Willie was a bank robber, and someone once asked him why he robbed banks. His answer was "You go where the money is."

Core needle biopsy of the thyroid

If the FNAB doesn't provide an accurate diagnosis, the next step may be a core needle biopsy. The needle in a core needle biopsy is significantly larger than in a fine needle aspiration biopsy. The nodule needs to be at least three-fourths of an inch in diameter to do a core needle biopsy, which you usually receive in the outpatient department of your hospital. The biopsy takes about 30 minutes, and you need to stay at the hospital for an additional 30 minutes to be observed for bleeding.

The skin over the area of the thyroid to be biopsied is cleaned with alcohol and is injected with a local anesthetic. A needle is inserted into the suspected tissue several times to obtain a sample of thyroid tissue. Unlike the fine needle biopsy, the suspected tissue maintains its structure so the pathologist can get a good view of it. The technique can be even more valuable if an ultrasound study guides the needle, allowing it to go exactly where the abnormal tissue is.

Sometimes you experience a little tenderness after a core needle biopsy. You can take Tylenol but nothing that prolongs your bleeding time, such as aspirin.

Part II
Diagnosing and Treating Thyroid Conditions

The 5th Wave   By Rich Tennant

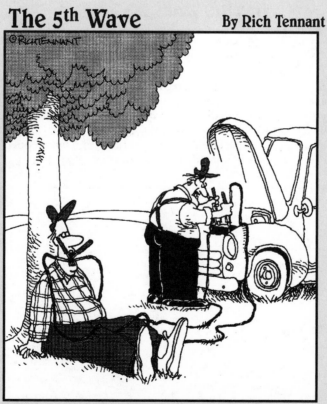

"Okay boy, I think you're so tired all the time because your thyroid needs jump startin'. Hang on, we're about ready for contact."

In this part . . .

The thyroid can be overactive or underactive. It can be too large or too small. It can be bumpy or smooth. The chapters in this part introduce you to all kinds of thyroid abnormalities. You discover how to recognize them and how to differentiate one from another. For those of you with thyroid disorders, I explain how they occur, which of the common signs and symptoms you have, how a particular disorder damages your body, and what you can do to cure it so no damage occurs.

Chapter 5

Dealing with Decreased Thyroid Function

*T*he most common form of thyroid disease throughout the world is *hypothyroidism,* or low thyroid function (also known as *myxedema*). Hypothyroidism has numerous causes, but worldwide, iodine deficiency probably leads the list (see Chapter 12). In the United States and Europe, however, iodine deficiency is rare, and the leading cause of hypothyroidism is autoimmune thyroid disease.

In this chapter, I introduce you to the immensity of hypothyroidism, show you how hypothyroidism affects the body, and explain the proper treatment for the various forms of hypothyroidism. In the last few years, some key changes in our understanding of hypothyroidism have developed. I include new medical information here so you can be up to date when you talk with your doctor about your symptoms and treatment.

Living with Autoimmune Thyroiditis

Stacy Dummy is a 46-year-old woman who is the cousin of Sarah and Margaret Dummy, whom you meet in Chapter 15. She has generally been healthy but recently noticed some swelling in the lower part of her neck. The swelling seemed to develop very slowly, and she didn't notice it until she tried to button a collar over her neck. Other than the swelling, she really doesn't have any physical problems. She isn't gaining weight. She sleeps well at night and isn't overly tired. She isn't feeling unusually hot or cold.

Her appetite is normal, as are her bowel movements. She has no discomfort associated with the growth in her neck.

Stacy's cousin Sarah, who recently received a diagnosis of hypothyroidism, tells Stacy that she knows a good thyroid specialist who told her that other members of her family may have thyroid disease. Stacy goes to see Dr. Rubin, who examines her and finds that her thyroid gland is twice as large as normal. He finds no other significant abnormalities. He sends Stacy to the laboratory for two tests — a thyroid-stimulating hormone (TSH) test and a free thyroxine (FT4) test — both of which return within the normal range (see Chapter 4). Because of his clinical suspicion, Dr. Rubin also obtains thyroid autoantibody tests. Stacy's autoantibodies are very elevated, particularly her thyroid peroxidase autoantibodies, but also her antithyroglobulin autoantibodies (see Chapter 4).

Dr. Rubin tells Stacy that she has a condition called autoimmune thyroiditis, also known as chronic thyroiditis. He tells her that treatment is optional for the present. If she's unhappy with the tissue sticking out on her neck, she can take thyroid hormone to shrink it. If not, she need only return in six months or a year to check to see whether the disease progresses to hypothyroidism.

Stacy's condition is a typical illustration of chronic thyroiditis, also called *Hashimoto's thyroiditis, autoimmune thyroiditis,* or *autoimmune thyroid disease.* She is currently free of symptoms of hypothyroidism such as coldness and fatigue, and her only abnormality is a *goiter,* an enlargement of the thyroid. The blood tests that reflect her thyroid function are normal. The high levels of thyroid autoantibodies in her system determine her diagnosis.

Most studies indicate that 10 percent of the world's population tests positive for elevated thyroid autoantibodies (see Chapter 4). If the U.S. has a population of approximately 296 million people, about 29.6 million of them would test positive. Many experts (including me) believe that these 29.6 million people have chronic thyroiditis. The good news: Chronic thyroiditis will never bother the vast majority of folks who have it.

Only about 1 in 1,000 people who test positive for elevated thyroid autoantibodies develop symptomatic chronic thyroiditis, which means that about 29,600 new cases of symptomatic chronic thyroiditis occur in the United States each year. A woman is 20 times more likely to have symptomatic chronic thyroiditis than a man. The typical patient is 30 to 50 years old, but chronic thyroiditis also affects children.

Chronic thyroiditis is a familial disease that mothers usually transmit to their daughters (see Chapter 14). Even members of a family who show no symptoms of chronic thyroiditis often have thyroid autoantibodies in their blood (especially the females) and may develop hypothyroidism later on.

Signs and symptoms

The classic picture of chronic thyroiditis is a very gradual, painless swelling of the entire thyroid gland in a woman between 30 and 50 years of age. Over time, destruction of thyroid cells may occur, and if it does, the end stage of chronic thyroiditis is hypothyroidism (see the following section, "Approach to treatment"). Alternately, hypothyroidism may develop from chronic thyroiditis when autoantibodies that block thyroid-stimulating hormone (TSH) prevent TSH from reaching the thyroid. In this case, the hypothyroidism can reverse itself when the antibodies that block TSH decline, a reversal that occurs for up to 25 percent of patients with chronic thyroiditis.

Other autoantibodies form in chronic thyroiditis that may stimulate the thyroid in a way similar to thyroid-stimulating hormone. If such autoantibodies predominate, the chronic thyroiditis leads to hyperthyroidism rather than hypothyroidism. Some patients can alternate between hypothyroidism and hyperthyroidism, depending on which autoantibodies are most active. (Turn to Chapter 6 for more information on hyperthyroidism.)

Some people with chronic thyroiditis do have symptoms, even when their thyroid function tests are normal. In addition to neck swelling, symptoms include

- ✔ Pain in the neck (which is unusual)
- ✔ Chest pain (which occurs in about 25 percent of patients)
- ✔ Trouble swallowing or a sensation of fullness in the neck

Chronic thyroiditis is one of several autoimmune conditions that can affect an individual. If you have chronic thyroiditis, you have a greater chance of contracting other autoimmune conditions, including type 1 diabetes, rheumatoid arthritis, celiac disease, adrenal insufficiency, and pernicious anemia (see the "Coexisting autoimmune diseases" section, later in the chapter).

Approach to treatment

Because it's so benign, doctors usually don't treat chronic thyroiditis that hasn't progressed to hypothyroidism. If you have neck pain because of chronic thyroiditis, aspirin can generally control it. In rare cases, the neck pain responds to nothing but removal of the thyroid gland.

If the swelling in your neck is unsightly or you have difficulty swallowing, your doctor will prescribe thyroid hormone to block the production of thyroid-stimulating hormone (TSH). Your thyroid gland then shrinks. Thyroid hormone works better to shrink the thyroid in younger people with chronic thyroiditis because permanent changes like scarring may occur as the patient gets older. The shrinkage may take place within two to four weeks after starting thyroid. Usually, you should stop the hormone treatment after a few years, because up to one quarter of patients with chronic thyroiditis have a remission and no longer need thyroid treatment.

Transient symptoms of hyperthyroidism as a result of chronic thyroiditis usually require no treatment either. The symptoms usually last a few weeks, and then you return to normal. In especially severe cases, you can take drugs that block the action of thyroid hormones (see Chapter 6).

Coexisting autoimmune diseases

Occasionally, a patient with autoimmune thyroid disease has other autoimmune diseases, many of which involve other glands of the body. For example, diabetes mellitus type 1 sometimes occurs together with autoimmune thyroid disease. The cause is the autoimmune destruction of the insulin-producing cells of the pancreas. Another example is Addison's disease, the autoimmune destruction of the adrenal gland. Addison's disease is associated with severe fatigue and low blood pressure and is especially important to identify because giving thyroid hormone without adrenal hormone to a patient who is hypothyroid and has Addison's disease can be dangerous.

Autoimmune destruction of the ovaries in women or the testicles in men may also occur when a patient has autoimmune thyroiditis. The result for women is failure to menstruate; for men it is infertility and impotency.

Another gland that autoimmune disease may affect is the *parathyroid* (which actually consists of four parathyroid glands), sitting behind the thyroid in the neck. Loss of parathyroid function results in low blood calcium and the possibility of severe muscle spasms and psychological changes.

Some autoimmune diseases that affect the joints of the body occur together with autoimmune thyroiditis. Rheumatoid arthritis is the most common example, but other diseases with names like *Sjogren's syndrome* and *systemic lupus erythematosis* may also be present.

Lastly, be aware of a blood disease called *pernicious anemia,* an autoimmune disease that accompanies autoimmune thyroiditis on occasion. In pernicious anemia, autoimmunity destroys cells of the stomach that produce acid. The patient is unable to absorb vitamin B12 and develops anemia along with symptoms in the nervous system.

On occasion, when different autoimmune diseases occur together, treatment of one of them treats the other at the same time. For example, treating your hypothyroidism with thyroid hormone may greatly improve your diabetes.

Identifying Hypothyroidism

Karen Dummy is Stacy's younger sister. Over the last few years, she has noticed the gradual enlargement of her neck — a symptom similar to the one Stacy experienced. But Karen has a number of other problems as well. She has gained a few pounds, and her legs appear swollen but don't retain an indentation when she presses on them. She feels cold when her husband feels comfortable and is constantly asking for more heat. Her skin is dry, and her nails are brittle. She has dry hair and notices that she is losing more hair than before. The outer third of her eyelashes seems to have disappeared. She used to love to sing in her choir, but her voice is husky lately. She has trouble seeing to drive at night and notices trouble hearing as well. When her periods occur, the amount of bleeding is much greater than it used to be. She and her husband are trying to become pregnant without much success.

Dr. Rubin, who is rapidly becoming the Dummy family doctor, examines her in his office. He finds that in addition to all the symptoms Karen explains to him, she also has a slow pulse and an enlarged thyroid gland. He sends her for thyroid function tests (TSH and FT4) as well as thyroid autoantibody tests.

Karen's tests show that she has a low FT4 and a high TSH. Her autoantibody levels are elevated. Dr. Rubin makes a diagnosis of hypothyroidism due to chronic thyroiditis. He starts her on thyroid-hormone replacement. Within six weeks, Karen is her old self. Full of gratitude, she puts Dr. Rubin in her will.

The preceding stories of Stacy and Karen illustrate that although thyroid disease runs in families, especially the female members of a family, it doesn't have to manifest itself the same way in each person.

Although Stacy doesn't show evidence of hypothyroidism, Karen is clearly hypothyroid.

Signs and symptoms of hypothyroidism

The classic signs and symptoms of hypothyroidism include

- ✔ A slow pulse and enlarged heart
- ✔ An enlarged thyroid *(goiter),* unless prior removal of the thyroid gland is the cause of hypothyroidism
- ✔ Dry, cool skin that's puffy, pale, and yellowish
- ✔ White patches of skin where pigment is lost (a condition called *vitiligo)*
- ✔ Brittle nails and dry, brittle hair that tends to fall out excessively
- ✔ Swelling that doesn't retain an indentation, especially of the legs

✔ Hoarseness and slow speech with a thickened tongue

✔ An expressionless face

✔ Slow reflexes

Patients with hypothyroidism complain of many different symptoms, and each patient has unique complaints. Among the most common are

✔ Intolerance to cold

✔ Weight gain

✔ Tiredness and a need to sleep

✔ Weakness

✔ Pain and stiffness in the joints and muscles

✔ Constipation

✔ Increased menstrual flow

✔ Trouble with memory and decreased concentration

✔ Trouble hearing and a ringing in the ears

✔ Trouble seeing at night

The symptoms of hypothyroidism develop over many years and are so gradual that most folks don't recognize the fact that the same disease causes them all. Plus, the signs and symptoms of hypothyroidism are fairly nonspecific, and you can easily confuse them with signs and symptoms of other common conditions. The three major sources of confusion are menopause, normal aging, and stress. All three are common occurrences for women, and men experience at least two out of the three (some people are now arguing that male menopause exists). You can see how a person with low thyroid function could easily neglect to check for hypothyroidism, which is a major reason why doctors, including me, advise routine thyroid testing starting at age 35 and continuing every five years thereafter, especially for women.

People who smoke cigarettes suffer much worse degrees of the symptoms of hypothyroidism than people who don't. Older people experience much less severity of symptoms than younger people.

Diagnosing the disease

The physician who sees a patient with the signs and symptoms of hypothyroidism obtains several tests to confirm the diagnosis. As I cover in Chapter 4, the two tests essential to the diagnosis are

✔ **Free thyroxine (FT4) level:** Lower than normal

✔ **Thyroid-stimulating hormone (TSH) level:** Higher than normal

If central hypothyroidism is present (see the "Absence of brain hormones," section, later in the chapter), the TSH is low when the FT4 is low. If you have subclinical hypothyroidism (see the "Managing Subclinical Hypothyroidism" section, later in the chapter) or nonthyroidal illness (see "Understanding the Nonthyroidal Illness Syndrome," later in the chapter), your TSH is slightly elevated but FT4 is normal.

Other tests that support the diagnosis include

- ✔ **Red blood cell counts:** A mild anemia (decrease in red blood cells)
- ✔ **Cholesterol count:** An increased cholesterol count
- ✔ **Thyroid autoantibody levels:** Elevated levels of thyroid autoantibodies (if the patient has autoimmune hypothyroidism)
- ✔ **Blood glucose level:** A blood glucose level that's lower than normal

After your doctor makes the diagnosis of hypothyroidism, he or she needs to check the various causes of your hypothyroidism (see the "Pinpointing the Causes of Hypothyroidism" section, later in the chapter) because many of them are reversible without treating the thyroid directly.

Related conditions

Hypothyroidism leads to a number of consequences that aren't good for the patient. This section describes the most important of them.

Fat abnormalities

As a result of the metabolic changes in hypothyroidism, the blood contains levels of total cholesterol and "bad" (LDL) cholesterol that lead to *atherosclerosis,* hardening of the arteries. The changes your doctor may find include the following:

- ✔ Increased total cholesterol
- ✔ Increased LDL, or "bad cholesterol"
- ✔ Decreased HDL, or "good cholesterol"
- ✔ Increased triglycerides

The result of hypothyroidism is an increased tendency toward heart attacks or strokes, which reverses when you receive proper treatment for your hypothyroidism.

Changes in reproductive function

Both men and women have major changes in their reproductive function due to lack of thyroid hormone. Their libido is reduced. Men may be impotent but can have normal semen production and make their partner pregnant. Hypothyroid women can get pregnant, but their rate of miscarriage increases. They tend to have high blood pressure with their pregnancy at a much higher rate. If hypothyroid pregnant women don't receive adequate treatment, their babies have a reduction in IQ.

Usually, hypothyroid women who are premenopausal suffer from increased bleeding during menstruation but occasionally have no menstrual flow at all. Both conditions reverse with treatment.

Pinpointing the Causes of Hypothyroidism

The two most common causes of hypothyroidism are iodine deficiency and autoimmune (chronic) thyroiditis. Iodine deficiency is rare in the United States and Europe but very common throughout the rest of the world. I discuss iodine deficiency in detail in Chapter 12. As I discuss earlier in this chapter, chronic thyroiditis is an inherited condition your doctor diagnoses by checking the levels of thyroid autoantibodies in your blood.

In addition to iodine deficiency and chronic thyroiditis, people become hypothyroid for many other reasons. Your doctor should rule out the causes I detail in the following sections before starting to treat your condition with thyroid-hormone replacement.

Removal of the thyroid

If you've had your thyroid removed because of cancer or an infection or in the course of treatment for hyperthyroidism (see Chapter 6), you are probably hypothyroid. Only if some tissue remains can the thyroid possibly continue to function.

Absence of brain hormones

Anything that destroys the *hypothalamus* (the part of the brain that secretes *thyrotrophin-releasing hormone*) or the *pituitary gland* (the part of the brain that secretes thyroid-stimulating hormone) produces *central hypothyroidism* — hypothyroidism originating in the control center of the body, the brain. A trauma, infection, or infiltration (a replacement of brain tissue with other tissue, which can occur when a patient has cancer) can cause this type of destruction. The same result can also occur if the pituitary is involved with a destructive lesion, such as radiation treatment to the area of the pituitary gland, that prevents the production and release of TSH.

If a problem with the hypothalamus or pituitary causes your hypothyroidism, your doctor won't be able to find some of the signs and symptoms associated with chronic (autoimmune) thyroiditis. In particular, hoarseness and a thickened tongue occur in autoimmune hypothyroidism but not in hypothyroidism associated with a lack of brain hormones. In addition, in hypothyroidism caused by the absence of brain hormones, the thyroid isn't usually enlarged because TSH isn't stimulating it. Also, the patient's hair and skin aren't coarse (as they are if the patient has autoimmune hypothyroidism).

Symptoms that result from a lack of other pituitary hormones also help to differentiate central hypothyroidism from failure of the thyroid gland. Symptoms include fine wrinkling of the skin of the face and a more pronounced loss of underarm, pubic, and facial hair.

Foods that cause hypothyroidism

Many common foods can cause hypothyroidism if you eat them in sufficient quantities, especially if you have an iodine deficiency or are already mildly hypothyroid. Foods that can cause hypothyroidism are called *goitrogens,* because they can trigger the enlargement of the thyroid (a goiter) as well as hypothyroidism. They block the conversion of T4 hormone to T3, the active form of thyroid hormone (see Chapter 2). They also prevent the formation of thyroid hormone by binding iodine so your body can't use it. Among the more common foods that may cause hypothyroidism are

- ✔ Almond seeds
- ✔ Brussels sprouts
- ✔ Cabbage
- ✔ Cauliflower
- ✔ Corn
- ✔ Kale
- ✔ Turnips

Soybeans can increase the need for thyroxine by increasing the loss of T4 in bowel movements. Soybeans also may contain a substance that blocks thyroid hormone production.

If consuming the preceding foods is the cause of your hypothyroidism, you can cure your hypothyroidism by simply removing them from your diet. It takes between three and six weeks for your thyroid to return to normal after you stop eating these foods.

Drugs that cause hypothyroidism

Many different medications cause hypothyroidism in the same way as the goitrogens I list in the previous section: They block the conversion of T4 to T3. The drugs you are most likely to run into include

- ✔ Adrenal steroids like prednisone and hydrocortisone, which treat inflammation
- ✔ Amiodarone, a heart drug
- ✔ Antithyroid drugs like propylthiouricil and methimazole (see Chapter 6)
- ✔ Lithium, for psychiatric treatment
- ✔ Propranolol, a beta blocker (see Chapter 6)

Diagnosing Severe Hypothyroidism

The United States rarely sees hypothyroidism in its severest form within its borders, but if the disease goes untreated and total thyroid failure occurs, the patient may die. The clinical picture that develops is one of extreme worsening of the signs and symptoms I describe earlier in the chapter. The skin becomes extremely dry and coarse, and the patient's hair falls out. The patient may lose all of his or her eyelashes, and body temperature may fall to a low level, 92 degrees or lower. The patient is less and less active and may lapse into a coma called *myxedema coma,* which can last for many days until the patient dies of heart failure or infection. (An infection or heart disease may precipitate the myxedema coma in the first place in an elderly person with very low thyroid function.)

Because a patient with the severest form of hypothyroidism may not be taking in food or, if the patient is, absorbing the food extremely slowly, treatment may require injections of thyroid hormones (which I describe in the following section).

Treating Hypothyroidism with Hormones

The treatment of hypothyroidism, once thought to be very complicated, is now fairly simple after a doctor makes a diagnosis. However, a number of newer thoughts on the subject are worth considering as you and your doctor discuss treatment.

Patients with hypothyroidism caused by chronic thyroiditis or removal of the thyroid take daily thyroid-hormone replacement pills. If the cause of your hypothyroidism is something other than autoimmune failure of the thyroid or removal of the thyroid, your physician must address the cause of your hypothyroidism along with replacing the thyroid hormone that's deficient.

For example, if you have a pituitary tumor responsible for a loss of TSH, your doctor must treat the tumor and replace other hormones in addition to thyroid hormones. If a drug or food is causing your hypothyroidism, removal of the responsible drug or food usually cures the condition. Sometimes you can't quit taking the drug causing your hypothyroidism, in which case you receive thyroid-hormone replacement to alleviate your hypothyroidism.

Turning to the right hormones

The first treatment to replace absent thyroid hormone came from the thyroids of animals and was called *desiccated thyroid*. For many decades, it was the only treatment available. When it became possible to make T4 hormone in the laboratory, T4 (also called *L-thyroxine*) replaced desiccated thyroid. Several reasons were behind the change. First, the amount of hormone in a given animal's thyroid differs from animal to animal, so the dose delivered could never be standardized. Second, desiccated thyroid contained both T4 and T3 in amounts significantly different from the way the normal thyroid gland secretes it. No logical reason now justifies using desiccated thyroid for the treatment of hypothyroidism.

Because 80 percent of the T3 thyroid hormone in your body comes from the conversion of T4 into T3 (at sites other than the thyroid), doctors believe that you can take T4 alone, and the body takes care of producing the T3 it needs. A number of recent studies confirm that you can safely take T4 alone. For example, a study reported in *The Journal of Clinical Endocrinology and Metabolism* in May 2005 reviewed nine controlled clinical trials that compared T4 alone to combinations of T4 and T3. No difference in mood, quality of life, or mental functioning existed between the two groups.

Almost all people in the world who are currently receiving replacement thyroid hormone to treat hypothyroidism are taking T4 alone.

Determining the right amount

Lifelong treatment with thyroxine subjects you to no medical complications if you're on the correct dose. A TSH test determines the amount of thyroid hormone you receive (assuming that central hypothyroidism isn't the diagnosis).

The normal blood level of TSH is 0.5 to 5.0 mU/ml (microunits per milliliter) in most laboratories.

Keep in mind that some doctors question whether 0.5 to 5.0 mU/ml is actually the normal range for TSH. We know that 10 percent of the population tests positive for thyroid autoantibodies and probably has autoimmune thyroid disease. Most of these 10 percent don't receive the diagnosis of hypothyroidism. When a laboratory creates a normal range, it tests several hundred or more people considered free of thyroid disease, usually because they have no signs or symptoms. The laboratory measures their TSH and produces the range for TSH in the normal population. But is the laboratory really measuring a normal population when one in every ten people tested may have a subclinical thyroid disease (see the "Managing Subclinical Hypothyroidism" section, later in the chapter)?

In my practice, I've had several patients who didn't feel normal with a TSH between 3 and 5. I've given these patients enough thyroid hormone to lower their TSH to under 3 with gratifying results. I believe that future studies will indicate that the normal range for TSH is more like 0.5 to 2.5.

If you're receiving treatment for hypothyroidism and don't feel right on your current dose of replacement thyroid hormone, ask your doctor to check your TSH. If it's above 3, ask your doctor to prescribe more thyroid hormone to lower it below 3.

Another important point is that hypothyroidism isn't necessarily permanent. Up to 25 percent of patients with autoimmune hypothyroidism may return to normal thyroid function at a later date. The reason is that the autoantibodies that block the action of TSH may decline over time.

If you've been receiving treatment for several years for autoimmune hypothyroidism, ask your doctor if you can stop the thyroid-hormone replacement for four to six weeks to see whether your TSH remains low. (Don't stop taking your hormone replacement without your doctor's supervision, however.)

On the other hand, a thyroid gland that's failing due to autoimmune thyroiditis goes through several levels of failure. At first, you may need little thyroid hormone to replace what you're missing. With time, more of your thyroid tissue may fail, or the antibodies that block TSH may increase, and you need more thyroid hormone. Seeing your doctor on a regular basis to check for the increasing (or decreasing) failure of your thyroid is important. Making routine appointments to check your thyroid function is especially important if your hypothyroidism develops as a result of radioactive iodine treatment for a hyperactive thyroid gland — in which case your thyroid gland gradually loses its function, and your dose of thyroid may not stabilize for several years.

After your thyroid function stabilizes, see your physician every six months or every year to check your TSH level and alter your dosage of thyroid hormone if necessary. Checkups are important, because you may not feel different even if your thyroid function gradually declines.

Filling your prescription and taking your medication

The various brands of thyroxine aren't necessarily biologically equivalent. You therefore need to get the same brand every time you renew your prescription. For example, if you're on Levoxyl, make sure your pharmacy gives you Levoxyl every time you get more pills. Small differences in dosage may result in overtreatment or undertreatment. If your pharmacy switches your brand for any reason, your doctor must be retest you in 8 to12 weeks on the new preparation.

Thyroxine (T4) comes in many different dose sizes so doctors can tailor it to the patient. The sizes include 25, 50, 75, 88, 100, 112, 125, 137, 150, 175, 200, and 300 micrograms. The correct dosage for you should be among the many choices I list.

Take thyroid hormone on an empty stomach.

Doctors have long recommended that people over 60 who have to start taking thyroid hormone start with a very low dose and build up to the correct dose. No evidence in the medical literature supports this assertion. A recent study published in the *Archives of Internal Medicine* in January 2005 shows that building seniors' dosage of thyroid hormone isn't necessary. The study gave 25 patients over 60 half the starting dose of another group of 25 patients over 60. None of the patients had symptomatic cardiac disease, and no one in the group given the larger dose voiced cardiac complaints. Therefore, doctors should start most patients on the full dose.

For many years, doctors suspected that generic forms of thyroid-hormone replacement pills didn't consistently provide a known level of the hormone, so doctors recommended brand-name products. Recent studies, however, show that generic thyroid hormone has the same potency as brand-name thyroid hormone and is, of course, much cheaper.

Testing hormone levels

About four to six weeks must elapse for a change in your dose of replacement thyroid hormone to make a difference in your lab tests. If your doctor changes your dose, he or she should retest you in about four to six weeks to make sure you're on the correct dose.

Treating Myxedema Coma

Mxedema coma, the severest form of hypothyroidism, is a medical emergency. Mxedema coma isn't something you can manage outside a hospital. Large medical centers may see one case a year, so no one has much experience treating it. About 20 percent of cases don't survive.

The person with myxedema coma may be unarousable. Her body temperature may be extremely low even though she has an infection. Usually some event, such as an infection, a drug overdose, some trauma, a stroke, or a heart attack, trips the patient over from severe hypothyroidism to coma. When doctors test the TSH, it may be 100 or 200, and the free T4 may not be measurable. However, the patient receives treatment for myxedema coma before the results of blood tests return.

The doctor checks all aspects of the patient, including respiration, blood glucose, body temperature, presence of a precipitating event, and so forth, and treats all aspects at the same time. The key treatment is thyroid hormone given by injection.

Managing Subclinical Hypothyroidism

In a way, subclinical hypothyroidism is one extreme of hypothyroidism, and myxedema coma is the other. In *subclinical hypothyroidism,* the free T4 is normal while the TSH is only slightly elevated. A value of 6 for the TSH is common. Knowing whether the slight fatigue or dry skin the patient complains about (if she complains about anything) has anything to do with her thyroid function is very difficult.

When doctors follow patients with subclinical hypothyroidism without treating them, very few of the patients, less than 20 percent, develop overt hypothyroidism later on. If they receive treatment, proving that they have improved in any way is difficult because they're mostly not symptomatic. Even if they do improve with treatment, saying whether their improvement is because of the thyroid hormone or a placebo effect is similarly difficult.

Though less than 20 percent of folks with subclinical hypothyroidism develop overt hypothyroidism later, the fact is that the presence of thyroid autoantibodies makes patients with subclinical hypothyroidism more likely than people without autoantibodies to go on to develop overt hypothyroidism.

Although the current consensus is that people with subclinical hypothyroidism don't need treatment because the consequences of the condition are minimal, the newest studies appear to reverse this assessment. See Chapter 19 for more information on recent studies that show that subclinical hypothyroidism should be treated. Thyroid doctors will be reviewing this new information over the next several months.

I believe that patients with subclinical hypothyroidism should generally be treated with thyroid hormone to make the TSH normal. Selected patients with more symptoms should definitely undergo a trial of six months of thyroxine therapy with a review of their clinical response after that.

Understanding the Nonthyroidal Illness Syndrome

Falling thyroid hormone levels aren't always due to hypothyroidism. Nonthyroidal illness syndrome may be to blame. The syndrome can cause confusion with hypothyroidism, so it requires understanding. A number of conditions cause nonthyroidal illness syndrome:

- ✔ Starvation
- ✔ Severe infection
- ✔ Severe trauma
- ✔ Severe illness

The first change in thyroid blood levels in a patient with nonthyroidal illness syndrome is a fall in the serum free T3. The fall is due, at least in part, to a failure of conversion of T4 to T3. As the condition gets worse, the free T4 falls as well. The fact that the free T4 falls is a very bad prognostic sign. Most people die when their free T4 is below a certain level. The TSH is usually normal in people with nonthyroidal illness syndrome.

When a doctor examines a patient with nonthyroidal illness syndrome for signs of hypothyroidism, the doctor usually can't find any, but the patient is so sick that the syndrome may be masking signs like low body temperature; plus, the signs of nonthyroidal illness syndrome usually take weeks to develop. However, a patient with the syndrome does have low tissue levels of T3 and T4 in addition to the low blood level of T3. The question is whether the low T3 and T4 tissue levels are beneficial for the very sick individual or need treatment.

When patients with nonthyroidal illness syndrome are givenT4, they show no improvement in their clinical condition or their mortality compared to patients with the syndrome who are not given T4, even though the measured T4 in their body increases. However, the measured T3 doesn't increase. When T3 is given, it does seem to improve the clinical situation to a mild degree and doesn't seem to make it any worse.

Much more study of this unique syndrome is required, but for now, the recommended treatment consists in giving the patient T3 while treating all the other features of the particular illness, such as infection, at the same time.

Chapter 6

Taming the Hyperactive Thyroid

● ●

In This Chapter

▶ Recognizing the symptoms of hyperthyroidism

▶ Linking hyperthyroidism and Graves' disease

▶ Deciding on treatment

▶ Battling severe hyperthyroidism

● ●

*H*yperthyroidism refers to the excessive production of thyroid hormones, which leads to many signs and symptoms that suggest your body is, in effect, speeding up. Hyperthyroidism is fairly common. Each year, about 100 per 100,000 people receive a diagnosis, which adds up to more than 296,000 new cases in the United States every year.

Most people with hyperthyroidism (about 80 percent) have an autoimmune disorder called *Graves' disease,* which I discuss in detail in this chapter. In addition to causing signs and symptoms of hyperthyroidism, Graves' disease also causes eye disease and skin disease. Hyperthyroidism and eye and skin disease are all the result of *autoimmunity* (your body, in essence, rejecting your own tissue; see Chapter 4). In some circumstances, a patient has hyperthyroidism but no eye disease or skin disease, and blood tests show no evidence of autoimmunity. Such patients don't have an autoimmune disorder, but the medical picture their hyperthyroid state produces is the same as if they had Graves'.

In this chapter, I show you how to recognize hyperthyroidism, what the treatment options are, and what possible complications may occur as a result of your treatment or the disease itself. You also discover how I would treat you if you came to me with Graves' disease. Hyperthyroidism has special features in various physical states and at different ages. Therefore, I devote more space to hypothyroidism during pregnancy (Chapter 17), in children (Chapter 18), and in the elderly (Chapter 19) later in this book. If this coverage applies to you, check out these chapters when you're finished here.

Many people believe that if you have hyperthyroidism, you're lucky because it makes weight control or weight loss easier. By the time you finish this chapter, I hope you realize why that thinking is flawed.

Detecting the Signs and Symptoms of Hyperthyroidism

Tami Dummy is the mother of Stacy and Karen. Stacy has recently received a diagnosis of autoimmune (chronic) thyroiditis and Karen a diagnosis of hypothyroidism (see Chapter 5). Tami has always been a very active person, but lately she has noticed a lot of things wrong with her, and they're getting worse.

Tami feels warm all the time, and her skin is moist. A few months ago, she lost some weight without trying and was delighted, but the weight loss has continued despite the fact that she has a strong appetite and is eating more than usual. She often feels her heart racing, which makes her very nervous. She notices that her hands shake when she just sits quietly. She goes to the bathroom more frequently than usual, both to urinate and to move her bowels.

The changes in Tami aren't lost on her husband, Patrick, or her daughters. They notice that she's constantly staring at them, though when they question her, she denies it. Patrick, in the course of giving her a massage, notices a bump on the front of her neck that wasn't there before. Tami's family insists that she see their favorite doctor, none other than (did you guess?) Dr. Rubin.

Dr. Rubin asks a number of questions and does a physical examination. He discovers that Tami's thyroid is enlarged, and he finds a skin abnormality on her lower legs. He tells the family that Tami almost certainly has hyperthyroidism due to Graves' disease. The final diagnosis requires only some confirmatory blood tests, and the outcome of the tests is so certain that Dr. Rubin gives Tami a prescription for antithyroid pills at the first office visit.

The tests confirm the diagnosis. Tami immediately starts taking a pill three times a day. After three weeks, she feels better, and after eight weeks she's her old self. She's a bit disappointed when the pounds start coming back, but she feels so good that she returns to her health club and sheds several of them in no time. Patrick is delighted to have his wife back at moderate rather than high speed. He has been wanting to go to the Oregon Shakespeare Festival, and he knew that she wouldn't sit through a play in her previous condition.

Tami continues taking the pills for the next year, with monthly visits with Dr. Rubin to confirm that she remains healthy. Blood tests show that her production of thyroid hormone is declining, and Dr. Rubin reduces her dose to two pills daily, which she can take all at once after three months. A few months later, he reduces her dose to one pill daily.

The abnormality on her lower legs doesn't get any worse but doesn't get much better either. Tami isn't particularly bothered by it, so no treatment is given. At the end of the year, Tami stops taking the medication entirely.

Tami comes in for follow-up visits every six weeks, then every two months, and then every three months. She has now gone four years without taking the antithyroid drug and remains in good health.

Hyperthyroidism, whether caused by Graves' disease or another condition, produces consistent signs and symptoms that affect every part of your body. In the following sections I describe the major abnormalities, grouped according to the organ system of the body hyperthyroidism is affecting.

The body generally

Although the signs and symptoms of hyperthyroidism seem distinctive, most occur in people who don't have hyperthyroidism as well. For example, although palpitations occur in 75 percent of people with hyperthyroidism, they also occur in 26 percent of people who don't have hyperthyroidism. While 73 percent of people with hyperthyroidism prefer the cold, so do 41 percent of people without hyperthyroidism. Therefore, you must use laboratory tests to confirm a diagnosis of hyperthyroidism.

Hyperthyroidism can cause your body temperature to be persistently high. As a result, you may prefer wearing fewer clothes and sleeping with no covers at night. You may prefer to take your vacations in Alaska rather than Mexico. You may sweat when everyone else is comfortable.

You may lose weight despite an increased appetite. The weight loss is due to the loss of lean body tissue like muscle, not a loss of fat. In rare cases, a patient gains weight because she's eating so many calories. Hyperthyroidism can cause you to feel weak. You may feel lymph glands all over your body, because Graves' disease is an autoimmune disease and the lymph system is a key player in autoimmunity. Your tonsils, which are part of the lymph system, also enlarge.

Your face may appear to be anxious or frightened. If you lose a lot of weight, your face may be thin or emaciated. But you may also have fairly severe hyperthyroidism without any obvious change in facial appearance. Your elbows may be red.

Other possible reasons, which are more serious than Graves' disease, such as cancer in the lymph glands, may explain the enlargement of your lymph glands, so if you experience enlarged lymph glands, see your doctor.

The thyroid

When Graves' disease is the cause of hyperthyroidism, your thyroid is enlarged in a symmetrical way and the entire gland is firm. When a single overactive *nodule* (a bump on your thyroid) is to blame for hyperthyroidism, the nodule is large, but it often causes the rest of the gland to shrink. (See Chapter 7 for a discussion of nodules.) When a multinodular goiter is responsible (see Chapter 9), you can feel many lumps and bumps on your thyroid. Figure 6-1 shows a comparison of the size of the thyroid gland before treatment with antithyroid drugs and six weeks after beginning treatment in one of my hyperthyroid patients. This figure also shows the before and after affects of treatment on the appearance of your eyes, which you can read about later in the chapter.

Before treatment

After treatment

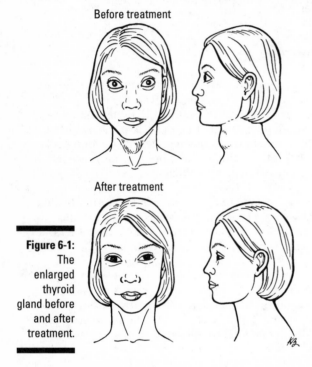

Figure 6-1:
The enlarged thyroid gland before and after treatment.

If you put your hand over an enlarged thyroid, you can often feel a buzz, or *thrill,* that results from the great increase in blood flow in the overactive thyroid. You can hear the thrill with a stethoscope; the sound is called a *bruit.* You may also have trouble swallowing and the sensation of a lump in your throat if your thyroid is large enough.

The eyes

Any form of hyperthyroidism results in reversible changes to your eyes. Your eyes appear more prominent than usual. Figure 6-1 shows an example. Your upper eyelids may be higher so that more of the white above your pupil is visible, which makes you appear as if you're staring and pop-eyed. When someone asks you to look down, your upper eyelid may not follow your eye, which exposes even more white, a phenomenon called *lid lag.* Graves' disease can cause more serious eye problems, which I discuss later in the "Thyroid eye disease" section of this chapter.

The skin and hair

The sweat glands depend upon thyroid hormone. Too much of the hormone causes them to work excessively so that the skin all over the body is moist. Because the blood vessels in the skin are widened in hyperthyroidism, the skin also feels warm. Moist and warm skin are often most notable in the hands and feet, which may appear red. You may experience a loss of skin pigmentation (a condition called *vitiligo*) in places, which is another sign of autoimmunity. Other areas of your skin may appear darker.

Your hair may be fine, straight, and unable to hold a curl. Hair growth also depends on thyroid hormone. Therefore, some loss of hair is common as the disease loses its grip. The same autoimmune process that affects the eyes and the skin affects the hair follicles.

Sometimes the nails of the fingers and toes undergo a distinctive change called Plummer's nails — a rising up of the end of the nails so that dirt and other substances can get underneath them, which makes keeping your nails clean very difficult. Plummer's nails begins on the fourth finger of each hand and spreads to the rest of the fingers and toes.

The heart

Hyperthyroidism can cause a rapid pulse, which you feel as heart palpitations. You may feel your heart beat very vigorously and may find it very uncomfortable, especially when trying to sleep. The first sign of Graves' disease is sometimes *atrial fibrillation,* an irregular heart rhythm. If a patient is older and already has heart disease, hyperthyroidism can induce heart failure. Heart pain (angina) may appear or worsen because the heart beats too rapidly. You may experience shortness of breath.

Even very mild increases in thyroid hormone may cause a decreased ability to exercise, because the heart is less able to respond to exercise. Make sure your dose of thyroid is correct if you're receiving treatment for hypothyroidism.

The nervous system and muscles

If you have hyperthyroidism, your fingers have a fine tremor when you hold your hands out. The loss of muscle tissue leads to weakness, especially in the muscles that are closer to the center of the body. Your reflexes increase; some patients can't sit still. In Chapter 15, I discuss the psychological changes associated with hyperthyroidism. Basically, if you're hyperthyroid, most likely you're nervous, you don't sleep as much as you used to, and you have rapidly changing emotions, from exhilaration to depression.

You may find that you can't perform mentally at the high level that you did before you developed hyperthyroidism. Several of my patients, law students and medical students, couldn't take examinations successfully and had to take several months off of school to recover before they could return to their studies. You may also tire much earlier than you used to.

The reproductive system

Hyperthyroidism can cause a decrease in fertility, because it interferes with ovulation. However, pregnancy can occur. Miscarriage is more common, especially if the hyperthyroidism goes uncontrolled. Menstrual flow decreases as well and may cease. I discuss more about hyperthyroidism and pregnancy in Chapter 17.

Males with hyperthyroidism have trouble having an erection in half the cases. They often experience infertility with reduced sperm count. The sperm appear abnormal when looked at under a microscope. All changes in the reproductive system disappear with successful treatment.

The stomach, intestines, and liver

If you're hyperthyroid, food moves more quickly through your intestines than it used to, and you have more frequent bowel movements or even diarrhea. You may experience nausea and vomiting. Your appetite greatly increases, and you eat more but don't gain weight. Your doctor may tell you that your liver is enlarged. Blood tests of the liver suggest a picture of hepatitis, but when the thyroid is under control, the liver returns to normal.

The bones

Your bones lose calcium and become less dense, especially if you're past menopause and aren't taking estrogen. Despite loss of bone density and calcium, bone fractures aren't common in hyperthyroid patients. When your doctor measures your blood calcium, it's elevated, but kidney stones don't occur. All bone changes return to normal with treatment of your hyperthyroidism.

The urinary system

As more blood flows, your kidneys filter more, and your body produces more urine, so you go to the bathroom more frequently. In turn, you feel thirstier than usual.

Confirming a Diagnosis of Hyperthyroidism

The signs and symptoms I describe in the previous section usually lead to a conclusive diagnosis of hyperthyroidism, which blood tests confirm. The definitive tests for hyperthyroidism are as follows:

- **Free thyroxine (FT4) level:** The levels of free T4 in your blood are elevated.

- **Thyroid-stimulating hormone (TSH) level:** The thyroid-stimulating hormone (TSH) level is suppressed (see Chapter 4).

Other tests that support the diagnosis include

- **Total T3 and Free T3 levels:** Less than 5 percent of patients with hyperthyroidism have a normal free T4 but an elevated total T3 and free T3, a condition called *T3 thyrotoxicosis,* which behaves just like T4 thyrotoxicosis. T3 thyrotoxicosis can be a source of confusion when the patient has all the symptoms of hyperthyroidism but has a normal T4. The TSH is still low in cases of T3 thyrotoxicosis.

- **Thyroid autoantibody levels:** If Graves' disease is the cause of hyperthyroidism, the levels of peroxidase autoantibody and antithyroglobulin autoantibody are elevated (see Chapter 4). They decline when the treatment is antithyroid drugs (see the "Antithyroid pills" section later in the chapter) but not when the patient receives radioactive iodine.

- **Blood glucose level:** Your blood glucose (sugar) level is elevated, because your body is absorbing food so rapidly. You may have insulin resistance, and your doctor may find that you have diabetes or that it's worsening if insulin resistance is already present. (Diabetes improves after you receive treatment for your hyperthyroidism.)

- **Liver function tests:** Blood tests of your liver function (such as the alkaline phosphatase and bilirubin levels in your blood) may be elevated.

- **Cholesterol count:** Blood tests for cholesterol and other fats may be lower than normal.

The radioactive iodine uptake and scan study (see Chapter 4) used to be a common test in the diagnosis of hyperthyroidism, but the free T4 and TSH results generally make radioactive iodine uptake unnecessary.

Determining Whether Graves' Disease Is the Culprit

Most cases of hyperthyroidism result from Graves' disease, an autoimmune condition. Graves' disease is most common in women; it occurs 10 to 20 times more often in women than in men. Symptoms tend to start between the ages of 30 and 60, but they can occur at any age. Graves' disease consists of any one or all of three parts: hyperthyroidism, eye disease, and skin disease.

Most of the signs and symptoms of Graves' disease are the result of hyperthyroidism, which in turn results from the excessive production of thyroid hormones. Doctors can distinguish Graves' disease from other forms of hyperthyroidism because blood tests identify autoimmunity. In addition to the symptoms of hyperthyroidism I detail earlier in the chapter, autoimmunity can lead to eye disease and skin disease.

Causes of Graves' disease

In Chapter 5, I explain that about 10 percent of the world's population has thyroid autoantibodies, and these autoantibodies can lead to both hypothyroidism (underactive thyroid function) and hyperthyroidism. Some autoantibodies suppress the thyroid, and others stimulate it. If you have Graves' disease, the stimulating antibodies are in control in your body. Just why a person develops Graves' disease isn't clear, but doctors and researchers have a number of theories:

✔ Your body makes many cells to prevent foreign tissue from invading and other cells that recognize your body's own tissue. When you have an autoimmune disorder, your body may have lost the cells meant to prevent other cells from reacting against the body's own tissue.

✔ Invading organisms such as viruses may share characteristics of normal body tissue. When your body creates antibodies to fight the invaders, the antibodies may react against normal tissue as well.

✔ Certain drugs can change the immunity of your body so that your body's immune system reacts against itself. The class of drugs that does this is called the *cytokines*. Doctors use cytokines to treat hepatitis and leukemia, for example. Their effect is to activate or increase immunity. As a side effect, they may activate thyroid-stimulating immunity.

✔ Women, especially, may have genes that promote autoimmunity. The frequent occurrence of Graves' disease in mothers, daughters, and sisters confirms the genetic association (see Chapter 14).

✔ When your thyroid suffers an injury, for example by a viral illness, it releases chemicals into your blood that aren't normally found there. The protective immunity cells may make antibodies against the chemicals, which then act to stimulate the thyroid.

✔ Iodine, given to a person with a large thyroid gland not making enough thyroid hormone (such as a person with a multinodular goiter; see Chapter 9), can cause a sudden production of a lot of thyroid hormone, leading to hyperthyroidism.

✔ Stress can produce a rapid heart rate, sweating, and other signs similar to hyperthyroidism. Its role in the onset of hyperthyroidism is unclear.

Symptoms specific to Graves' disease

Eye disease and skin disease associated with Graves' disease may be apparent even when a person has no overt symptoms of hyperthyroidism. Eye disease may be present long before the hyperthyroidism begins. Sometimes eye and skin problems progress even after hyperthyroidism is under control. Severe forms of thyroid eye and skin disease are rare, but thyroid eye disease can lead to blindness.

Thyroid eye disease

Thyroid eye disease, called *infiltrative ophthalmopathy* or *exopthalmus,* is present in almost all patients with Graves' disease. An ultrasound or MRI of the eye area can determine whether a patient has thyroid eye disease. Usually the condition is mild and doesn't progress after hyperthyroidism comes under control. Sometimes — in no more than 5 percent of Graves' patients — it does progress despite controlling the hyperthyroidism.

Although Graves' disease is much more common in women than in men, the ratio of women to men decreases as the eye disease worsens. About nine women for every man has mild thyroid eye disease, but the ratio of women to men is almost equal in cases of severe eye disease.

A strong association exists between eye disease in Graves' disease and cigarette smoking. Smokers have larger thyroid glands and higher levels of autoantibodies than nonsmokers, so thyroid damage may be the cause of this association.

Thyroid eye disease presents a clear-cut clinical picture. The eye, with its muscles and coverings, sits in a bony part of the skull called the *orbit.* When eye disease is present, the skin covering the eye and the muscles within the orbit are swelled and puffy. The limited room within the orbit forces the swollen skin and muscles to push forward. Usually thyroid eye disease affects both eyes, but the disease can start or progress more rapidly on one side. If your eye is pushed forward far enough, your eyelids cannot close fully. The result is irritation and redness of the eyeball.

Thyroid eye disease stretches and sometimes damages the optic nerve that carries the visual signal to your brain as well as the back of the eye, the *retina,* where your eye focuses what it sees. Eye disease may compromise the blood supply to the optic nerve and retinal tissues.

With eye disease, your eye muscles don't function properly, so your eyes don't move together; you may experience double vision as a result. Occasionally, blindness may be the end result of all the damage.

As a result of the abnormalities thyroid eye disease causes, the person with thyroid eye disease has the following complaints:

- ✔ **Injection:** The eye appears red much of the time.
- ✔ **Tearing:** Tears form without provocation.
- ✔ **Foreign-body sensation:** Pain like a dust particle in the eye.
- ✔ **Photophobia:** Sensitivity to bright light.

When a doctor examines the eye muscles of a patient with thyroid eye disease under a microscope, large numbers of autoimmune cells appear (similar to what appears in the thyroid itself).

Studies show that thyroid eye disease progresses more often when treatment is by radioactive iodine rather than antithyroid drugs (see the "Radioactive iodine treatment" section later in the chapter). In one typical study in the *New England Journal of Medicine* in January 1998, a group of 150 patients received radioactive iodine as treatment, and 148 patients took antithyroid drugs. After treatment, the eye disease was worse in 15 percent of the radioiodine patients but in only 2.7 percent of the antithyroid patients.

Treatment of thyroid eye disease usually occurs in steps; doctors apply severe measures only when milder measures fail. First, you receive local measures like methylcellulose-containing eye drops to treat the inflammation. Sunglasses manage your sensitivity to light. Prisms correct the double vision that sometimes occurs. If all these treatments fail to cure the problem, you take oral steroids to reduce your immunity. Doctors can also prescribe other drugs that suppress immunity.

If you've taken radioactive iodine for hyperthyroidism (see the "Radioactive iodine treatment" section) and are now taking thyroid hormone, adjusting the level of the thyroid hormone won't affect your eye disease.

Severe cases of thyroid eye disease usually respond to irradiation of the muscles in the orbit. If irradiation doesn't work or the case is severe enough, a surgeon can remove bone from the orbit, thus decompressing the tissues.

While the eye doctor is removing bone from the orbit, another surgeon also attempts to remove all your thyroid tissue to eliminate antigens against which antibodies can be made, and the immune cells decline. After a doctor removes your thyroid, you need to take thyroid hormone replacement pills. In theory, it would be helpful for you to take an antithyroid drug (which I describe later in "Antithyroid pills") along with thyroid hormone replacement, because the antithyroid drugs decrease immunity. But the effect of taking antithyroid drugs in conjunction with thyroid hormone hasn't received enough careful study to warrant a recommendation.

Thyroid skin disease

Thyroid skin disease, called *pretibial myxedema* and *thyroid acropachy,* occurs even less often than thyroid eye disease and is very severe in only 1 to 2 percent of patients with Graves' disease.

Pretibial myxedema is an abnormal thickening of the skin, usually in the front of the lower leg. Raised patches of skin are pink in appearance. Rarely, thyroid skin disease affects other parts of the body, such as the thighs, shoulders, and forearms. The skin problems may last for several months or longer, then gradually improve. If they become severe, they may respond to steroids applied under tight dressings. A study in the *Journal of Clinical Endocrinology* in February 2002 suggests that people who don't receive steroids as treatment have about the same clinical course as those who do, so steroids may not be of much value in treating skin disease.

With *thyroid acropachy,* a patient's fingers become wider, and she may experience arthritic damage to the joints of her fingers. Fortunately, arthritic lesions usually cause only unsightly fingers and no symptoms. Patients with these finger changes don't receive any particular treatment.

Recognizing Other Causes of Hyperthyroidism

Although the vast majority of patients with hyperthyroidism have Graves' disease, about 20 percent don't. Hyperthyroid patients without Graves' disease may have one of several other conditions that lead to the increased production of free T4 and T3 (thyroid hormones). The treatment of these conditions may differ from the treatment of Graves' disease, so recognizing them is important.

Factitious (false) *hyperthyroidism* occurs when a patient is consuming large amounts of thyroid hormone without a doctor's knowledge. Usually some kind of psychological disturbance causes this behavior. The way to distinguish between factitious hyperthyroidism and other causes of hyperthyroidism is to check the size of the thyroid gland; someone with factitious hyperthyroidism has a small thyroid gland. The large amount of thyroid hormone suppresses the gland. If a doctor does a radioactive iodine uptake (see Chapter 4), this patient's thyroid gland won't absorb a great deal of the iodine.

A large thyroid with many nodules that's exposed to a lot of iodine may become hyperthyroid (see Chapter 9). Sometimes a single nodule may produce excessive amounts of thyroid hormone and cause the rest of the thyroid to shrink. A doctor can feel whether nodules are present on the thyroid, which an ultrasound study or a thyroid scan can confirm (see Chapter 4). A number of situations exist in which consuming iodine may precipitate "iodine-induced hyperthyroidism":

- ✔ You take iodine for a goiter caused by iodine deficiency (see Chapter 12).
- ✔ You take iodine after being hyperthyroid but are normal after taking antithyroid pills.
- ✔ You take iodine and have multiple nodules but aren't hyperthyroid (see Chapter 9).
- ✔ You take iodine without having iodine deficiency, aren't hyperthyroid, but have a large thyroid.

Occasionally the thyroid produces large amounts of T3 but normal or even low levels of T4, a condition called T3 *thyrotoxicosis.* T3 thyrotoxicosis is an autoimmune condition and produces the same signs and symptoms as Graves' disease. If you have T3 thyrotoxicosis, you receive exactly the same treatment as people with Graves' disease (which is associated with a high free T4 level). T3 thyrotoxicosis is really just Graves' disease with a predominance of T3. Doctors don't yet know why T3 is elevated in these cases rather than T4. If you have the signs and symptoms of hyperthyroidism but your free T4 level is normal or even low, your doctor should measure your T3 level.

Subacute thyroiditis (see Chapter 11) may cause the release of a lot of thyroid hormone from the thyroid and briefly cause hyperthyroidism. It results from the breakdown of thyroid cells rather than overproduction of thyroid hormone. The thyroid is usually tender, and the hyperthyroidism doesn't last because the disease is usually brief in duration and the cells stop breaking down. In fact, a period of hypothyroidism may also occur as thyroid hormone stores in the thyroid gland build up again.

Certain (not very common) tumors called *choriocarcinomas,* which arise from the placental tissue between a fetus and its mother, produce a lot of the *human chorionic gonadotrophin* hormone, which stimulates the thyroid. Your doctor can measure this hormone in your blood.

Finally, *central hyperthyroidism* may also cause hyperthyroidism, although it occurs much less frequently than Graves' disease. Central hyperthyroidism has two causes: too much thyrotrophin-releasing hormone from the hypothalamus in the brain and too much thyroid-stimulating hormone (TSH) from the pituitary gland in the brain (often as a result of a tumor). In this condition, the patient's TSH level is high (whereas with Graves' disease, TSH level is low). The patient may experience symptoms of a brain tumor, such as headaches or loss of part of the visual field.

Your doctor shouldn't have difficulty differentiating any of the conditions I discuss in this section from Graves' disease, especially if he or she looks for signs that your eyes and skin are changing and orders tests that check for thyroid autoantibodies.

Choosing the Best Treatment for Graves' Disease

The treatment of Graves' disease has evolved over the years as doctors and researchers have come to understand it better and additional tools have become available. As soon as doctors understood that the thyroid was responsible for the excessive production of thyroid hormones, their obvious response was to cut out the offending tissue — a practice that produced an era of great thyroid surgeons, along with a lot of unexpected problems, which I describe in the next section, "Thyroid surgery." Around 1950, the administration of radioactive iodine began to replace surgery, which cured many patients but brought its own difficulties. Finally, antithyroid drugs became available.

Each form of treatment has its pros and cons. I find it interesting that doctors in Europe generally prefer antithyroid pills, while doctors in the U.S. choose radioactive iodine more often. In the following sections, I explain the advantages and disadvantages of each treatment, and I share with you my own bias regarding the best treatment options.

No useful or proven homeopathic methods exist for the treatment of Graves' disease; none withstand scientific investigation. A certain number of patients go into remission without any treatment, which may be the reason that some have thought that certain treatments besides surgery, RAI, and antithyroid drugs can cure hyperthyroidism.

Thyroid surgery

Thyroid surgery involves the removal of part of the thyroid gland. Surgery quickly reduces the symptoms of hyperthyroidism by removing the source of those symptoms: the thyroid that was producing too much hormone. With the availability of nonsurgical treatments, patients rarely undergo surgery today for hyperthyroidism. Some situations, however, leave surgery as the only choice:

✔ You refuse to take radioactive iodine and develop an allergy or a bad reaction to antithyroid pills (or simply fail to take them).

✔ Your thyroid gland is extremely large, which means that radioactive iodine or antithyroid pills may not be effective.

✔ You receive a diagnosis of hyperthyroidism during pregnancy that antithyroid drugs cannot control, causing problems for you or the fetus. (Women can have surgery safely any time in the second trimester of pregnancy.)

✔ Your thyroid has a nodule that suggests a possible cancer. Ultrasound and other studies I describe in Chapter 7 can evaluate you if you have nodules indicating cancer.

One reason doctors rarely perform surgery to treat thyroid conditions these days is that surgery carries certain risks. I list them here in no particular order:

✔ Any surgical operation requiring anesthesia involves risk.

✔ A person with severe heart or lung disease can't undergo surgery.

✔ Women in their third trimester of pregnancy can't undergo surgery, because it can induce labor.

✔ Surgery can damage one or both *recurrent laryngeal nerves,* which can lead to hoarseness or permanent damage to your voice with vocal cord paralysis.

✔ Surgery can damage the *parathyroid glands,* which lie behind the thyroid, leading to a severe drop in blood calcium.

✔ Although a surgeon's goal is to leave enough thyroid tissue to keep your thyroid function normal, low thyroid function may begin immediately after surgery or develop during the next few years.

✔ If you've had previous neck surgery, attempting another operation is risky because there's so much scar tissue from the previous surgery and the nerves, glands, and blood vessels are no longer in their usual positions.

✔ The surgery is intricate, and a highly experienced surgeon isn't always available. See Chapter 3 for help finding a highly competent thyroid surgeon.

Some specialists believe that surgery releases thyroid *antigens* (tissue or chemicals that the body isn't normally exposed to) into the blood stream and leaves a lot of thyroid tissue intact, which can worsen the autoimmune condition, possibly resulting in worse eye disease. Whether this is true is unclear.

Thyroid surgery controls hyperthyroidism in 90 percent of patients. The rest have a recurrence, usually due to the fact that doctors didn't remove enough thyroid tissue. Just as determining the exact dose of radioactive iodine to eliminate hyperthyroidism but avoid hypothyroidism (see "Radioactive iodine treatment" below) is impossible, determining the exact amount of thyroid tissue to remove is also impossible. The fact that thyroid tissue can regrow further complicates the question of how much thyroid tissue to remove.

For more information about thyroid surgery, see Chapter 13.

Radioactive iodine treatment

In radioactive iodine treatment, a patient swallows a capsule containing radioactive iodine (RAI). Because the thyroid uses more iodine than any other organ or gland in your body, the RAI concentrates in your thyroid and slowly destroys the overactive thyroid cells. Radioactive iodine may seem like an ideal solution to the problem of hyperthyroidism. Decades of experience with radioactive iodine have lain to rest a number of the fears surrounding this treatment. Here are some of its benefits:

- ✔ Adults who receive RAI experience no increase in thyroid cancer.

- ✔ After RAI, no increase in cases of leukemia occurs.

- ✔ RAI doesn't affect reproductive ability.

- ✔ RAI is effective and safe for small children and adolescents with hyperthyroidism.

- ✔ Children of mothers who previously received RAI have normal thyroid function and no congenital defects at birth (though doctors never give RAI to women during a pregnancy or during breast feeding). Children of mothers who received RAI can, however, still develop Graves' disease later in life because it's hereditary.

In addition, RAI is inexpensive and avoids the risks of surgery.

But RAI does have its share of drawbacks:

- ✔ Pregnant women can't take RAI, because it crosses the placenta and enters the baby's thyroid, possibly destroying it.

- ✔ RAI should not be used in babies because of the possible incidence of thyroid cancer when babies are exposed to it. (For example, thyroid cancer was rampant among children exposed to RAI outside the Russian nuclear plant at Chernobyl.)

- ✔ Finding the exact dose to cure your hyperthyroidism but leave you with normal thyroid function is impossible. If you take too little RAI, you need another treatment. Most patients who receive enough RAI to cure their hyperthyroidism eventually become hypothyroid and need to take thyroid hormone replacement (possibly for life). You can receive even a third treatment with RAI if necessary.

Hypothyroidism caused by RAI may feature three unusual symptoms doctors don't find in other causes of hypothyroidism: joint aches, stiffness, and headaches. The headaches may be due to swelling of the pituitary gland.

- ✔ By slowly destroying the thyroid, RAI releases a large amount of thyroid antigens into the patient's circulation, similar to what occurs in surgery, which may greatly increase autoimmunity and make eye disease worse.

✔ A patient must have follow-up blood tests for years to monitor for the development of hypothyroidism.

You must take some precautions after RAI:

✔ Because some iodine appears in saliva, you shouldn't kiss someone for two or three days after receiving RAI.

✔ Stay away from very close contact with your baby or spouse for two days, including sleeping in the same bed, dancing, and other very close interactions.

After you receive RAI, it takes about three weeks to begin to have an effect, and it has its maximal effect about two months after treatment. (Timeframes can vary depending on how large the gland is when the treatment occurs.)

Antithyroid pills

Doctors use two antithyroid pills in the United States to control hyperthyroidism, *propylthiouricil* (PTU) and *methimazole*. In other countries, doctors also use a third drug, *carbimizole*. All three pills block the production of thyroid hormones, but propylthiouricil also blocks the conversion of T4 to T3, giving it a theoretical advantage over methimazole. (The advantage doesn't seem to matter so much in practice unless you're trying to control the hyperthyroidism very rapidly.)

A major advantage of antithyroid pills is that, unlike surgery or radioactive iodine, they help to treat all complications of Graves' disease, including eye disease, by reducing autoimmunity. Very soon after you start taking the pills, levels of thyroid-peroxidase autoantibody and thyroid-stimulating antibody (see Chapter 4) begin to fall and stay down after you stop taking the drug. Also, taken in correct dosages, they don't lead to hypothyroidism.

When these drugs are given, you usually begin to feel better after three weeks, and the hyperthyroidism comes under control within six weeks. Then monitoring your free T4 level at least every six to eight weeks becomes important, because treatment can lower the T4 into the hypothyroid range. This may be detected if your thyroid starts to enlarge even though you have no more symptoms of hyperthyroidism.

Follow-up should continue for years after successful treatment, because your thyroid gland is unstable once you've had hyperthyroidism, especially if you're under severe stress. In the absence of symptoms, a visit to your doctor every six months to a year is appropriate.

The TSH can't be used to monitor the effect of treatment with antithyroid drugs. It will remain suppressed for many weeks to months after normal thyroid function is restored.

One way to speed up your return to normal — by as much as one to two weeks — is to use the drug cholestyramine. This drug has been used to lower cholesterol by binding the cholesterol in the intestine so it can't be absorbed into the blood stream. Thyroxine circulates between the liver and the intestine in a similar way. Cholestyramine can bind thyroxine and keep it in the intestine so it doesn't get absorbed, just like cholesterol. The dose (in case any doctors might be reading this) is 4 milligrams twice daily for the first four weeks of treatment.

Most patients start taking 5 milligrams of methimazole three times daily or 50 milligrams of propylthiouricil three times daily. The major advantage of methimazole is that doctors can prescribe it in a once-a-day regimen from the very beginning, because it lasts longer in the body. As your T4 level falls, your doctor can reduce the dose to two pills or even one pill daily. The current standard is to keep the drug going for a year and then to stop it to see whether the disease recurs.

The hyperthyroidism of about 50 percent of patients taking antithyroid pills remains under control after they stop taking the propylthiouricil or methimazole. For the others, the symptoms recur after they stop taking the pills, usually within three to six months of stopping the drug. These patients can continue on antithyroid drugs or undergo surgery or take RAI. A study in the *European Journal of Endocrinology* in May 2005 shows that methimazole is a safe and effective treatment for more than ten years for patients with hyperthyroidism caused by Graves' disease.

Like surgery and RAI, antithyroid drugs carry some risks. The major risk is that they can cause a reduction in white blood cells and, very rarely, a complete lack of white blood cell production *(agranulocytosis)*. Although this usually occurs early in treatment when patients take especially large doses of medication, diminished white blood cell production occasionally occurs later on and in patients taking low doses. This problem goes away when the patient stops taking the antithyroid drug. Some patients develop a rash when using one of the antithyroid drugs. You can try one of the other antithyroid drugs if you develop a rash. Rarely, the pills affect the liver, and blood tests become abnormal. Make sure your doctor checks your liver function every few visits when you take antithyroid drugs. Once your liver function remains normal for several tests, this problem will likely not recur. These abnormalities in your liver also respond to withdrawal of the offending drug.

If you're on methimazole or propylthiouricil and develop a cold, sore throat, or other illness usually associated with a virus, contact your doctor, who should do a white blood cell count. One way to avoid severe loss of white blood cell production is to have white cell count done each time you visit your doctor while you're on the antithyroid pills.

My choice of treatment

For most patients with Graves' disease, methimazole is my first choice of treatment (or propylthiouricil for pregnant women). Although not all (about 70 to 80 percent) patients have a permanent remission after taking antithyroid drugs, the fact that antithyroid drugs suppress the immune reaction (thus helping to reduce eye disease in hyperthyroidism) is an important reason for my choice. Methimazole and propylthiouricil (plus carbamizole in Europe) are the only choices of treatment that may be truly curative and not simply destructive. The largest thyroids I've seen have eventually responded to antithyroid drugs.

Many doctors cite the need to take a pill every day as a reason not to recommend antithyroid drugs. Most of these doctors give their patients radioactive iodine, and the patients often end up hypothyroid and needing to take daily thyroid hormone replacement pills, so I don't agree with this argument.

For other chronic illnesses, such as diabetes or hypertension, patients take pills for a lifetime. I've never understood the reluctance to do the same thing with Graves' disease to avoid surgery and radioactive destruction of the thyroid gland. No rule says that a patient can't take pills for more than a year. Patient can also stop

taking the pills on a yearly basis and not start them again until the disease recurs, if it does.

I have a number of patients in my practice who've gone more than five years with normal thyroid function after a course of antithyroid therapy. They haven't had to take any pill. Many of them are in the 30-to-50 age group and are quite happy to be free of medications.

If a patient is very symptomatic at the beginning of treatment, I use the beta blocker propranolol to control her symptoms until methimazole takes effect (in three to four weeks).

I can see a patient who is stable on pills every few months, as long as she knows that she should contact me if she experiences any symptoms of a virus, which may mean a reduction in her white blood cell count that the medication causes.

I've had occasion to use radioactive iodine on only a few patients in the last ten years, who were generally elderly patients with other severe complicating conditions. The vast majority I treated with antithyroid medication. A few of them required a second treatment with antithyroid drugs or needed treatment for longer than one year because their thyroid gland took a long time to shrink. Several patients have gone five years or longer with no further treatment and are doing fine.

Other helpful considerations and medications

You need to take into account two further general considerations in the treatment of your hyperthyroidism:

✔ **Rest:** As a result of the hypermetabolism of hyperthyroidism, you may be exhausted both mentally and physically. You're certainly unable to do an eight-hour job while you're still hyperthyroid and for some time thereafter. Your doctor should provide you with a note for your employer or your school asking for time for you to rest or to delay test taking until you're functioning more normally. Don't try to continue any heavy exercise routine until your thyroid tests are normal and you regain your muscle strength.

✔ **Nutrition:** In terms of nutrition, hyperthyroidism is a state of catabolism, which means you're losing muscle, bone, and even some fat while the disease is still active. Your lost muscle, bone, and fat needs restoring, which happens fairly quickly, especially if you continue to eat when your thyroid function is normal as you did when you were hyperthyroid. During hyperthyroidism, everything in your body is used up, including your vitamins and minerals. You may have to pay special attention to restore your body's levels of vitamins and minerals. You can read a lot more about this topic in Chapter 20.

Certain pills can reduce the symptoms of hyperthyroidism without treating the condition. They're valuable for controlling the disease while antithyroid pills or radioactive iodine has a chance to work. They don't affect the underlying disease, and you shouldn't take them alone in treatment. The major class of drugs is called *beta blockers,* and the most commonly used drug is *propranolol.* When taken in a dose of 20 to 40 milligrams three to four times a day, propranolol slows the heart, decreases anxiety, and reduces tremors. You can continue taking it for a few weeks until the other medications take effect or it can be used as preparation for surgery. Preparations of iodine temporarily block thyroid hormone production and reduce the blood flowing to the thyroid in preparation for surgery.

Treating Other Causes of Hyperthyroidism

People who have hyperthyroidism not caused by Graves' disease may need other treatment options:

✔ Factitious hyperthyroidism is treated by removing the thyroid pills from the patient and starting some form of psychotherapy.

✔ A thyroid with one or more nodules that produce too much thyroid hormone responds best to radioactive iodine because an autoimmune condition doesn't cause the nodules, so no concern exists about thyroid eye disease lingering after the treatment. In the case of a single nodule causing the hyperthyroidism, after RAI eliminates the nodule, the rest of the thyroid often functions normally. When single or multiple overactive nodules are present, antithyroid drugs almost never cause a permanent remission.

✔ T3 thyrotoxicosis responds to antithyroid medication just like Graves' disease caused by excess T4.

✔ The hyperthyroid phase of subacute thyroiditis doesn't last very long. If necessary, the beta blocker propranolol can control symptoms until the hyperthyroidism subsides.

✔ A surgeon must remove a choriocarcinoma-that is making hormones that stimulate the thyroid.

✔ Surgery or radiation therapy is the treatment for a tumor in the brain causing excessive production of thyroid-stimulating hormone.

Surviving Thyroid Storm

Fortunately, *thyroid storm* is rare, because doctors almost always diagnose hyperthyroidism at a much earlier stage. However, the condition may be fatal. It is primarily a disease of the elderly, so as the population ages, doctors will see more cases. The clinical picture is one of extreme signs and symptoms of hyperthyroidism. The patient has a high fever, as high as 103 to 104 degrees Fahrenheit, and a very rapid heart rate, 130 beats per minute or more. She may be vomiting, have diarrhea, and become dehydrated. She may be in heart failure and have an uncontrollable heart rhythm. She can be delirious and lapse into a coma.

Just as in myxedema coma (see Chapter 5), a precipitating event usually produces thyroid storm in someone who already has hyperthyroidism. The most important such events are:

✔ Heart failure

✔ Diabetic ketoacidosis

✔ Bowel loss due to loss of circulation

✔ Surgery or labor and delivery

✔ Trauma

✔ Clot in the lung

✔ Infection

✔ Mental disturbance

The preceding kinds of events are already dangerous and often fatal to an elderly patient. When thyroid storm adds to the illness, the outlook is grim, with a mortality rate of between 25 and 60 percent.

Thyroid storm is a true medical emergency that should be managed by a physician who is very aware of the treatment of severe hyperthyroidism.

The doctor usually starts a number of treatments all at once. The patient is given fluids, one of the antithyroid drugs (such as propylthiouricil), potassium iodide, steroids, and a beta blocker like propranolol. This can lower the level of T3 hormone to normal in a day, although the patient takes many more days to fully recover.

Chapter 7

Thyroid Nodules

• •

• •

*I*n some ways, the thyroid is really an annoying gland. If it weren't so important to our health, there would be good reason to get rid of it, just like doctors used to get rid of tonsils. The thyroid is forever forming bumps and growths that turn out to be of little or no significance but that doctors have to evaluate on the outside chance that they're cancerous. Even if a thyroid growth turns out to be cancerous (see Chapter 8), it's rarely fatal.

The reason doctors pay so much attention to bumps on the thyroid is the same reason a piece of property is valuable: location, location, location. If the thyroid gland weren't located so prominently in the front of the neck, you wouldn't notice all its little growths, and most people would be no worse off for it. Instead, your thyroid got put right up front, thus providing a lifetime source of work and income for specialists who call themselves thyroidologists (like me).

This chapter tells you what you need to know about all your thyroid's bumps and lumps. I explain whether you should be concerned about or just ignore a nodule on your thyroid, as well as what to do if you must get rid of it. By the end of the chapter, I think you'll appreciate that most thyroid nodules are minor inconveniences and that knowing what to do about them keeps them that way.

What's a Thyroid Nodule?

Kenneth Fine is a 35-year-old man in excellent health. While shaving one day, he notices a bump on the front of his neck that he hasn't seen before. He ignores it for several months but finally decides that he ought to have someone check it out. He goes to his doctor, who does thyroid function tests. His free T4 and thyroid-stimulating hormone (TSH) levels are normal (see Chapter 4). His doctor then sends him to a thyroid doctor for evaluation.

The thyroid doctor asks Kenneth if the lump has grown noticeably and if it causes any trouble swallowing or breathing. Kenneth answers "no" to these questions. The specialist then proposes that Kenneth have a fine needle aspiration biopsy (see Chapter 4). When this test is done, the report comes back affirming Kenneth has a *benign thyroid adenoma,* which means that the lump isn't cancerous. The doctor tells Kenneth to come back in a year for a reexamination.

A year later, no change in the lump has occurred, and the specialist asks him to return a year after that. Kenneth forgets about his appointment, and the doctor's receptionist has a poor bookkeeping system, so Kenneth lives happily ever after.

Kenneth is a very good example of the typical case history of a person with a thyroid nodule. He illustrates the unexpected finding of a bump, the tendency to ignore it, and the fact that it generally isn't a problem in the long run.

Kenneth's story isn't meant to minimize the fact that some nodules, about 5 percent, do turn out to be cancerous and that doctors must deal with them in the proper way. Kenneth's example simply illustrates the most common course of events.

The thyroid is ordinarily a smooth, butterfly-shaped gland (see Chapter 2). Whenever something grows that alters its smoothness, the growth is considered a *nodule.* Nodules can be *benign,* that is, free of cancer, in which case they're called *adenomas,* or they can be *malignant.* When ultrasounds are done routinely on a group of people, as many as 20 percent of them have nodules. That 20 percent represents 60 million people in the United States alone. Picking out the few who have cancer provides full-time work for a lot of people.

Exactly why nodules form isn't clear, but a number of theories exist:

- ✔ Because they're most common in women, some people think that hormonal changes, especially through the menstrual cycle or during pregnancy, cause alternate growth and shrinkage of thyroid tissue. When shrinkage isn't complete, thyroid nodules result.

- ✔ Another cause of thyroid nodules is the growth of thyroid tissue that occurs when you have part of your thyroid removed.

✔ Chronic thyroiditis (see Chapter 5) may enlarge the thyroid in an irregular fashion, leading to nodules.

✔ The condition called subacute thyroiditis (see Chapter 11) may also enlarge the thyroid irregularly.

A *neoplasm* is any new growth on the thyroid. Despite its harsh-sounding name, the term simply means "new growth." A person's thyroid may have one or several growths, and multiple explanations exist for why they appear. Physicians identify the various possibilities according to the appearance of the nodule tissue under a microscope. This is known as the *pathological appearance* of the tissue. For our purposes, we just want to know whether the nodule is benign (not cancerous) or malignant (cancerous).

Most thyroid nodules — *more than 95 percent* — are benign.

Evaluating Cancer Risks

A number of facts about a patient's history, signs, and symptoms can help sway the balance toward or away from a diagnosis of cancer:

✔ **Gender:** Doctors find nodules less often in men than women, but nodules are cancerous more often in men.

✔ **Age:** Nodules found in children are cancerous more frequently than they are in adults. However, a nodule in a child is still benign more often than it's malignant.

A nodule in a person over age 70 is also highly suspicious for cancer. Whether a person over 70 should have surgery for such a generally nonaggressive cancer is another issue.

✔ **Number of nodules:** If a patient has many nodules, this suggests that a cancer isn't present. Most multinodular thyroids are benign.

✔ **Growth rate:** A nodule that grows rapidly is probably a cancer, but if it pops up suddenly and is tender, it may be a hemorrhage. A hemorrhage that suddenly occurs isn't usually a serious problem, but it does cause discomfort.

✔ **Additional growths:** Finding growths in the neck away from the thyroid suggests cancer that has spread, and those growths must be evaluated by a biopsy.

✔ **Hoarseness and trouble swallowing:** These symptoms suggest cancer, especially if they're of recent onset.

✔ **Movement:** If the thyroid doesn't move freely, it's a sign of fixation, which suggests cancer.

> ✔ **Previous exposure to irradiation:** (This doesn't include the use of radioactive iodine in the treatment of hyperthyroidism — see Chapter 6.) A significant increase in reports of thyroid cancer occurred among children exposed to the radiation from the Chernobyl nuclear plant in Russia. In this case, multiple nodules don't rule out cancer. Almost half the nodules in an irradiated gland turn out to be cancer. Doctors may find the cancer 10 to 30 years after the irradiation. Even today, doctors use radiation to treat tumors in the head and neck, which will result in a certain amount of cases of thyroid cancer.

Virtually no family or hereditary connection pertains to nodules, either benign or cancerous. The exception is a condition called *multiple endocrine neoplasia,* in which many members of a family have nodules on several different glands, such as the thyroid, the pancreas, the parathyroids, and the adrenal glands. When such a family history is present, doctors should perform a blood test for calcitonin levels because the tumor that is found in the thyroid, medullary thyroid cancer (see Chapter 8), produces a lot of calicitonin. Although the thyroid tumor is malignant, the tumors in the other glands may be malignant or benign.

Securing a Diagnosis

If the factors in the previous section don't provide enough evidence suggesting whether a nodule is cancerous, your doctor can use several tests to make a diagnosis.

Thyroid function tests

Thyroid function tests that suggest hyperthyroidism (see Chapter 6) or hypothyroidism (see Chapter 5) usually mean that a thyroid nodule is benign. However, the possibility exists for two different conditions to be present in the thyroid at the same time. Therefore, your doctor should examine the nodule occasionally to guarantee that it isn't growing.

The thyroid scan

A thyroid scan (see Chapter 4) distinguishes a nodule that takes up radioactive iodine from one that doesn't. A nodule may be actively concentrating the iodine even though the thyroid function tests are normal. A "warm" nodule takes up radioactive iodine like the rest of the gland. If the nodule concentrates most of the iodine (while the rest of the gland is less active) and the thyroid function tests are elevated, it's a "hot" nodule. Cancerous nodules are usually "cold," meaning they don't concentrate the radioactivity. However, most cold nodules aren't cancerous.

Figure 7-1 shows the typical appearance of a cold nodule and a hot nodule.

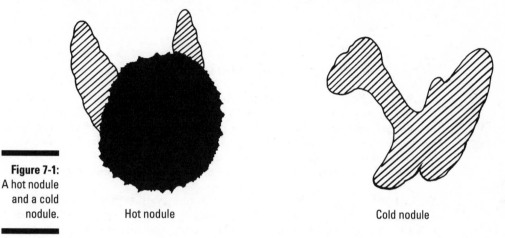

Figure 7-1:
A hot nodule
and a cold
nodule.

Hot nodule

Cold nodule

In addition, the thyroid scan sometimes shows multiple nodules when a doctor sees or feels only one. Multiple nodules argue against a cancer.

The thyroid ultrasound study

The thyroid ultrasound study (see Chapter 4) also gives a picture of the entire thyroid and demonstrates if more than one nodule is present. More helpful than that, the ultrasound can distinguish between a solid mass and a cyst. A *cyst* is a nodule that is either filled with fluid or contains some solid tissue. A cyst filled with fluid is generally believed to be a benign growth. A cyst that contains some solid tissue may be a cancer.

The thyroid ultrasound can also be performed on several occasions to provide a continuous picture of the status of the nodule — whether it's shrinking, growing, or remaining the same. A nodule that shrinks or remains the same is less likely to be a cancer. Because thyroid cancer doesn't tend to be aggressive, an ultrasound every few months to follow the growth of a nodule is reasonable, particularly if the patient doesn't want a biopsy.

Abnormalities may be seen in an ultrasound study that helps to identify cancers, including tiny bits of calcium and greatly increased blood flow in the nodule, but these abnormalities aren't total proof of cancer. They simply help doctors in choosing which nodule to biopsy first when several nodules are present in a thyroid gland.

Another important use for thyroid ultrasound is guiding the needle when doctors perform a fine needle biopsy. Doctors can place the tip of the needle so accurately that no doubt exists whether the tissue of interest is being biopsied.

The fine needle aspiration biopsy

The fine needle aspiration biopsy is the gold standard for the diagnosis of a thyroid nodule. Often specialists skip the other steps and go right to this simple, painless, and very specific procedure. The test involves sticking a tiny needle into the nodule and removing bits of tissue from it. Doctors believe that this test gives the correct diagnosis 98 percent of the time, especially when an ultrasound guides it, as I explain in the preceding section.

When a person has a fine needle aspiration biopsy, the organization of the tissue as it exists in the body is lost. Cells that would've been found next to other cells in the intact tissue are broken apart. The pathologist is looking for the presence of certain cells and the appearance of the cells to make a diagnosis. A hallmark of cancer, which is invasion of surrounding tissues, isn't visible during a fine needle aspiration biopsy, but usually it doesn't matter.

Ever since doctors have used the fine needle aspiration biopsy, the number of surgeries for possible thyroid cancer has dropped dramatically. Fine needle aspiration biopsies allow doctors to place their diagnosis of a nodule into one of four possible categories and then take the appropriate actions:

- **Benign adenoma (about 65 percent of the time):** Benign nodules require no further treatment. They don't turn into cancers at a later date.

- **Suspicious nodule (about 15 percent of the time):** Suspicious nodules are probably the most difficult of the categories to deal with. They evince no definite sign of cancer but exhibit changes that are sometimes observable in cancer but also observable when cancer isn't present. Doctors usually remove a suspicious nodule and examine it in a more intact state under a microscope. However, you can avoid surgery if you have a thyroid scan with radioactive iodine and the nodule demonstrates it's active by concentrating iodine. Active nodules are generally not malignant.

- **Malignant nodule (about 10 percent of the time):** Doctors must remove malignant nodules (cancers) along with the rest of the thyroid gland, because cancer is often in other parts of the gland, especially if you have a history of irradiation.

- **Nondiagnostic (about 10 percent of the time):** Doctors find nondiagnostic nodules when the tissue consists of follicular cells (see Chapter 2). In order to know if they're cancerous, invasion of surrounding tissues must be visible. As I note above, the normal architecture of the tissue is lost with fine needle aspiration biopsies, so doctors can't detect invasion with this technique. If the nodule is nondiagnostic, the patient will usually go to surgery so the nodule can be examined in a more intact state. If cancerous, the thyroid is removed.

Thyroid cancers tend to grow either very slowly or so fast that they're obvious. If they grow fast, you have the biopsy done immediately. If they grow slowly, you can have the fine needle aspiration biopsy done a year or more after you discover a slowly growing nodule, still leaving plenty of time to treat a newly discovered cancer. Of course, your doctor must check for evidence of changes in the key findings I discuss previously (see the "Evaluating Cancer Risks" section) each time he sees you, such as the development of hoarseness, the finding of a new growth away from the thyroid in the neck, or fixation of a thyroid that previously moved freely.

You can also have a fine needle aspiration biopsy if you have any lymph nodes that are suspicious in the area of the nodule. Finding thyroid cancer in a lymph node verifies a diagnosis of thyroid cancer in the thyroid gland, even if the nodule is negative.

Treating Cancerous Nodules

Every so often, one of the anonymous nodules turns out to be a cancer (see Chapter 8), and treatment becomes necessary. (Sometimes all the tests available to a doctor don't provide a definitive diagnosis, in which case I believe treating the nodule as if it were cancer is wise.) The treatment of choice for a cancerous thyroid nodule is surgery. (Even benign nodules may sometimes require surgery if they're unsightly or cause compression or trouble swallowing.)

When you and your doctor determine that surgery is necessary, you need to find two additional competent and experienced physicians:

✔ **Surgeon:** A surgeon with plenty of experience in thyroid surgery must be available. I discuss the potential complications of thyroid surgery in Chapter 13. No general surgeon who does only occasional thyroid cases should undertake thyroid surgery for potential cancer, because the cancer may be very extensive. Furthermore, a surgeon must do the right procedure the first time around, because a second surgery is much more difficult and complicated.

If you need to have thyroid surgery, check the qualifications of the surgeon. Don't accept a referral without checking the surgeon's experience and rate of complications. See Chapter 3 for help in finding a good thyroid surgeon.

✔ **Pathologist:** A *pathologist* is a doctor trained to diagnose disease by looking at the abnormal tissue under a microscope. The hospital where you're having your surgery must have an experienced pathologist because the pathologist gives a diagnosis of the tissue that the surgeon removes as surgery proceeds. The pathologist's opinion determines whether the surgeon does a complete removal of the thyroid (called a *total thyroidectomy*) and then goes on to remove lymph nodes in the neck around the thyroid to see if the cancer has spread. Your surgeon should not perform this extensive (and expensive) operation unless the pathologist gives the surgeon a precise diagnosis. Ideally, the final diagnosis of the tissue, made after surgery is complete, won't contradict the diagnosis made during the operation.

You probably won't find highly experienced pathologists at community hospitals, even though doctors discover many thyroid cancers at these hospitals. Do yourself or your loved one a major favor and go to a referral center to get this special care.

A few thyroid specialists argue that even if a doctor diagnoses your nodule as cancerous, you're better off leaving the nodule alone. They base this argument on the fact that although doctors detect about 15,000 new cases of thyroid cancer in the United States each year, only 1,500 to 2,000 people in the U.S. die from thyroid cancer each year. Furthermore, the 15,000 new cases of thyroid cancer derive from as many as 15 million people with nodules of one kind or another. Because death from thyroid cancer is such a rare event, some specialists reason that treatment may not matter. Most evidence doesn't support not treating cancerous nodules, however.

I believe that surgical removal should be the treatment for nodules that contain thyroid cancer.

Dealing with Nodules That Aren't Cancer

Hot nodules and benign cysts may require some treatment but not necessarily surgery.

Dealing with the thyroid nonsurgically is almost always preferable if the results will be satisfactory because of the potential for surgical complications, not to mention the cost and the trauma that surgery brings with it.

Fortunately, other treatment choices are available for nodules that aren't cancerous, and specialists are discovering new ones regularly.

Hot nodules

A hot nodule produces hyperthyroidism, so it must be treated. Hot nodules represent about 10 percent of the nodules doctors find. One choice of treatment is to take radioactive iodine (RAI), as patients with Graves' disease do (see Chapter 6). However, up to 40 percent of the patients who receive RAI develop hypothyroidism (underactive thyroid) later in life. Those who don't develop hypothyroidism usually return to normal thyroid function.

A second choice of treatment for a hot nodule is surgical removal of the lobe of the thyroid in which the nodule is found. Surgeons perform a surgical removal on younger individuals and those who refuse radioactive iodine. Antithyroid drugs help prepare patients for surgery. When thyroid function is normal, patients undergo surgery. In the hands of a good surgeon, you experience few problems with the surgical approach. However, about half the patients who have this kind of surgery become hypothyroid later on.

A newer treatment that eliminates the hot nodule while not destroying the rest of the thyroid gland is the injection of ethanol into the nodule. Injections take place several times over several days. Complications include pain in the thyroid area and fever. Doctors may use this treatment more and more often in the future as they gain experience with it. Doctors can inject ethanol into the nodule very precisely using guidance by ultrasound. One big advantage is that patients who receive these injections don't develop hypothyroidism later. Doctors in Europe first used this treatment. Although it is done in the United States, it is not the treatment of first choice here. My own opinion is that it can be successful at a medical center with experience in the technique and that it will become the treatment of first choice as more and more doctors gain that experience.

Benign cysts

A nodule filled with fluid shrinks when a doctor inserts a needle and removes the fluid. Unfortunately, the cyst often fills right up again. Repeated removal of the fluid sometimes cures the problem. Doctors can inject ethanol into a cyst just as into a solid nodule; they then remove the ethanol by the same needle they use to inject it. The cyst often shrinks after one ethanol treatment.

Then again, you can leave the cyst alone if you're willing to live with it.

Warm or cold nodules

Doctors sometimes treat nodules that don't produce excessive thyroid hormone and aren't cancer by giving you thyroid hormone in an attempt to shrink the nodule. Little evidence supports that this treatment actually works. Very rarely have I found these nodules to respond to thyroid hormone. The risk involved is that giving too much thyroid hormone can cause bone loss or abnormal heart beats.

Sometimes, when even a fine needle biopsy doesn't produce a definite diagnosis, a doctor suggests using *thyroid hormone suppression,* having patients take thyroid pills to shrink the nodule. If a patient consumes thyroid hormone and the nodule shrinks, then the doctor assumes that the nodule isn't a cancer. If the nodule doesn't shrink, the suspicion of a cancer is greater. I disagree with this method, because most nodules don't respond to thyroid hormone, yet most nodules aren't cancer.

Your doctor should examine your warm and cold nodules every six months or every year. Should your nodule grow, you have a fine needle biopsy done again. Otherwise, a nodule can be left alone.

Ignoring small nodules

Every so often a study, such as an ultrasound of the neck, reveals one or more very small nodules on the thyroid. The best specialists probably can't feel a nodule that's less than one centimeter in size. The ultrasound may detect a half-centimeter or smaller nodule. My advice is to ignore a bump this small, which has been termed an *incidentaloma* (a thyroid specialist's agonizing attempt at humor).

Chapter 8

Thyroid Cancer

*F*or me, this chapter is probably the hardest one to write. The word *cancer* evokes a number of images, and none of them are particularly positive. The fact is that people do die of thyroid cancer. For this reason, you must know what thyroid cancer is, how it grows, how you treat it, and how you follow up after treatment if you or a loved one has thyroid cancer. Putting thyroid cancer into perspective is also important.

Researchers estimate that as much as 6 percent of the world's population has cancer in the thyroid gland. Based on this percentage, about 16.5 million people in the United States may have evidence of thyroid cancer. Yet in the U.S., doctors find only 15,000 new cases each year, and the total deaths due to thyroid cancer each year are 1,500 to 2,000. The vast majority of people with thyroid cancer live and die without ever knowing they had it. Only when doctors carefully examine the thyroid under a microscope can they detect the cancer.

Thyroid cancer doesn't appear among the top 75 causes of death in the United States. Among cancers, thyroid cancer isn't in the top 15 causes of death, which suggests that compared to most other cancers, thyroid cancer is one of the least dangerous. If you have to have a cancer, this may be the one to choose.

The relatively benign course of most thyroid cancers makes it difficult to say which treatment is best. Perhaps certain treatments are very effective, or perhaps any number of treatments works just as well because the disease itself is so mild. For this reason, much difference of opinion prevails among thyroid specialists. If you ask two thyroid specialists how to treat a certain type of thyroid cancer, you may get three opinions. In this chapter, I give you my recommendations based on the best and most recent investigations of thyroid cancer treatment.

Determining What Causes Thyroid Cancer

John D'Mee is 40 years of age and has noticed that he has a lump in the front of his neck on the left side. His family has no history of thyroid cancer. The lump is painless and moves when he swallows. He doesn't know how long it has been there. John goes to see his doctor, who does thyroid function tests and finds that John's TSH and free T4 are normal. The doctor does a thyroid scan and finds that the area of the nodule on John's thyroid doesn't take up any radioactivity — it's a *cold nodule.* John's doctor sends him to see Dr. Rubin, who does a fine needle aspiration biopsy (see Chapter 4). The pathologist diagnoses a *papillary carcinoma,* the most common type of thyroid cancer. Dr. Rubin sends John to a head and neck surgeon who has done more than 2,000 thyroid surgeries.

The surgeon, Dr. Stark, recommends removing the thyroid gland while carefully retaining the tissue around the parathyroid glands and the recurrent laryngeal nerves that pass along the thyroid. Dr. Stark performs the surgery successfully, and no other suspicious nodes or nodules appear during the procedure.

John has no other treatment initially. He returns to Dr. Rubin, and three weeks after surgery he has a TSH test. The result is very high — 45 — indicating that little thyroid tissue remains in his body. He has another scan that shows no uptake of radioactive iodine except for in a small area of the thyroid tissue the surgeon left intact. Dr. Rubin gives John a large dose of radioactive iodine to eliminate that small bit of tissue. A follow-up scan shows that all the thyroid tissue is gone. Dr. Rubin places John on thyroid-hormone replacement and continues to monitor him. John will probably live a normal life span with no further trouble associated with the thyroid cancer other than the periodic visits for follow-up.

John is representative of the majority of people who develop thyroid cancer. The cancer shows itself as a thyroid nodule (see Chapter 7). Keep in mind that the vast majority of thyroid nodules aren't cancerous.

Our understanding of why cancer occurs is becoming clearer and clearer. We know that genes (part of our hereditary makeup) called *oncogenes* cause a cell to grow and divide without control. Oncogenes exist in all our cells. Just exactly what permits certain oncogenes to begin to be active isn't clear, but a mistake in cell division (a *mutation*) or some chemical or radiation in the environment could be to blame. Scientists have found other genes called *tumor suppressor genes* in the human chromosome (the *DNA*). Some people lack tumor suppressor genes and can develop tumors. Doctors have actually found loss of the tumor suppressor gene in some thyroid cancers.

TECHNICAL STUFF

Experimental thyroid cancer

Two conditions are necessary for scientists to successfully produce thyroid cancer in animals. The first is some abnormal change in the chromosomes, the nuclear material in the thyroid cells. Exactly what kind of damage is necessary isn't clear. As a result of the change in the chromosomes, the cells aren't able to produce enough thyroid hormone, provoking the second condition, which is overstimulation of the thyroid cells. Scientists have caused an abnormal change in the chromosomes with radiation to the thyroid. By giving the animals goitrogens, the chemicals that further block thyroid hormone production, scientists cause increased thyroid-stimulating hormone, resulting in the second condition. In human children, irradiation of the neck for acne, enlarged tonsils or adenoids, or other reasons results in a hundredfold increase in the occurrence of thyroid cancer. The higher the dose of radiation, the greater the number of cases of thyroid cancer. Adults who received radiation in Hiroshima or Nagasaki also developed thyroid cancer, but their incidence wasn't as high as in children who also received radiation.

The best-known initiator of thyroid cancer is irradiation, which has been the source of many cancers in children who lived in the area of Chernobyl in Russia during the nuclear disaster. The children drank milk from cows that ate the grass upon which radioactive substances (including radioactive iodine) fell. Within a few years, many of the children had multiple sites of cancer in their thyroid glands. Adults exposed to radioactive iodine also developed thyroid cancer, though not as often as children, who seem to be more sensitive.

Children who have received neck and face irradiation for benign conditions such as acne or enlarged tonsils have also developed thyroid cancer — as many as 40 years after the irradiation. The size of these cancers isn't different from cancers that have no association with radiation, but they usually exist in multiple places in the thyroid, and often the thyroid shows several benign adenomas as well.

Doctors who analyze the chromosomal content of thyroid tumor cells find that all cells in one tumor have exactly the same genetic makeup. This uniformity indicates that thyroid cancers start in one cell, which multiplies over time to form the thyroid cancer that you can feel.

Exactly why radioactive iodine treatment for hyperthyroidism doesn't cause thyroid cancer isn't clear. It may be that the very high dose used destroys the thyroid cells before they can develop cancer.

Some cancers of the thyroid run in families, especially *medullary thyroid cancer.* I discuss this hereditary connection later in the "Medullary thyroid cancer" section. In some places like Hawaii and Iceland, thyroid cancer occurs at an unusually high rate. In Hawaii, it's especially high among Chinese males and Filipino females, much higher than in their country of origin. Many believe that something in the environment is the cause, though no one knows exactly what.

Identifying the Types of Thyroid Cancer

Although it can be discovered in different ways and follow several different courses, most thyroid cancer can be expected to approach the following history:

✔ Discovery occurs by accident by the female patient who notices a lump in her neck or the male patient who notices a lump in his neck while shaving. Or an ultrasound performed for other reasons detects the lump as an unexpected finding.

✔ Occasionally a cancerous thyroid lump may appear as an enlarging mass with hoarseness, trouble swallowing, or trouble speaking.

✔ When your doctor examines your neck, she finds a painless lump on one side of your thyroid.

✔ If you find a cancerous lump before the age of 45, it takes a more benign course than if you find a lump later on.

The rest of the course depends on the particular type of tumor.

A pathologist identifies thyroid cancer according to the appearance of the tissue that she examines. If she diagnoses a nodule as cancer, identifying the particular cancer is important because each one follows a different course. Treatments that work for one type of thyroid cancer may not work at all for a different type.

As a patient, you don't need to know how to identify types of thyroid cancer — that's the pathologist's job. But a basic understanding of the types of cancer helps you know what the future holds if your doctor identifies a thyroid cancer. When your doctor tells you the name of the cancer, you then have an idea of what to expect.

The descriptions for each type of thyroid cancer are true for most patients with that type of cancer, but exceptions exist. Occasionally, people with the most aggressive type of thyroid cancer find that their cancer isn't as aggressive as expected. By the same token, once in a while, a more benign form of thyroid cancer (based upon its appearance) takes a more aggressive turn. Medicine isn't an exact science.

How a pathologist identifies a cancer

Pathologists look for a number of abnormalities that separate normal tissue from cancerous tissue. They study thousands of tissue slides and know the difference in appearance between tissue that suggests cancer and tissue that's benign. The key elements that pathologists look for are as follows:

✔ A malignant appearance to the tissue — very large, abnormal-looking cells containing abnormal-looking parts.

✔ The presence of even normal-looking tissue in an area where it doesn't belong, which suggests that it has invaded the area. Examples are thyroid cells in a lymph gland, in bone, or in the lung.

Papillary thyroid cancer

Papillary thyroid cancer is the most common form that thyroid cancer takes, accounting for more than 70 percent of thyroid cancers in both adults and children. Fortunately, this form of thyroid cancer also tends to take a benign course, meaning it's not very aggressive. Although it spreads to the local lymph glands in the neck as often as half the time, the spread doesn't seem to make the cancer more aggressive. The following are the most important characteristics of papillary thyroid cancer:

✔ It rarely spreads away from the neck. Spread to lymph nodes in the neck may even be protective in younger patients, while it's a bad sign in patients over 45. Why this is so is not known.

✔ Diagnosis occurs most commonly between the ages of 30 and 50.

✔ Females have papillary cancer three times as often as males.

✔ It's the thyroid cancer most often associated with radiation exposure.

✔ It may be present for decades without harming you.

✔ It can also spread to bone and the lungs, but without causing problems for years.

✔ It concentrates radioactive iodine, which doctors can use to destroy it.

✔ Patients over age 45 may have a more aggressive course, especially if the tumor is larger than 1 centimeter.

✔ It's especially mild in younger patients, very rarely causing death.

Follicular thyroid cancer

Follicular thyroid cancer makes up another 20 percent of all thyroid cancers. It's a little more aggressive than papillary cancer but still usually takes a benign course. It doesn't tend to spread locally to lymph glands but goes to bone and the lungs more often than papillary cancer. The following are its central features:

- Diagnosis occurs most often between the ages of 40 and 60.
- It affects females three times as often as males.
- Local spread to lymph nodes is uncommon.
- It concentrates radioactive iodine, which makes treatment easier.
- It invades blood vessels, accounting for its tendency to go to distant sites, especially bone and lung.
- When it's more aggressive, it invades local structures like the trachea and nearby muscles, blocking the airway.
- It tends to be more aggressive in older patients.

Another cancer follows a course similar to follicular cancer but has a different appearance under the microscope: *Hurthle cell tumor.* It doesn't tend to concentrate radioactive iodine, so doctors can't use radioactive iodine in treatment. Despite not being able to use radioactive iodine, patients with Hurthle cell tumors survive the cancer at a rate almost identical to people with follicular thyroid cancer.

Medullary thyroid cancer

Medullary thyroid cancer makes up only about 5 percent of all cancers of the thyroid gland. This cancer doesn't arise in the cells that produce thyroid hormones; rather, it arises in another type of cell found in the thyroid, the *C cell.* The C cell produces a chemical (a hormone) called *calcitonin,* which doesn't affect metabolism. After doctors treat this cancer by completely removing the thyroid, they can measure the calcitonin level. If calcitonin levels are measured at regular intervals, a recurrence of cancer can be diagnosed easily.

Medullary thyroid cancer differs from the other thyroid cancers in its occasional tendency to run in families. Eighty percent of the time no other family member has it. Twenty percent of the time it's hereditary. Either another member of the family also has medullary thyroid cancer or the patient has medullary thyroid cancer as part of a condition called *Multiple Endocrine Neoplasia* (MEN) *Syndrome.* Two different types of MEN exist:

- Patients with MEN type II-A have tumors of the adrenal medulla (called *pheochromocytoma*) and the parathyroid glands in the neck. The adrenal medulla makes a hormone called *epinephrine,* so these patients have high blood pressure. They also have elevated levels of calcium as a result of the parathyroid tumor.

- MEN type II-B also includes the adrenal tumor that produces excessive amounts of epinephrine but not the parathyroid tumor. People with MEN II-B also have tumors in the mouth.

If your diagnosis is medullary cancer of the thyroid, a doctor must check to see if you have tumors in the adrenal medulla, because medication must control such tumors before surgery. Otherwise, your blood pressure can be high, making surgery on your neck extremely dangerous.

The important characteristics of medullary thyroid cancer include the following:

- It occurs in women more often than in men, but the difference between the sexes is smaller than for other tumors that begin in the thyroid.

- It's not associated with exposure to radiation.

- It's more aggressive than papillary or follicular thyroid cancers, especially if it spreads to the lymph glands in the neck or to the bone and liver. More than 50 percent of people with medullary thyroid cancer have local or distant spread at the time of their diagnosis.

- The medullary thyroid tumors secrete other hormones besides calcitonin. While calcitonin can cause diarrhea, the other hormones can cause constipation.

- Drinking alcohol may cause secretion of calcitonin by the tumor, and the patient may have flushing and diarrhea.

- If one family member receives a diagnosis of medullary thyroid cancer, other family members should have their calcitonin levels checked. If a family member's calcitonin is elevated, he or she should have the thyroid removed; elevated calcitonin almost always indicates cancer is present or, if not yet present, will develop later.

- Even when the calcitonin isn't elevated in a family member, genetic testing can determine whether the family member may eventually get a medullary thyroid cancer (see Chapter 14).

- Measuring calcitonin levels reveals whether a tumor has spread or recurred after the removal of the thyroid.

Some thyroid specialists advocate measuring calcitonin as a screening test for all nodules suspected to contain thyroid cancer. So far, doctors aren't practicing this kind of screening.

After ten years, about 70 percent of patients with medullary thyroid cancer who receive treatment are still alive.

Undifferentiated (anaplastic) cancer

Fortunately, *undifferentiated cancer* is very rare, accounting for about only 2 percent of all thyroid cancers. This type of cancer is very aggressive and rarely cured. Although 95 percent or more of patients with papillary or follicular thyroid cancer will be alive and doing well after ten years, less than 10 percent of patients with undifferentiated thyroid cancer will be alive after three years.

This cancer is aggressive and invasive. Although lymph node invasion by papillary cancer isn't a bad sign, lymph node invasion by undifferentiated cancer predicts a bad outcome.

The cancer tends to attach to local structures like the nearby muscles, the trachea, the esophagus, and the blood vessels, making surgery very difficult, if not impossible. The outlook is so bad that little justification exists for extensive surgery that just mutilates the patient without accomplishing a cure.

Important features of undifferentiated cancer include the following:

- The ratio of people with undifferentiated cancer is 60 percent female and 40 percent male.
- It presents itself most often with a rapidly enlarging neck mass.
- It usually occurs in patients over the age of 65.
- It may occur in patients with a distant history of radiation to the neck or face.
- By the time a person receives a diagnosis, the cancer has already spread to local nodes and distant structures like the lungs, bone, brain, and liver.
- The average survival period following diagnosis is three months, and most people die of this cancer within six months or a year of diagnosis.

Undifferentiated cancer is most probably the kind of thyroid cancer that Chief Justice William Rehnquist suffered from beginning in October 2004. The fact that he needed a tracheotomy, an opening from the outside into his windpipe, very early suggests a very aggressive tumor that had spread into his trachea. The fact that he was able to continue his work to the extent that he did while being treated for this disease is surprising. He lived about one year with the tumor, which is the most that you can expect under current methods of treatment.

The Stages of Thyroid Cancer and the Treatment Options

For purposes of treatment, thyroid cancers are *staged* (divided into stages). Cancers divide up by whether the cancer remains within the thyroid, whether and where spread has taken place, and whether the tumor moves or is attached to surrounding tissues. Knowing which stage a cancer is in is important, because a follicular cancer in the same stage as a papillary cancer responds to treatment in the same way, while two follicular cancers at very different stages respond differently.

- ✔ **Stage I:** The tumor is entirely within the thyroid gland with no spread to other areas.

- ✔ **Stage II:** A tumor is in the thyroid but also has spread to the local lymph nodes. Both the thyroid and the lymph nodes are freely movable. The tumor hasn't become attached to surrounding tissues.

- ✔ **Stage III:** The tumor and/or lymph nodes are attached to the surrounding tissues.

- ✔ **Stage IV:** The tumor has spread outside the neck.

Most treatment of thyroid cancer initially involves surgery. The experience and competence of the surgeon is extremely important, no matter what stage of cancer you're in.

The most controversial treatment involves stage I of thyroid cancer, because knowing if the treatment itself or the benign course of the disease is responsible for a good outcome is difficult. General agreement exists about the best way to treat the other stages, but even there some disagreement exists. In the following sections, I try to offer the most generally accepted treatment recommendations, but of course anyone facing treatment must talk with an internist and surgeon to get their perspective.

Stage 1

Because the size of the tumor plays a role in the prognosis, doctors recommend different levels of surgery depending on whether the tumor is less than or greater than 1 centimeter.

Surgeons treat a tumor smaller than 1 centimeter by removing the lobe of the thyroid in which it's found, plus partially removing the other lobe, leaving some tissue intact (including the tissue next to the parathyroid glands and the recurrent laryngeal nerve). Surgeons usually treat a tumor larger than 1 centimeter by removing the entire thyroid, with the exception of the tissue adjacent to the parathyroid glands and recurrent laryngeal nerve. Both operations are intended to ensure that the patient's parathyroid glands continue to function and that his or her speech won't be damaged after surgery. The difference between the two is that the first operation leaves part of the thyroid intact because the chance that the cancer has spread to the other lobe is small.

Some thyroid specialists recommend the smaller operation for any stage I thyroid tumor, regardless of size, due to the generally good prognosis of any stage I tumor. No one has proved that more surgery is better for stage 1 tumors.

If even a small tumor has developed as a result of receiving radiation to the thyroid, you should have the larger operation (removal of the entire thyroid) because usually cancer is present in both lobes.

In the previous edition of this book, I suggested that a patient who has most of his or her thyroid removed (the larger operation) is kept off thyroid hormone treatment in order to prepare him for evaluation of remaining tissue. If any thyroid cancer remains, a radioactive iodine scan detects it, which a large dose of radioactive iodine can treat. The radioactive iodine destroys all remaining thyroid tissue, which a subsequent scan can prove, and makes it easier to diagnose and treat a recurrence of the thyroid cancer in the future.

However, more recent evaluation of patients with stage I thyroid cancer suggests that doing post-operative radiation treatment to ablate (remove) the remaining thyroid isn't necessary. Patients who don't have post-operative ablation with radioactive iodine do just as well as those who do. In a publication in the *World Journal of Surgery* in August 2002, the 25-year survival rate of 636 low-risk thyroid cancer patients at the Mayo Clinic who didn't take radioactive iodine after surgery was 100 percent. No difference existed between the survival of patients not given radioiodine therapy in the 1940s and those given radiotherapy in later decades when the cancer was stage I or II. Radioactive iodine treatment can't improve on that.

Giving large doses of radioactive iodine isn't completely free of side effects, especially if metastases (cancerous spread away from the original site of the cancer) of the thyroid cancer are in critical places, which concentrate the iodine and expose the tissue to a lot of radioactivity. Some of the possible damage from radioactive iodine includes the following:

✔ Radiation sickness

✔ Pain in the tissues surrounding the radioactivity

✔ Damage to the salivary glands with decreased saliva and loss of teeth

✔ Suppression of ovulation or even sterilization if metastases are in the ovaries

✔ Suppression of sperm formation

✔ Fibrosis of the lung with severe difficulty breathing

✔ Decreased white blood cells, platelets, and red blood cells

✔ Suppression of the bone marrow and even bone marrow failure

I highly advise using radioactive iodine only when definite proof supports that it will be beneficial.

Stage II

Thyroid doctors generally agree about the correct treatment for stage II thyroid cancer: An experienced surgeon should remove as much of the thyroid as possible, preserving the parathyroid glands and the recurrent laryngeal nerves. The surgeon also looks for enlarged nodes in the neck, which he removes. If the surgeon finds cancer in these nodes, he removes as many of the nodes in the local area of the neck as he can find. Doing a neck ultrasound, which can detect enlarged, suspicious nodes, before surgery makes detecting cancerous lymph nodes easier.

After surgery, the doctor keeps a patient off thyroid hormone treatment for three weeks and then measures the level of TSH. If it's above 20, the doctor does a thyroid scan to look for any residual thyroid tissue. A large dose of radioactive iodine removes any tissue found. The doctor then places a patient on enough thyroid hormone to keep the TSH at the bottom of the normal range (around 0.3). The patient takes thyroid hormone, because even thyroid cancer responds to TSH stimulation, and the object is to prevent further growth of the cancer.

Stage III

Because the tumor has invaded the local structures, treating stage III thyroid cancer requires more extensive surgery. The need for a highly experienced surgeon is even greater. An invasion of the tumor into the wall of the *trachea* (windpipe) may have occurred, and a surgeon must remove part of the trachea. If a tumor is in the muscle, the surgeon removes the involved muscle. The surgeon must remove as much of the tumor as possible without disfiguring the patient. Because the cells of this stage III tumor are so abnormal, they often don't take up radioactive iodine, so radioactive iodine can't treat patients in stage III. Instead, patients often receive external irradiation if much of a tumor has to be left in the neck during the surgery.

Stage IV

If possible, the surgeon removes any distinct areas where the tumor has spread away from the thyroid outside the neck. In addition, the surgeon completely removes the thyroid as well as the lymph glands in the neck. If the spread of cancer is very wide, the doctor makes an attempt to get the distant tumor to take up radioactive iodine after removing the thyroid. If the tumor doesn't take up radioactive iodine, doctors use external irradiation to treat it.

Only about 5 to 10 percent of stage IV patients have successful removal of all the tissue in the neck that contains the thyroid tumor. For these patients, their survival is longer. The rest, unfortunately, won't survive more than a year.

If the tumor is more like normal thyroid tissue in appearance but has distant metastases or is of the anaplastic variety, chemotherapy can also be a treatment. For chemotherapy, you need the help of an oncologist, a specialist in cancer chemotherapy who should be aware of the various protocols developed for aggressive thyroid cancer treatment.

Medullary thyroid cancer

This type of cancer isn't a tumor that originates in thyroid-producing cells, so its treatment is a little different. A surgeon removes the entire thyroid, because the fact that medullary thyroid cancer, or medullary carcinoma, doesn't concentrate iodine means radioactive iodine can't eliminate thyroid tissue. The surgeon also removes lymph nodes in the neck that contain the tumor. External irradiation may be a treatment for medullary thyroid cancer. The doctor measures a patient's calcitonin level at intervals to check for any regrowth of the tumor.

Family members of a patient with medullary carcinoma should have their calcitonin levels checked, and if their levels are high, they should seek treatment as well. Genetic testing can also rule out medullary thyroid cancer in other family members.

Following up on Cancer Treatment

Any patient who has most or all of her thyroid removed must start taking a thyroid-hormone replacement after surgery and needs to continue that treatment for the rest of her life. As I discuss in Chapter 5, thyroid-hormone replacement simply involves taking a daily pill. The current technique is to give enough thyroid hormone to keep the TSH between 0.1 and 0.3, which is supposed to suppress the growth of new thyroid tissue, including cancer.

Patients who receive treatment for stage I or II thyroid cancer should have their blood levels of thyroglobulin (see Chapter 2) checked regularly after surgery. If their levels start to rise, their doctors stop thyroid-hormone replacement for several weeks. The doctor does a full body scan with radioactive iodine, looking for any evidence of thyroid tissue. If the body scan finds thyroid tissue, the patient receives a much larger treatment dose of radioactive iodine, which destroys the remaining thyroid tissue. The patient resumes replacement thyroid hormone a few days later.

Stopping the thyroid hormone allows the body to produce thyroid-stimulating hormone (TSH), which stimulates uptake of radioactive iodine by thyroid tissue. Instead of stopping thyroid-hormone replacement, your doctor can give you synthetic TSH injections for several days prior to a thyroid scan with almost as good a result. Another approach that works is to reduce your usual dose of thyroid hormone to half of the daily dose for several weeks. If the TSH rises above 20, you can do the radioactive treatment.

Patients with stage III or IV thyroid cancer probably show regrowth of their tumor. Their tumor may respond to more external irradiation or to chemicals known to kill the tumor. The outlook is poor for patients who have recurrent stage III or IV thyroid cancer.

Chapter 9

Multinodular Goiters: Thyroids with Many Nodules

*M*ultinodular goiters — large thyroids with many nodules — may well be the most common of all thyroid disorders. In various studies of thyroid glands of people who died of any cause, between 30 and 60 percent of the glands had multiple nodules. This means as many as 165 million people in the United States alone have multinodular goiters. What a bonanza for thyroid specialists! (With numbers like that, you have to wonder whose idea it was to place the thyroid gland so prominently in the front of the neck, near so many vital structures, and to make it so important. I call it bad planning.)

Fortunately (or unfortunately, depending on which side of the desk you're sitting on), doctors never see or treat most people with multinodular goiters for their thyroid nodules. Only a small fraction of people with multinodular goiters develop the signs and symptoms I discuss in this chapter and need an evaluation.

A Multinodular Goiter Grows Up

Ryan Fine (a distant cousin of Kenneth from Chapter 7) is 46 years old. He goes to his doctor for a routine physical examination, and the doctor tells him that his thyroid feels bumpy. He has no symptoms of pain or difficulty swallowing in his neck. His doctor obtains thyroid function tests, which are normal, and thyroid autoantibody tests, which are negative. His doctor refers him to the specialist, the venerable Dr. Rubin.

Dr. Rubin examines Ryan and tells him that he can feel several distinct nodules, all of them soft and freely movable. He sends Ryan for a thyroid scan, which shows that all the nodules can concentrate radioactive iodine (none of them are "cold"; see Chapter 7). Dr. Rubin assures Ryan that he has a multinodular goiter and that he needs no treatment as long as he is free of symptoms. He asks Ryan to return in six months so that he can examine the thyroid again.

Four months later, Ryan suddenly feels pain in his neck and notices that one area has gotten larger. He goes to see Dr. Rubin, who inserts a needle in that area and removes a small amount of blood. He tells Ryan that a hemorrhage has occurred in one of the nodules, forming a *cyst* (a fluid-filled nodule) that requires no more treatment than evacuation of the blood. A hemorrhage occurs once more, and then it stops. Ryan returns every six months thereafter and experiences no further change.

Ryan is an excellent illustration of the way that someone typically discovers a multinodular goiter, how a specialist evaluates it, and the most common outcome of the condition. Doctors believe that multinodular goiters result from some or all of the following circumstances:

- ✔ Starting around puberty, sometimes related to a deficiency of iodine (see Chapter 12), the thyroid is stimulated to grow. It grows a certain amount and then enters a resting state. This growth-resting cycle repeats itself many times.

- ✔ The cells in the thyroid, though they almost all perform the same task of making thyroid hormone, aren't identical and grow at different rates.

- ✔ Some thyroid cells develop and multiply that aren't under the control of thyroid-stimulating hormone (TSH). They form the autonomous nodules that are often found in a multinodular goiter and can lead to hyperthyroidism.

- ✔ Certain stresses to the body, such as a pregnancy, increase the need for iodine, leading to more stimulation of the thyroid.

- ✔ Some foods called *goitrogens* (see Chapter 5) prevent the production of thyroid hormone and lead to more stimulation of the thyroid.

- ✔ Certain drugs, such as amiodarone (taken for heart rhythm irregularities), block production of thyroid hormone, which leads to more growth of the thyroid to compensate.

- ✔ Genetic connections may cause multinodular goiters to occur more often in some families than in others.

Figure 9-1 shows what a multinodular goiter looks like in comparison to a normal thyroid.

Ryan illustrates one way you can discover a goiter, but you may find goiters in many ways, including the following:

✔ Your neck suddenly gets much larger, leading to a visit to the doctor.

✔ You feel a sudden pain in your neck, and one side of your neck becomes larger because of bleeding in a nodule.

✔ A doctor feels a large thyroid with many nodules during a routine examination.

✔ Symptoms develop, such as a cough, difficulty swallowing, a feeling of pressure in the neck, or a lump in the throat.

✔ Your doctor discovers the goiter incidentally when you have other testing done, like an ultrasound study of the neck or an X-ray of the chest.

✔ Occasionally, particularly in older people, the patient has a heart irregularity or signs and symptoms of hyperthyroidism (see Chapter 6). Rarely if ever do patients with a multinodular goiter become hypothyroid. When they do, the diagnosis is probably Hashimoto's thyroiditis (see Chapter 5).

Figure 9-1:
A multi-nodular goiter compared to a normal thyroid.

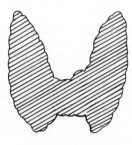

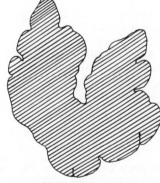

Normal thyroid   Multinodular goiter

Multinodular goiters are very common throughout the world, but they're especially common in places where iodine is deficient in the diet.

Making a Diagnosis

Depending on how you discover a multinodular goiter, a doctor does a number of studies to determine exactly what is going on in the thyroid gland. A good pair of expert hands can feel the presence of many nodules (although no one can feel nodules smaller than a centimeter). An examination by a specialist is very important, because it serves as a baseline for future thyroid exams. The doctor notes the size of the thyroid so he can compare what he feels during future examinations to determine if the thyroid is growing.

The first study of a multinodular goiter consists of thyroid function tests to see whether your thyroid is making enough thyroid hormone. These test results are usually normal, but occasionally they show excess production of thyroid hormone. You should always have thyroid function tests done if you have a multinodular goiter. Depending on the stress you feel from the growth in your neck and how much the doctor values leaving no stone unturned, your doctor may do many, all, or none of the following tests.

- ✔ **Thyroid autoantibody tests:** Your doctor sometimes does these tests, especially if you have a family history of goiters. These test results are usually negative unless autoimmune thyroiditis is present (see Chapter 5).

- ✔ **Fine needle aspiration biopsy:** When one nodule stands out or is harder than the others, the doctor often does a fine needle aspiration biopsy to rule out cancer, even though the study has a poor sensitivity in this situation. But the test is so benign that it's worth doing despite the rare positive finding of cancer. A thyroid scan may precede the biopsy to see whether the nodule is functional (warm or hot) or if it's cold (see Chapter 7). Cancers are usually cold. However, keep in mind that the majority of cold nodules aren't cancer. If cancer isn't present, the fine needle biopsy doesn't add any information that points to a diagnosis of the multinodular goiter.

- ✔ **Thyroid scan:** A thyroid scan gives a general picture of the thyroid, showing the size of the gland, the many nodules, and the position of the gland, which is particularly important if it's below the sternum (as I explain in the previous section).

- ✔ **Thyroid ultrasound:** A thyroid ultrasound picks up very small nodules. This test can show whether a tender nodule is a cyst (a fluid-filled nodule).

- ✔ **Barium swallow:** If you feel significant pressure in your neck or have trouble swallowing, your doctor may order a *barium swallow:* You swallow barium, and your doctor takes X-rays as it passes down. This test may show that the thyroid gland is putting pressure on the *esophagus,* the swallowing tube from the mouth to the stomach. A plain film (without barium) of the neck reveals if the mass of the thyroid is deviating the trachea.

If thyroid function tests indicate hyperthyroidism, your doctor looks for other signs of hyperthyroidism due to Graves' disease. Thyroid eye and skin disease, which I describe in Chapter 6, support a diagnosis of Graves' disease. A patient who has hyperthyroidism in a multinodular goiter may instead have a condition called *toxic multinodular goiter,* also known as *Plummer's disease.* Plummer's disease doesn't involve eye disease. A thyroid scan can differentiate the two conditions (see Chapter 4). Graves' disease shows increased activity throughout the gland, while Plummer's disease shows a few hyperactive nodules.

Choosing to Treat It or Ignore It

Multinodular goiters generally proceed along the same path in most patients. When thyroid function tests are done, the results are either normal or the thyroid hormone levels are possibly elevated, suggesting hyperthyroidism; the thyroid hormone levels are rarely low. If a patient experiences sudden pain in one area of the thyroid, the doctor performs a *fine needle aspiration biopsy* (see Chapter 4). Usually that area of the thyroid contains blood as a result of a hemorrhage in one of the nodules. When a doctor removes the blood, the nodule shrinks.

If a particular nodule stands out or is harder than the others, it is biopsied and usually found to be benign. If the nodule is cancerous, treatment for cancer is begun (see Chapter 8). The problem is that a fine needle biopsy of a dominant nodule in a multinodular gland rarely discovers a cancer, even when cancer is present.

If the only problem is the large gland, most of the time the doctor doesn't treat it. If you experience other symptoms in the neck, or if the thyroid gland is particularly unsightly, the doctor treats the gland.

Sometimes the thyroid, instead of growing up and out, grows downward behind the chest bone (the *sternum*) and is said to be *substernal.* In a substernal position, where the goiter has little room to grow, it can squeeze other organs like the *trachea,* the air pipe from the nose to the lungs. Treatment may be necessary to reduce symptoms that arise from substernal goiters.

Most people with a multinodular goiter don't realize they have it, and even if they're aware that it exists, they don't find treating it necessary. Even very large goiters don't seem to disturb patients other than the cosmetic abnormality. Goiters that compress the trachea and push it sideways don't seem to cause any problem in breathing.

Treating a Multinodular Goiter

Therapy for a multinodular goiter differs somewhat depending on whether the goiter is toxic and causing hyperthyroidism.

The nontoxic goiter

If the nodules of a multinodular goiter aren't causing symptoms of hyperthyroidism and don't contain cancer, and if you have no symptoms, your doctor usually leaves the multinodular goiter alone. Doctors used to think that you could shrink a multinodular goiter with thyroid hormone. This hasn't proven to be the case. In fact, thyroid hormone may be dangerous for an elderly patient, who may become overtreated.

If you dislike the appearance of your neck, or if you're hyperthyroid, your doctor uses radioactive iodine to destroy some of the thyroid tissue (see Chapter 6). This treatment works even for large goiters but sometimes results in hypothyroidism. Also, in the course of destroying thyroid tissue, a lot of thyroid hormone flows into the bloodstream, inducing temporary hyperthyroidism if it isn't present already. Older people, especially, need to receive antithyroid drugs before using radioactive iodine (see Chapter 6).

Some people (less than 10 percent) who take radioactive iodine to shrink a large multinodular goiter develop Graves' disease, which I discuss in Chapter 6. Graves' disease happens because thyroid tissue is released into the bloodstream, and the body forms antibodies against it.

Doctors rarely perform surgery for a multinodular goiter unless they find a cancer. Radioactive iodine is able to treat most thyroid glands, even the large ones that grow in a downward direction. Some reasons to do surgery include the following:

✔ Sudden growth of the goiter

✔ Bleeding in the goiter with compression of vital tissues

✔ One very firm nodule suspicious for cancer

✔ Paralysis of the vocal cords, suggesting cancer

✔ Suspicious lymph nodes, again suggesting cancer

If you have surgery for a benign multinodular goiter, you have enough thyroid tissue left to keep functionally normal. You don't take thyroid hormone pills. Even if you did take them, they wouldn't prevent a multinodular goiter from growing again. If more growth of the goiter occurs, then you can have radioactive iodine.

If you have a multinodular goiter, you should return to your doctor at least annually to have an examination of your thyroid. Visit your doctor earlier when you see new growth or pain develops.

The toxic goiter

Doctors treat hyperthyroid multinodular goiters in a similar fashion to non-hyperthyroid glands. But hyperthyroid multinodular goiters usually require more radioactive iodine to control the hyperthyroidism, which generally leads to hypothyroidism later on.

Some patients have a worsening of their hyperthyroidism when they take radioactive iodine. This is because the thyroid cells are breaking down and release a large amount of the hormone stored in the thyroid. To avoid worsening hyperthyroidism, patients can take antithyroid drugs to make them normal and diminish the amount of stored thyroid hormone for several weeks before their doctor administers radioactive iodine.

Dealing with a Goiter Behind the Sternum

A goiter behind the sternum occurs when the nodules form at the lower part of the thyroid and grow in a downward direction. Because little room exists in this area for further growth, the thyroid begins to compress vital structures like the trachea and the swallowing tube, the esophagus. The symptoms come from this compression, but hyperthyroidism can also occur.

Some of the complaints of people with goiters behind the sternum include the following:

✔ A severe choking sensation

✔ Severe shortness of breath during a respiratory infection

✔ Sudden increase in symptoms due to bleeding in a nodule

✔ A cough and hoarseness

A doctor can make the diagnosis just by a chest X-ray that shows the large goiter behind the sternum. A thyroid scan also reveals a lot of thyroid tissue below the neck, where it doesn't belong.

The treatment is like that for a multinodular goiter above the sternum — radioactive iodine. The radioactive iodine shrinks the thyroid and sometimes permits it to return to the neck position when the large amount of thyroid that prevents upward movement is gone.

Occasionally, doctors perform surgery if the patient doesn't want radioactive iodine or the gland is in a particularly difficult position. Antithyroid drugs prepare the patient for surgery. Surgery is more complicated than radioactive iodine, but the surgeon can raise up the thyroid fairly easily once it's separated from the tissues surrounding it.

Chapter 10

Drugs That Impact Your Thyroid

. . . .

In This Chapter

▶ Realizing the impact of food and drugs on your thyroid

▶ Knowing the effects of specific drugs

▶ Avoiding drug interactions

▶ Determining whether you are taking one of these drugs

. . . .

*I*t should come as no surprise that a ton of drugs are going to have some effect on your thyroid, because thyroid hormones affect every cell in your body. Drug scientists haven't yet reached the stage where they can produce a drug that hits only the target they're aiming at without banging a few other, unexpected targets along the way. These undesired hits are *side effects*. You must understand side effects so that you don't draw wrong conclusions about the state of your thyroid health from changes in your thyroid hormone levels or your metabolism that result from using the drugs I discuss in this chapter. Certain drugs in our food and in the environment also change thyroid function. You need to understand and perhaps avoid these substances, too.

Whether you have high blood pressure or a headache or heart failure, at some point you're bound to run into drugs that impact your thyroid function. In this chapter, you meet most of the important drugs that interact with your thyroid in one way or another. By absorbing the information in this chapter, you can probably tell your doctor a thing or two. Just try not to embarrass your doctor.

With so many drugs effecting thyroid function in one way or another, avoiding drug interactions is difficult, particularly if one of the drugs you're taking is thyroid hormone. If you're taking thyroid hormone, your body isn't able to make the subtle changes in thyroid function necessary to compensate for the other drug you're taking, which is most likely reducing the thyroid hormone available to your system. The best solution is to ask either your doctor or druggist to run a computer program that looks at multiple drugs and determines interactions. If your doctor doesn't have the capability to do this check, she can ask her hospital pharmacy to do it.

Revealing the Drug-Food-Thyroid Connection

The following cases illustrate the broad spectrum of effects that various drugs and foods can have on thyroid function. Some drugs affect thyroid function tests while the thyroid itself is still normal. Other drugs can create hypothyroidism or hyperthyroidism. As if these effects aren't confusing enough, the same drug given to two different people may cause opposite effects, depending on their particular clinical situation.

Natasha Smart is a 36-year-old woman who is healthy and wants to avoid having any more children. She asks her gynecologist to put her on oral contraceptive tablets. One day, while browsing in a bookstore, she comes upon Dr. Rubin's book *Thyroid For Dummies, 2nd Edition* (Wiley). (She can't miss it; the "Must Read" section of the bookstore features it.) She opens it and reads on the Cheat Sheet at the front of the book that thyroid testing is advised for people over age 35 every five years. After buying several copies of the book for herself and her friends, she returns to her gynecologist and asks to be tested. Her gynecologist, unfortunately, hasn't read the book and still tests thyroid function with a total thyroxine test (see Chapter 4). The result is high. He tells Natasha that she may have hyperthyroidism. Natasha reads further in the book and finds that the estrogen in oral contraceptive pills raises the amount of thyroid-binding protein in her system. Meanwhile, the *free thyroxine,* the form of the thyroid hormone that can enter cells and therefore actually have an effect, remains normal. She informs her (embarrassed) gynecologist, who does a free thyroxin test and a TSH (thyroid-stimulating hormone) test, both of which are normal. Nothing further is done.

Leonard Bright is a 72-year-old man who is having trouble with a very irregular heartbeat. His physician places him on a relatively new drug called *amiodarone* that is used to correct irregular heartbeats.

About two months later, Leonard's heartbeat has become regular, but he is beginning to feel cold and sleepy. He has gained a few pounds and notices that his skin is dry. His doctor recognizes the symptoms of hypothyroidism (see Chapter 5), sometimes associated with amiodarone. The doctor orders thyroid function tests to confirm the diagnosis and starts Leonard on thyroid hormone. In a month, he returns to his normal state of health.

Dr. Rubin has followed Kathy Brilliant for many years because of a multinodular goiter. No treatment has been necessary. At the age of 68, she develops a rapid heartbeat and sees a cardiologist, who places her on amiodarone (the same medication that Mr. Bright takes), and her heart problem resolves itself. However, after six weeks she notices that her heart is beating rapidly again. Not only that, she is losing weight and having trouble sleeping. She feels warm all the time, though she is well past her menopause.

Kathy returns to the cardiologist, who recognizes that her symptoms are a side effect of amiodarone and sends her back to Dr. Rubin. He tells Kathy that she has hyperthyroidism due to the effect of amiodarone on her multinodular goiter. He suggests that she take pills to control the thyroid and stop taking the amiodarone if the cardiologist can substitute another drug.

Kathy stops the amiodarone and takes pills called *methimazole,* but her condition doesn't improve. After two months, Dr. Rubin recommends thyroid surgery. When the surgery is done, Kathy improves dramatically. She is now able to take the amiodarone and feels fine.

George Shrub absolutely loves broccoli and consumes prodigious quantities, even at breakfast. He finds that he is often sleepy and cold. He has trouble thinking and making appropriate decisions. He goes to his doctor, who runs blood tests that show a high TSH. The doctor tells George that he is hypothyroid and puts him on thyroid medication.

One night, George and his wife invite Natasha Smart and her husband to dinner. As Natasha watches George consume huge quantities of broccoli, she remarks that she has read in Dr. Rubin's book that broccoli contains a substance that reduces thyroid function. George is very surprised to hear this news, but he sharply reduces his broccoli intake after that night. After talking the situation over with his doctor, he also gradually reduces his thyroid-hormone replacement. After he's been off broccoli for a month, George's thyroid tests are normal.

Each year, all the various drug companies get together to produce a huge book called the *Physicians' Desk Reference* (PDR). The purpose of this book is to provide, in one convenient place, current information about all the drugs that require prescriptions (a separate book covers nonprescription drugs). Every physician receives a copy of the PDR annually. The edition for the year 2005 contains more than 3,400 pages, describing more than 2,000 drugs. To say that most of these drugs affect the thyroid in one way or another isn't an exaggeration. Fortunately, in most cases, the effect is nothing to worry about. But plenty of drugs are a source of concern.

Do I know all the details about how each of these 2,000-plus drugs affect the thyroid? No way, Renee! But I know about the ones that folks use most frequently and the ones that have the greatest effect on thyroid function or thyroid function tests. These are the products I discuss in this chapter. I deal with them in terms of how they affect thyroid function.

At the end of the chapter, I group these drugs according to their main clinical purpose so that you can check if you need to be concerned about your blood pressure pill or the pill you take for diabetes or fluid retention. Although I use only the generic (nontrademarked) name in the earlier sections, I give you all the various drug company names at the end of the chapter so you can recognize the particular drug you're taking. For example, *nifedipine* is the generic name for Adalat, Procardia, and Nifedipine capsules, all the same drug made by different manufacturers. Pretty confusing, huh?

How drugs affect your thyroid hormones

Chapter 2 explains how your body makes and releases thyroid hormones, how they're carried around the body, how cells take them up, where they do their work, and how they work within the cells. Drugs can affect thyroid function at any one or more of these levels.

✔ **Thyroid hormone production:** Thyroid hormone forms when iodine is added to a compound called *thyronine*. When four iodine molecules are attached to this compound, the result is *thyroxine* (T4). When three molecules of iodine are attached, the resulting compound is *triiodothyronine* (T3). Removing one iodine molecule from thyroxine can also produce T3. Many drugs and food substances block the production of both T4 and T3.

✔ **Amount of thyroid-binding proteins present:** After your body produces T3 and T4, they must travel in the body to get to their site of action. Thyroid-binding proteins carry them in the bloodstream (see Chapter 2). Drugs can affect thyroid function by increasing or decreasing the amount of binding protein in the blood. Drugs can affect thyroid test results even while the thyroid function remains normal. This occurs because the *free thyroid hormone* (hormone not bound to protein) is active in the body, not the hormone that is attached to protein.

✔ **Cell receptor sites:** The free hormone arrives at the cell where it needs to do its work. It must get into the cell by attaching to a substance called a receptor on the membrane of the cell. The receptor is another place where certain drugs can prevent thyroid hormone from doing its job. They can block the receptors so that no hormone can enter. The situation may be almost like diabetes, in which plenty of glucose (sugar) is available in the bloodstream for energy, but it can't enter the cell where it does its work.

✔ **Hormones' effects inside of cells:** Once inside the cell, the thyroid hormone attaches to the nucleus, where the genetic material is stored. Thyroid hormone then encourages a certain action to take place within the cell. Here, various drugs block the hormone's attachment to the nucleus or alter it so that it doesn't produce the desired effect.

You should know that new medications come on the market at least hourly. These products get better and better at curing the latest diseases, but initially, drug companies rarely know their other effects from the few thousand people who test them before they come to market. The side effects of many drugs don't become clear until hundreds of thousands of people take them. Many if not all new drugs affect the thyroid in one way or another. The people who must pay particular attention to the side effects of new drugs are those who have some underlying thyroid disease to begin with. For example:

✔ If you've had hyperthyroidism (see Chapter 6) and it's under control with antithyroid drugs, a drug containing a lot of iodine will probably cause a recurrence of your disease.

✔ If you've had a multinodular goiter (see Chapter 9), iodine will possibly bring on hyperthyroidism.

✔ If you're borderline hypothyroid (see Chapter 5), iodine or one of the drugs that block thyroid hormone production will bring on clinical hypothyroidism.

✔ If you have mild subacute thyroiditis (see Chapter 11), some drugs make it worse to the point that you experience more severe symptoms of thyroiditis.

Identifying the Effects of Specific Substances

In this section, you encounter particular drugs that affect the thyroid. I group them together according to their potential impact on your thyroid. I don't provide brand names of medications here — only generic names. If you're wondering whether your specific brand of medication is something that may affect your thyroid, check out the listings in the "Discovering Whether You're at Risk" section later in the chapter, where I group these drugs according to their primary purpose.

Initiating or aggravating hypothyroidism

Many drugs have the potential to cause or intensify hypothyroidism. In the following sections, I introduce you to the most commonly prescribed medications that have these potential side effects.

Drugs and chemicals that compete with iodine

If iodine can't enter the thyroid, your body can't make thyroid hormone, and you experience hypothyroidism. Some drugs compete with iodine for entry into the thyroid. Usually the effect is mild, and hypothyroidism doesn't occur. But if your diet is limited in iodine, these drugs can cause low thyroid function. The most important drugs in this category include:

✔ **Lithium,** for the treatment of manic-depressive psychosis. In one study, as many as 10 percent of patients who took lithium became hypothyroid. This effect is much more common in women than in men and occurs within the first two years of treatment. Most likely, the large population of women with autoimmune thyroid disease (see Chapter 5) is most susceptible to the antithyroid effect of lithium. Not only does lithium block the uptake of iodine, but it also inhibits the production and release of thyroid hormone. Some people being treated with lithium develop a goiter. Curiously (and rarely), lithium can cause hyperthyroidism rather than hypothyroidism.

✔ **Ethionamide,** for the treatment of tuberculosis. A goiter may or may not accompany the hypothyroidism that results.

Minerals such as **fluorine,** which is found in the diet (especially in fluoridated water), have a similar effect on the thyroid. If you consume substantial amounts of fluorine, your thyroid decreases its production of T4. Your pituitary gland then makes more TSH to stimulate the thyroid, and you can end up with a goiter.

Drugs and chemicals that prevent the addition of iodine to form thyroid hormones

Another large group of medications blocks the production of thyroid hormones in a slightly different way. They keep iodine from combining with thyronine to form either T4 or T3, the two thyroid hormones. This group of medications includes the following:

✔ **Aminoglutethimide,** for the treatment of breast and prostate cancer. As many as one-third of patients treated with this medication develop hypothyroidism.

✔ **Ketoconazole,** used as an antifungal drug. Hypothyroidism is a rare side effect of this agent.

✔ **Para-aminosalicylic acid,** for the long-term treatment of tuberculosis.

✔ **Sulfonamide drugs,** which eliminate excess water from the body and act as antibiotics. These include **sulfadiazine, sulfasoxazole,** and **acetazoleamide.** If you use these diuretics and antibiotics for prolonged periods of time, they can cause hypothyroidism.

✔ Certain **sulfonylureas,** used in the treatment of diabetes, such as **tolbutamide** and **chlorpropamide.** Doctors rarely prescribe these drugs today.

✔ The **thionamide** drugs, including **propylthiouricil, methimazole,** and **carbimazole.** With the exception of carbimazole, I discuss these drugs extensively in Chapter 6, because they're the primary drugs used to treat hyperthyroidism. Carbimazole is used in the United Kingdom especially.

Two chemicals found in food have an impact similar to the medications in the preceding list. They are

✔ **Isoflavins,** found in soybeans. Children who eat large amounts of soy products may develop a goiter.

✔ **Thiocyanate,** which is in many common foods like Brussels sprouts, cauliflower, cabbage, horseradish, kale, kohlrabi, mustard, rutabaga, and turnips. If cattle consume foods like these and you drink milk from those cattle, thyiocyanate can affect your thyroid as well.

Drugs that affect the transport of thyroid hormone

Many drugs affect how thyroid hormones are transported in your bloodstream. Chances are you'll take one of these drugs at some point in your life. If you have normal thyroid function, your thyroid simply makes more or less thyroid hormone to compensate for the effects of these drugs. But if you're hypothyroid and taking a thyroid-hormone replacement, your doctor may need to increase or decrease your dose if you have to take one of these drugs.

The following drugs increase thyroid-binding protein, resulting in an increase in total (but not free) thyroxine, unless you get your thyroid hormone as a medication:

✔ **Estrogens** are the most commonly used drugs in this category. For years, estrogens caused confusion about thyroid function, because doctors used to measure how much total thyroxine was in your system, not just the amount of free thyroxine (see Chapter 4). Estrogens are found in birth control pills and hormone replacement therapy. Some animals are fed estrogens to fatten them up, so as you consume those animals, you get estrogen that way as well. The list of medications that contain estrogens is huge.

✔ **Clofibrate** is a drug used for lowering blood fats, especially cholesterol and triglycerides. There are now better drugs for this purpose, but some doctors still use this one. Not only does it increase thyroid-binding protein, but it may act like thyroid hormone, attaching to proteins that thyroid hormone normally attaches to, and stimulating thyroid function. It can lead to muscle breakdown.

✔ **Perphenazine** is a treatment for psychotic disorders in the group of drugs called *phenothiazines*. This group includes a number of well-known medications, such as **prochlorperazine, trifluoperazine,** and **chlorpromazine.** Perphenazine is the main ingredient in a number of different preparations and can also treat nausea and vomiting.

The following drugs decrease thyroid-binding protein, resulting in a decrease in total (but not free) thyroxin, unless you get your thyroid hormone as a medication:

✔ **Anabolic steroids** promote weight gain after extensive surgery or severe illness, as well as assist in the treatment of anemia. Doctors rarely use them, because they frequently cause liver abnormalities.

✔ **Androgens** substitute for the male hormone, testosterone, when the patient can't make his own. They permit muscle growth and normal sexual function.

✔ **Glucocorticoids** are used very extensively to treat inflammation and to reduce immunity when the inflammation and autoimmunity are damaging to the body, such as in rheumatoid arthritis and many other illnesses. The list of glucocorticoids is a long one.

✔ **Nicotinic acid** is a vitamin used for the treatment of elevated fats in the blood.

If you're hypothyroid and your doctor puts you on one of the agents that decreases thyroid-binding protein for a long time, have your doctor check your thyroid function with a TSH test periodically.

The opiates **heroin** and **methadone** also impact the movement of thyroid hormones in the bloodstream.

Amiodarone

Amiodarone treats disturbances of the heart rhythm. This drug may cause hypothyroidism in up to 10 percent of the people who take it. The drug is also associated with a number of other side effects, including skin and corneal discoloration and fibrosis of the lungs. It may cause hepatitis and bone marrow suppression. Despite all these negatives, it's very useful in treating heart rhythm disturbances.

Amiodarone has received a great deal of study because doctors prescribe it so extensively. It contains a large amount of iodine and acts like other large sources of iodine. It blocks the production of the thyroid hormone T3 from T4 (see Chapter 2). It also has a structural resemblance to thyroid hormone and causes a reduction of thyroid hormone entering tissues where it does its work.

When amiodarone releases iodine, the iodine may block thyroid hormone production, causing hypothyroidism in areas of the world that are already iodine sufficient. Or it may form large amounts of thyroid hormone, causing hyperthyroidism in areas that are deficient in iodine.

The best way to determine the clinical state of the patient is to do a thyroid-stimulating hormone test. If you're hypothyroid, your TSH should be high. If you're hyperthyroid, your TSH should be low.

If amiodarone causes hypothyroidism, you require an unusually large amount of thyroid hormone to overcome the situation or, if possible, you stop taking the amiodarone. Radioactive iodine can't treat amiodarone-induced hyperthyroidism, because the large amount of iodine suppresses the iodine uptake of the thyroid. Therefore, you either have surgery or take antithyroid drugs if stopping the amiodarone is impossible.

Drugs that treat severe hyperthyroidism

The drugs in this group are very useful when a patient has severe hyperthyroidism and needs to reduce the T3 hormone level as soon as possible. However, these drugs have other primary purposes, and when doctors prescribe them for those other purposes (to patients who aren't hyperthyroid), they can create hypothyroidism.

- ✔ **Glucocorticoids** I discuss in the preceding "Drugs that affect the transport of thyroid hormone" section.

- ✔ **Iodinated contrast agents** assist in achieving better X-ray studies. Doctors have used such agents as **ipodate** and **iopanoic acid** in the treatment of hyperthyroidism. A single dose can last for ten days.

- ✔ **Propranolol** slows a rapid heartbeat, but doctors also use it to treat hyperthyroidism because it controls many of the symptoms, such as palpitations, shakiness, and nervousness.

- ✔ **Propylthiouricil** is one of the standard drugs for the treatment of hyperthyroidism.

Growth hormone

When the body doesn't make its own growth hormone, an injectable growth hormone restores growth. Doctors administer growth hormone to children who aren't growing properly because they lack this hormone. If someone is borderline hypothyroid, this hormone may push her into hypothyroidism by reducing the T4 hormone to abnormally low levels.

Drugs that remove thyroid hormone from your system

A number of drugs act upon the liver to speed up the metabolism of thyroid hormones into products that aren't active. Other drugs pull thyroid hormones out of the body with bowel movements. These drugs are very common.

If you're taking a thyroid-replacement hormone and you use one of the following drugs, you may develop hypothyroidism. Ask your doctor to check your thyroid hormone levels about a month after you start to take one of the following drugs:

- ✔ **Aluminum hydroxide** neutralizes the acid in patients with peptic ulcers.

- ✔ **Carbamazepine** and **diphenylhydantoin** treat convulsions.

- ✔ **Cholestyramine** and **colestipol** reduce fats.

- ✔ **Ferrous sulfate** is given to people who are deficient in iron and have anemia. At some point, the doctor stops the ferrous sulfate treatment when the patient's iron reserves are full. The patient may actually become hyperthyroid when she stops taking the ferrous sulfate if her doctor increased her thyroid hormone dose due to the initial effects of the drug.

✔ **Phenobarbital** treats convulsions as well as mild anxiety.

✔ **Rifampin** is one of the treatments for tuberculosis. This drug very rarely causes hypothyroidism in a person who takes thyroid hormone.

✔ **Sucralfate** treats peptic ulcer disease. It may result in hypothyroidism if you take it chronically.

Monitoring your thyroid function is important both during and after use of a short-term medication that lowers the levels of thyroid hormone in your blood, especially if you're taking oral thyroid medication.

Drugs that decrease your TSH

The following drugs can lower the level of thyroid-stimulating hormone in your system, potentially leading to lower thyroid function:

✔ **Acetylsalicylic acid** is commonly known as aspirin. People taking more than 8 or 10 aspirin daily may suffer a lower level of TSH.

✔ **Bromergocryptine** prevents lactation (milk production) and shrinks prolactin-secreting pituitary tumors.

✔ **Clofibrate** lowers the fat particles that contain triglycerides. It also lowers the TSH but doesn't seem to cause clinical problems.

✔ **Dopamine** lowers blood pressure, especially in an emergency setting. It lowers TSH, but patients usually don't use it long enough to cause problems with hypothyroidism.

✔ **Glucocorticoids** treat inflammation and reduce immunity.

✔ **Octreotide** treats certain tumors that produce hormones, especially *acromegaly,* which produces excessive growth hormone, and *carcinoid tumors,* which produce a chemical that causes severe diarrhea and flushing.

✔ **Opiates,** including morphine and heroin, control pain if taken legally and are taken illegally for a chemical high.

✔ **Pamidronate** (brand name Aredia) may cause hypothyroidism. Doctors prescribe it for building bone when a person has diminished bone formation.

✔ **Phentolamine** controls blood pressure in patients who have a tumor of the adrenal gland called a *pheochromocytoma.* This drug reduces TSH, but patients generally don't take it long enough to make a difference in thyroid function.

✔ **Pyridoxine** is vitamin B6. Doctors prescribe it to women during pregnancy and when evidence suggests that someone has a B6 vitamin deficiency.

✔ **Thyroid hormones** replace a deficiency or suppress thyroid cancer or a goiter. They suppress the production of TSH.

Creating false test results

Certain drugs can alter the thyroid hormone (T3 and T4) tests that measure total thyroid hormones (but not free thyroid hormones, which remain normal). If you're taking one of the drugs I list here, you and your doctor should keep that fact in mind if your total T4 test shows hypothyroidism but you aren't experiencing any symptoms of the condition.

- ✔ **Salicylates** such as aspirin are the most commonly used drugs in this group.

- ✔ **Diphenylhydantoin** and **carbamazepine** treat convulsions.

- ✔ **Furosemide** causes the loss of excess water through the kidneys.

- ✔ **Heparin** prevents blood clots. It doesn't change your thyroid function, but if you receive an injection of *low molecular weight heparin,* a measurement of free T4 taken within 10 hours of the injection will be falsely elevated.

- ✔ **Orphenadrine** relieves muscle spasms in a number of drug preparations. It isn't a muscle relaxant but may reduce pain.

Initiating hyperthyroidism

The following drugs increase the production of TSH, which can result in hyperthyroidism:

- ✔ **Amphetamine** reduces congestion, and some people also use it (inappropriately) as a weight-loss agent.

- ✔ **Cimetidine** and **ranitidine** reduce acid secretion to treat peptic ulcers. Both can raise the TSH, but studies don't show a change in thyroid function with these drugs.

- ✔ **Clomiphene** brings on ovulation to promote pregnancy. It has effects on several of the hormones in the pituitary gland, including TSH.

- ✔ **L-dopa inhibitors** such as **chlorpromazine** and **haloperidol** help to manage psychotic disorders. They raise TSH, although people who take them don't generally become hyperthyroid.

- ✔ **Metoclopramide** and **domperidone** control nausea and vomiting, especially after surgery. Metoclopramide also treats gastrointestinal disorders in diabetes mellitus.

- ✔ **Iodine** can raise TSH levels as it blocks the release of thyroid hormones.

- ✔ **Lithium** raises TSH, in addition to all its other effects on thyroid function. In very rare cases it causes hyperthyroidism. (It causes hypothyroidism much more frequently.)

Looking At the New Drugs

Since the first edition of this book, thousands of drugs have come on the market. The vast majority are drugs that have been around for years and have reached the point that the original drug company that made the drug no longer has the exclusive right to sell it. Any company can manufacture and sell it. Another large group of drugs are the "me-too" drugs. Me-too drugs are slightly different chemically from other drugs with exactly the same action, but because of the slight difference, the food and drug administration permits companies to sell them.

I've looked at most of these "new" drugs for the possibility that they interact with the thyroid and thyroid hormone. Doctors prescribe most of them so rarely that they aren't worth discussing. The new me-too drugs that affect the thyroid belong to classes of drugs that I cover in the previous "Identifying the Effects of Specific Substances" section.

A few new drugs deserve discussion, because doctors prescribe them very often, and they interact with thyroid hormone. Curiously, several of them are drugs used in type 2 diabetes mellitus (see my book *Diabetes For Dummies, 2nd Edition* [Wiley]). The drugs are as follows:

- ✔ **Rosiglitazone** (brand name Avandia), of the class of drugs called glitazones, interacts with thyroid hormone. The thyroid hormone reduces the effect of rosiglitazone. The glitazone drugs increase the activity of insulin in the body. They sensitize the body to insulin.

- ✔ **Pioglitazone** (brand name Actos) belongs to the same class of drugs as roziglitazone and has the same interaction with thyroid hormone.

- ✔ **Miglitol** (brand name Glyset) is affected in the same way as the two preceding drugs by thyroid hormone. Thyroid hormone reduces its effect. It is used to slow the digestion of carbohydrates, thereby reducing the blood glucose. Thyroid hormone interferes with this action.

- ✔ **Repaglinide** (brand name Prandin) also is affected by thyroid hormone, which reduces its effect. Repaglinide lowers glucose by stimulating insulin.

- ✔ **Nateglinide** (brand name Starlix) has the same effect as repaglinide.

Discovering Whether You're at Risk

You may not recognize many of the drugs I name in the previous sections, because I use their generic names. The generic name is the official name of the drug regardless of the name the manufacturer gives it. In this section, I list brand names of drugs that may affect your thyroid, and I group them according to their usage. If you have a specific medical problem that requires one or another of a class of drugs — for example, anemia drugs — go to the section below that refers to your problem, look at the drugs I list, and see whether the brand name is the same as the one you're using.

If one of the drugs I list below is something you take, asking your doctor to run thyroid function tests may be a good idea.

Anemia drugs

Ferrous sulfate: Feosol elixer and tablets, Fero-Folic 500 Filmtab tablets, Fero-Grad 500 Filmtab tablets, Iberet-500 liquid and tablets, Irospan capsules and tablets, Slow Fe tablets, Fe-50 caplets, Vi-Daylin/F multivitamin and iron drops with floride

Antiaddiction agents

Methadone: Dolophine Hydrochloride tablets, Methadone HCl powder, Methadose dispersible tablets, Methadose oral tablets

Antibiotics

Ethionamide: Trecator-SC tablets

Ketoconazole: Nizoral tablets, Ketoconazole tablets

Para-aminosalicylic acid: Paser granules

Sulfonamide drugs: Bactrim tablets, Septra tablets

Rifampin: Rifadin capsules, Rifater

Anti-inflammatory drugs

Glucocorticoids: Celestone, Decadron, Depo-Medrol, Hydrocortone tablets, Solu-medrol sterile powder

Aspirin: Darvon compound, Ecotrin Enteric coated aspirin, Excedrin, Fiorinal Halprin tablets, Norgesic tablets, Percodan tablets, Robaxisal tablets, Soma compound, Fiortal capsules, Gelpirin tablets, Propoxyphene compound, Roxiprin tablets

Antithyroid drugs

Propylthiouricil: Propylthiouricil tablets

Methimazole: Tapazol tablets, Methimazole tablets

Diabetes drugs

Tolbutamide: Orinase

Chlorpropamide: Diabinase

Diuretics (reduce body water)

Furosemide: Lasix, Furosemide tablets

Drugs to improve alertness

Amphetamine: Adderall tablets

Fat-lowering drugs

Clofibrate: Atromid-S capsules

Cholestyramine: LoCholest powder, Questran Light for oral suspension, Prevalite for oral suspension

Colestipol: Colestid tablets

Growth-hormone controlling drugs

Octreotide: Sandostatin

Heart rhythm drugs

Amiodarone: Cardarone tablets, Pacerone tablets

Propranolol: Inderal tablets, Propranolol HCl tablets

Phentolamine: Regitine vials

Hormone replacement

Estrogens (female hormones): Estinyl tablets, Estrace vaginal cream, Estratab tablets, Menest tablets, Ogen tablets, Premarin tablets, Vagifem tablets

Estrogen and progestin combinations: Activella tablets, Brevicon 28-day tablets, Demulen (many strengths), Desogen tablets, Estrostep 21 tablets, Levora tablets, Lo/Ovral tablets, Mircette tablets, Modicon tablets, Necon tablets (many strengths), Norinyl tablets (many strengths), Ortho Tri-Cyclen tablets (many strengths), Ortho-Cyclen tablets (many strengths), Ortho-Novum tablets (many strengths), Ovcon tablets, Premphase tablets, Prempro tablets, Trinorinyl-28 tablets, Triphasil tablets, Trivora tablets, Zovia tablets

Anabolic steroids: Anandrol-50 tablets, Oxandrin tablets, Winstrol tablets

Androgens (male hormones): Androderm transdermal system, AndroGel, Android capsules, Delatestryl injection, Testoderm transdermal systems, Testred capsules

Growth hormone: Geref for injection, Humatrope, Nutropin, Protropin, Saizen for injection

Clomiphene: Clomid tablets, Serophene tablets, Clomiphene Citrate tablets

Thyroid hormones: Synthroid, Levothroid, Levoxyl tablets

Nausea-controlling drugs

Metoclopramide: Reglan, Metoclopramide tablets

Pain medication

Morphine: Astramorph/PF injection, Duramorpf injection, Kadian capsules, MS Contin tablets, MSIR oral capsules, Oramorph SR tablets, Roxanol 100 concentrated oral solution, Morphine Sulfate, OMS concentrate CII, RMS suppositories CII

Peptic ulcer drugs

Aluminum hydroxide: Amphogel, Maalox, Mylanta, Alu-Cap capsules, Alumina and Magnesia oral suspension

Sucralfate: Carafate suspension and tablets, Sucralfate tablets

Cimetidine: Tagamet, Cimetidine tablets

Ranitidine: Zantac, Ranitidine HCl

Prolactin controlling drugs

Bromergocryptine: Parlodel capsules, Bromocryptine Mesylate tablets

Psychoactive drugs

Lithium: Eskalith capsules, Eskalith CR controlled-release tablets, Lithium Carbonate capsules, Lithobid slow-release tablets

Perphenazine: Estrafon 2–10 tablets, Estrafon tablets, Estrafon-Forte tablets, Trilafon tablets, Perphenazine tablets

Chlorpromazine: Thorazine, Chlorpromazine HCl

Haloperidol: Haldol

Chapter 11

Thyroid Infections and Inflammation

. . . .

In This Chapter

▶ Encountering subacute thyroiditis

▶ Dealing with postpartum and silent thyroiditis

▶ Suffering from acute thyroiditis

▶ Finding out about more rare forms of thyroiditis

. . . .

I use the term *thyroiditis* in this book (see Chapter 5) to denote Hashimoto's thyroiditis and chronic thyroiditis. In this chapter, I introduce you to causes of thyroiditis that are less common than autoimmune disorders but just as important to know about. Usually, but not always, non-autoimmune thyroiditis is associated with infection.

Fortunately, infection of the thyroid is rare, perhaps because of all the iodine and hydrogen peroxide in the thyroid gland. If you ever had a cut or boo-boo when you were young, your mother probably covered it with a solution containing iodine or hydrogen peroxide, both of which kill bugs.

Despite all the thyroid's natural protection, every so often people develop an infected thyroid. In this chapter, you discover how doctors tell one form of infection from another, as well as the method of treatment and the prognosis for each illness.

Putting a Face on Subacute Thyroiditis

Subacute thyroiditis has gone by many names in the past, including *de Quervain's thyroiditis, giant cell thyroiditis,* and *subacute painful thyroiditis.* It's called *subacute* to differentiate it from the condition I discuss later in the chapter, *acute* thyroiditis, which is usually much more painful and associated with more symptoms that make the patient sick. Subacute thyroiditis isn't very common. In my practice, which is about 60 percent diabetes mellitus and 40 percent thyroid disease, I see perhaps two cases per year.

Joan Sharp is a 40-year-old woman who has been suffering from a cold and a cough with a low-grade fever for about a week. One morning, she awakens and notices that her neck hurts. She can tell that the pain is located in the center of her neck beneath her Adam's apple. She goes to her doctor, Dr. Hammerbe, who notes that her thyroid is enlarged and tender. The doctor also finds that Joan is nervous, and her fingers are shaking slightly.

Dr. Hammerbe sends Joan to the lab for some tests. The lab results show that her free T4 is elevated, while her TSH is depressed (see Chapter 4), suggesting hyperthyroidism. The doctor does a test for inflammation called an *erythrocyte sedimentation rate,* and the result is elevated. Knowing that neck pain is unusual in hyperthyroidism due to Grave's disease (see Chapter 6), Dr. Hammerbe calls Dr. Rubin about what to do next.

Dr. Rubin suggests that she do a blood test for *serum thyroglobulin,* which comes back high, and a thyroid uptake (see Chapter 4), which comes back low. Joan finds out that she has subacute thyroiditis. Dr. Hammerbe starts her on aspirin, and Joan rapidly improves. The swelling of her neck declines, and the tenderness rapidly decreases.

As you can tell from the case of Joan Sharp, this condition often begins with an infection that suggests a virus. The person may have muscle aches and fever and then begins to feel neck pain in the area of the thyroid. This pain may be severe. The neck pain usually brings the patient to the doctor. When the doctor examines the patient, the thyroid isn't only painful but enlarged as well.

Causes and effects

Subacute thyroiditis has four stages in the more severe cases:

- ✔ **Stage 1** lasts one to three months, during which the thyroid is painful and tender. You experience fever and muscle aches and pains.

  As a result of the inflammation, the thyroid releases much of its stored hormone along with the stored thyroglobulin (see Chapter 4). The virus seems to temporarily damage thyroid cells at this point. The large quantity of released thyroid hormone produces hyperthyroidism. Because the thyroid cells are damaged and the production of thyroid hormone isn't ongoing, the hyperthyroidism lasts only a brief time, sometimes a few days, until the thyroid gland is depleted of hormone.

- ✔ **Stage 2** lasts one to two weeks. You experience a state of normal thyroid function as thyroid hormone levels fall. The acute infection releases thyroid hormone that clears from the body.

- ✔ **Stage 3** can last for months and is the stage of hypothyroidism because the thyroid suffers such severe damage that the gland is depleted of hormone.

✔ **Stage** 4 occurs when you return to a state of normal thyroid function. Because a viral illness usually doesn't last, the thyroid gland returns to normal, the pain goes away, and the thyroid function returns to normal. However, 5 percent of people with subacute thyroiditis remain permanently hypothyroid.

Evidence exists that a virus may cause subacute thyroiditis: Cases of this condition tend to be seasonal, and they sometimes occur in outbreaks like any infectious disease. Over the years, doctors have looked for a particular virus that may be the cause of all cases of subacute thyroiditis, but they've never been able to isolate any one virus in all cases. The only virus doctors have found with some frequency is the mumps virus. Subacute thyroiditis seems to occur more often in people who have decreased immunity from infection, such as AIDS patients or people who are getting bone marrow transplants for leukemia.

Like most thyroid conditions, subacute thyroiditis is more common in women than in men; the ratio of cases is three to one. This condition appears to have some genetic basis, because the same genetic marker — an antigen on human white blood cells — is present in about 75 percent of cases, suggesting that these patients are more susceptible to the disease because of their genetic makeup. In fact, scientists have described two different genetic markers for subacute thyroiditis. Each marker seems to be associated with the disease occurring at a particular time of the year, although in either case subacute thyroiditis generally occurs in a person's forties or fifties.

If you have subacute thyroiditis, you have a small (about 2 percent) but definite possibility of a recurrence some years later. A recurrence is generally milder than the original attack. Occasionally, a patient may experience repeated attacks of pain. Thyroid hormone helps to prevent such recurrences, but if you continue to have recurrences, removing the thyroid with surgery or radioactive iodine becomes necessary.

Laboratory findings

Lab tests are very helpful in pinning down a diagnosis of subacute thyroiditis. Some of the findings from lab tests are as follows:

✔ The *erythrocyte sedimentation rate,* a general blood test for inflammation, is often unusually high considering the relative mildness of the symptoms, sometimes reaching a value of over 100, when the normal is about 20.

✔ Shortly after the thyroid becomes infected, up to 50 percent of patients experience hyperthyroidism, so TSH level are low while FT4 levels are elevated.

✔ The inflammation causes the release of a large quantity of both T4 and T3. Because the thyroid contains so much more T4 than T3 compared to the blood, a drop in the ratio of T4 to T3 occurs as T4 and T3 escape into the bloodstream.

✔ Liver tests often reveal an elevated level of *alkaline phosphatase*. The infection appears to affect the liver in addition to the thyroid, though the impact on the liver is mild.

✔ Blood tests show that a lot of thyroglobulin is present in the blood.

✔ The test for thyroid autoantibodies (see Chapter 4) is negative.

✔ Some specialists suggest that a thyroid ultrasound study (see Chapter 4) is distinctive in subacute thyroiditis, but doctors usually don't run this test.

✔ The key test, the thyroid uptake of radioactive iodine, is very low, which differentiates subacute thyroiditis from other causes of hyperthyroidism.

When your doctor puts the results of all these tests and the clinical picture together, the diagnosis is fairly certain, although no one test proves that subacute thyroiditis is present. To prove the diagnosis, a biopsy of the gland is necessary, but the mildness of the disease means that your doctor rarely needs to do a biopsy.

The presence of generalized thyroid pain differentiates subacute thyroiditis from other forms of thyroiditis, though sometimes the pain may occur on one side of the thyroid only. Another cause of a painful thyroid is bleeding, producing a hemorrhagic thyroid cyst. This pain usually occurs on one side of the thyroid, and a viral illness doesn't precede it. Lab tests help to secure a diagnosis, particularly a radioactive uptake, which is normal for the cystic thyroid but low for subacute thyroiditis. In rare cases, chronic thyroiditis is painful (see Chapter 5). With chronic thyroiditis, levels of thyroid autoantibodies are high.

Treatment options

At the beginning of subacute thyroiditis, when you're hyperthyroid, a drug such as propranolol can reverse the symptoms of excessive thyroid hormone. *Propranolol* is a beta blocker that slows the heart, decreases anxiety, and reduces tremor. Antithyroid drugs like propylthiouricil and methimazole have no place in this treatment, because the thyroid isn't chronically making excessive hormones.

Aspirin or a nonsteroidal anti-inflammatory agent can manage thyroid pain. Once in a while, using a steroid like prednisone is necessary for a week or two. When the uptake of radioactive iodine returns to normal, the inflammation is finished, and you can stop taking steroids.

With the end of symptoms, the patient is back to normal permanently in almost every case. Like so much in medicine, rare exceptions exist where the disease goes away and then returns, or the pain is persistent. Patients who experience persistent pain or a return of the disease may need to have their thyroids removed to finally control the disease.

Coping with Postpartum and Silent Thyroiditis

Michelle Clever is a 29-year-old woman who gave birth to a healthy boy about five months ago. Recently she has noticed that her neck is larger than before, but it's not painful. She is feeling nervous, and her hands shake. She has trouble going to sleep, which makes her situation tough because the baby wakes her up at night. She can feel her heart beating rapidly at times.

Michelle goes to her obstetrician, who examines her and tells her that she is probably hyperthyroid. Her obstetrician sends her to see Dr. Rubin, who notes that she was pregnant recently. He obtains thyroid function tests, which are elevated. Dr. Rubin tells Michelle that he believes she probably has postpartum thyroiditis. He places her on the beta blocker propranolol, which controls her symptoms well. He also explains that she will probably go through a phase of low thyroid function before she returns to normal. A few weeks later she appears to be better.

Several weeks after that, Michelle notices that she is feeling cold and having trouble keeping awake. Dr. Rubin reassures her that this is the hypothyroid phase of postpartum thyroiditis. Within a few weeks, she feels normal. Two years later, after a second pregnancy, the problem recurs.

Doctors consider postpartum and silent thyroiditis to be variations of the same disease. Postpartum thyroiditis occurs usually three to six months after a pregnancy, while silent thyroiditis can happen to anyone at any time.

Understanding the disease

Doctors consider postpartum thyroiditis to be an autoimmune disorder, because high levels of peroxidase autoantibodies are present in the blood (see Chapter 4). In this condition, the antibodies seem to damage thyroid cells, causing a release of thyroid hormone that leads to temporary hyperthyroidism. So far, no one has found a single gene associated with postpartum thyroiditis.

Postpartum thyroiditis is very common; it occurs after 5 to 10 percent of all pregnancies. With this condition, unlike subacute thyroiditis, a patient has no symptoms of fever or weakness, although she may complain of feeling warm. A rapid heartbeat and palpitations are part of the condition. The thyroid itself isn't painful, although it's often abnormally large. However, the changes that occur in thyroid function are similar to those that occur with subacute thyroiditis. Postpartum thyroiditis usually occurs in the following stages:

1. **Hyperthyroidism for the first one to three months after giving birth.**

2. **Normal thyroid function for a month or two.**

3. **Hypothyroidism at four to six months after delivery.**

4. **The hypothyroidism may resolve, but the patient is at high risk for permanent hypothyroidism.**

Women who develop postpartum thyroiditis show a high rate of recurrence in later pregnancies, and 25 percent of them are permanently hypothyroid after three to five years. As many as 50 percent are hypothyroid after seven to nine years. The recurrence rate of silent thyroiditis is also very high.

Doctors used to think that postpartum thyroiditis was associated with depression in women who had given birth. Recent investigation has shown, however, that the depression occurs just as often when women don't have postpartum thyroiditis as when they do.

Interpreting lab results

The lab test that best distinguishes a patient with subacute thyroiditis from a patient with postpartum or silent thyroiditis is the test of *erythrocyte sedimentation rate*. With subacute thyroiditis, the rate is high, but with postpartum or silent thyroiditis, the rate is normal.

Thyroid function tests from patients with postpartum or silent thyroiditis are initially high, then normal, then low. As in subacute thyroiditis, the hyperthyroid phase of the disease is due to leakage from the thyroid. Because the ratio of T4 to T3 is much higher in the thyroid than it is in the blood, the ratio of T4 to T3 temporarily becomes high in the blood as well. The TSH and the radioactive uptake of iodine are also on the low side during the hyperthyroid phase.

If the hyperthyroidism is severe, it may mimic Graves' disease. But the hyperthyroidism is the result of damage to thyroid cells and release of thyroid hormone, so the uptake of radioactive iodine is low rather than high, as it is in Graves' disease.

Getting treatment

Treatment for postpartum and silent thyroiditis depends on the stage at which your doctor diagnoses the disease. If your doctor diagnoses you during the hyperthyroid phase, you take the beta blocker propranolol, which helps to control the symptoms of hyperthyroidism. Antithyroid drugs aren't useful, because they won't prevent hyperthyroidism caused by a leakage of thyroid hormone. When the hypothyroidism phase occurs, you take thyroid-hormone replacement with the understanding that you may not need it on a permanent basis.

Identifying Acute Thyroiditis

Patrick Clever is a 45-year-old man who has suddenly developed severe pain in his neck, fever, and chills. The pain is so severe that he has to bend his neck forward to cope with it. He can't swallow without pain. He also feels weak.

Patrick goes off to see his doctor, who notes that he is very sick. His thyroid gland is exquisitely tender, and he has a fever. The doctor sends him to his thyroid specialist friend, Dr. Rubin, who notes that the tender area is somewhat soft. He puts a fine needle into it and removes a quantity of pus. Dr. Rubin sends the pus for culture and for staining to determine the bug causing the infection and places Patrick on an antibiotic along with aspirin.

In a few days, Patrick is feeling much better. The pus grows out a bug that's sensitive to the antibiotic, which Patrick continues taking for ten days. Patrick recovers fully.

Acute thyroiditis is much rarer than subacute thyroiditis, but doctors can confuse the two, depending on the way the disease appears in the patient. In my 33 years in practice, I've seen only four cases of acute thyroiditis. However, because many more people have lost their immunity to infection as a result of the AIDS epidemic, doctors will probably see more cases in the near future.

Describing the disease

Doctors have found many different organisms in the thyroid glands of patients with acute thyroiditis. Bacteria are present about 70 percent of the time. The type of bacteria varies from *pneumococcus* (which often causes pneumonia) to *streptococcus* (associated with strep throat) to *staphylococcus* (which causes skin infections). About 15 percent of the time, a fungus is the infecting organism; tuberculosis is the cause 10 percent of the time, and various other bugs are the culprits much less frequently.

Besides the tender thyroid, nearby structures such as the trachea (voice box) and esophagus (swallowing tube) are inflamed, and local lymph glands in the neck are tender. In many patients, doctors find a connection from the outside (such as the throat) to the thyroid tissue, through which the infection invades. This connection is called a *fistula* and is a result of abnormal development from birth. It acts as an open pipe to the thyroid for the passage of the infection. If a doctor discovers a fistula in association with acute thyroiditis, a surgeon must remove it, or infection will recur. Acute infection of the thyroid is so rare that doctors should look for a fistula in every case.

If you have acute thyroiditis, you look obviously sick. You complain of the pain in your neck and may have to bend your neck forward to decrease it. You have a fever and chills. Your thyroid is enlarged (usually on one side), hot, and tender. Depending on how large your thyroid gets, you may have trouble swallowing or even breathing. Lymph nodes are often enlarged, swollen, and tender as well.

Confirming the diagnosis with lab tests

In a patient with acute thyroiditis, general blood tests for infection, such as the white blood count and the erythrocyte sedimentation rate, are abnormally high. These results confirm that an infection or inflammation is present.

When your doctor does thyroid tests such as the free T4 and the TSH, the results are generally normal, although once in a while the destruction of the thyroid is so great that enough hormone leaks to cause hyperthyroidism. Thyroid uptake of radioactive iodine is normal. Thyroid autoantibodies are negative.

The best test for acute thyroiditis is a needle biopsy. Usually the biopsy shows inflammation and the infecting organism, but occasionally no inflammation appears. Then the diagnosis is much more difficult. Sometimes the thyroid has an abscess, which the needle drains.

Treating acute thyroiditis

The treatment for acute thyroiditis is to give the appropriate antibiotic based on the suspected organism. The biopsy can provide a good idea of what type of organism is causing the infection, which a culture of the biopsy tissue can confirm. The right antibiotic generally cures the infection and restores normal thyroid function. Sometimes the infection doesn't respond, and surgery to remove the infected part of the thyroid or the whole thyroid is necessary.

When acute thyroiditis recurs, a doctor should suspect that a fistula is allowing bugs to get into the thyroid from the outside. In this situation, the patient does a barium swallow, which shows a trail of barium going from the throat into the thyroid gland. Surgery is necessary to eliminate a fistula.

Occasionally, acute thyroiditis causes such damage to the thyroid tissue that the patient needs to take replacement thyroid hormone.

A Rare Form of Thyroiditis

Christopher Dull is a 42-year-old man who comes to his doctor complaining of gaining weight and feeling tired, weak, cold, and sleepy. He also says that his neck feels very tight. He has trouble swallowing and breathing.

His doctor examines him and notes that his neck feels very dense. His thyroid barely moves when he swallows. The doctor doesn't feel swelling in the lymph nodes in his neck.

The doctor runs thyroid function tests, which show a low free T4 and a high TSH. At the same time, he obtains a calcium level, and this test result is low as well. The doctor runs a test of the hormone made by the parathyroid glands, called *parathyroid hormone,* and the result of the test is low. The doctor sends Chris for a barium swallow, which shows compression on the esophagus. He refers Chris to Dr. Rubin.

Dr. Rubin attempts to do a fine needle biopsy of Chris's thyroid but is unable to get tissue. Dr. Rubin makes a presumptive diagnosis of *Riedel's thyroiditis.* He starts Chris on steroids, thyroid hormone, and calcium. Chris's symptoms gradually decrease, but the hypothyroidism and the *hypoparathyroidism* (low parathyroid function resulting in low calcium) remain. Chris continues to take thyroid hormone replacement and vitamin D for the rest of his life.

To be thorough, I feel that I need to discuss this final form of thyroiditis even though I've seen only one case in my career. The disease is called Riedel's thyroiditis. The cause isn't known. Reidel's thyroiditis is associated with elevated levels of antithyroid autoantibodies, so autoimmunity probably plays some role, especially in view of the good response of people with the disease to steroids. Some specialists believe that Riedel's thyroiditis is a variant of chronic autoimmune thyroiditis (see Chapter 5). Both conditions are associated with autoantibodies, and both can coexist with other autoimmune diseases in the same person.

Some say Riedel's thyroiditis is twice as frequent in men as in women, but so few cases are recorded that it's hard to tell. It tends to occur between ages 30 and 60.

In Riedel's thyroiditis, the thyroid experiences a *fibrosis* — the replacement of thyroid tissue by hard fibers that can be so dense that the patient loses thyroid function and becomes hypothyroid. The fibrous tissue firmly attaches the thyroid to the trachea and the nearby muscles so that it doesn't move in the neck. A small needle can't penetrate the fibrous thyroid.

If the fibrosis continues, it involves the parathyroid glands, which sit behind the thyroid. The fibrosis can destroy them, and the patient develops hypoparathyroidism. Because the parathyroid glands are important for maintaining calcium levels, the result of this disease is a fall in calcium. Symptoms of tingling and numbness in the hands and feet and tingling around the mouth begin to occur. As the calcium falls, it can result in severe muscle spasms.

Sometimes the fibrosis stops, and the patient remains stable. Other times it continues, and the patient has trouble breathing, swallowing, and even talking. The fibrosis can extend into the chest, the eyes, the gall bladder, and other parts of the body.

When the doctor does thyroid function tests early in the disease, they may be normal. Later the patient becomes hypothyroid. The erythrocyte sedimentation rate is normal as well.

Because the fibrosis can be so invasive, people sometimes confuse Reidel's thyroiditis with anaplastic carcinoma, an extremely rapidly growing, invasive form of thyroid cancer that's usually fatal (see Chapter 8). A biopsy generally shows the difference. Sometimes doctors don't recognize the condition until the patient is in the operating room about to have surgery for what doctors think to be cancer.

If severe neck symptoms occur, surgery may be necessary to free the tissues. Sometimes so much fibrosis is present that surgery isn't successful in removing the tissue. A trial of steroids often slows or stops progression of the disease. The other agent that has shown some success is the drug tamoxifen.

Chapter 12

Iodine Deficiency and Excess Disease

*I*n the movie *Love and Death,* Woody Allen describes a convention of village idiots in Russia. If such a convention actually occurred, sadly, most of the people in attendance would probably be suffering from iodine deficiency disease.

This chapter gives you a greater appreciation of the major role of thyroid hormone in the growth and development of the human body, particularly mental development. As you discover in this chapter, iodine deficiency disease is the world's most common and preventable cause of mental retardation. What stops its elimination is more often politics than medicine. The situation is very similar to the problem of infectious diseases that immunization can prevent. Doctors clearly understand the science of the condition, including the treatment. Only the means to transfer that knowledge into action is missing.

A case in point is the story of the former East Germany. Prior to 1980, 50 percent of East German adolescents developed goiters. In 1980, the country began a program of adding minute amounts of iodine to common table salt, and the percentage of adolescents with goiters dropped to less than 1 percent. With the reunification of Germany, iodization became voluntary, and the goiter rate began to rise again.

When you finish this chapter, you won't have any chance of getting invited to that convention in Russia.

Consuming Iodine in the U.S., Canada, and the U.K.

The recommended intake of iodine daily is 150 to 200 micrograms. One teaspoon of salt contains about 400 micrograms of iodine, and a slice of bread contains about 150 micrograms of iodine. A recent study in *Thyroid* in July 2005 shows that the intake of iodine by the American population has stabilized at an acceptable level. In other words, most folks in the United States get a daily amount of iodine that is sufficient for the needs of the thyroid. But this hasn't always been the case — even in the recent past.

In Canada, all table salt is iodized, so there's no problem with deficiency. In fact, Canada has been a leading advocate for iodinization of salt throughout the world. In the U.K., there's no policy of iodizing table salt, and the soil contains little salt, but people in the U.K. get their iodine from cow's milk. The cows are fed iodine-enriched feed. There's no deficiency of iodine in the U.K. either.

With iodized salt and the addition of iodine to bread, there were no recognized cases of hypothyroidism due to lack of iodine in the U.S. for some time. In the 1970s and 1980s, in fact, doctors were concerned more about the overuse of iodine than the underuse. A study by the Michigan State Department of Health provided dramatic evidence of the benefit of the iodization of salt. The study indicated that in 1924, 39 percent of all children in several counties in Michigan were found to have a *goiter,* an enlarged thyroid. After salt was iodized, the numbers dropped to 10 percent by 1928 and 0.5 percent by 1951.

But a study in the *Journal of Clinical Endocrinology and Metabolism* in October 1998 showed that the urinary excretion of iodine, a well-established method for monitoring sufficient iodine intake, had fallen by half compared to earlier times in the United States. Twelve percent of Americans had low iodine concentration in their urine compared to 1974, when the percentage was less than 1. Europe has also seen an increase in cases of iodine deficiency that has resulted in adding more iodine to table salt and monitoring more carefully the population's iodine intake. The problem in Europe is now improving as well. The major reasons for the decline seem to be a reduction in the addition of iodine to salt as well as a reduction of amounts of iodine in bread.

Vegetarians are at risk if they eat vegetables grown in soil that has little iodine, which is the case in the U.K. They must be sure to use salt that has been iodized or eat iodine-rich seaweed. (Check out Chapter 20 for more information.)

Realizing the Vastness of the Problem

More than one-quarter of the world's population, or 1.6 billion people, suffer from some level of iodine deficiency disease. Of these people, 655 million have a goiter, an enlargement of the thyroid that can sometimes be debilitating. Twenty-six million people have brain damage, and 11 million of those 26 million are *cretins,* individuals so handicapped by their thyroid conditions that they're completely dependent on those around them to live. Some researchers believe that for each day we delay treating this vast problem, 50,000 infants are born with decreased mental capacity caused by an iodine deficiency.

The numbers of people affected with iodine deficiency are even more startling when you look at certain areas of the globe. For example, 99 percent of the people of Eastern Europe and Southeast Asia are iodine deficient, while 98 percent of the people of China and the Far East and 91 percent of the people of the Americas are iodine sufficient. (For more details on how many people iodine deficiency disease affects on each continent, go to the Web page of the International Council for the Control of Iodine Deficiency Disorders at http://indorgs.virginia.edu/iccidd.)

The reason so many people suffer from iodine deficiency is that the food they eat or the ground their food comes from contains little or no iodine. Chapter 2 explains that iodine is necessary to form *thyroxine* (T4) and *triiodothyronine* (T3), the two major thyroid hormones. Table 11-1 shows the usual sources of iodine in our diet.

Table 11-1	Where Our Iodine Comes From
Dietary Iodine	*Daily Intake in Micrograms*
Dairy products	52
Grains	78
Meat	31
Vegetables	20
Eggs	10
Iodized salt	380

All soil on earth used to contain iodine. However, over hundreds of thousands of years, the iodine has been leached out of the soil in two major areas of the earth: the high mountains and the plains. Far from oceans, water covered the plains in the past. Glaciers once covered the high mountains. As the glaciers melted, they carried iodine out of the soil, back to the ocean. In the same way, the flooded plains leached iodine from the soil and carried it back to the ocean as the water flowed away. As a result, high mountains and plains far from oceans are the areas where iodine deficiency disease occurs most often.

Crops that grow in soil low in iodine are iodine deficient. Animals that feed on crops grown in soil low in iodine become iodine deficient. If cows that provide milk feed on these crops, children who drink their milk may be iodine deficient. The meat from those cows is also iodine deficient. The result is a huge public health problem. Even pets such as dogs become iodine deficient.

If you look at a map of the world that shows the areas where iodine deficiency disease is most prevalent, you see that vast areas of China, Russia, Mexico, South America, and Africa are rife with the disease. Surprisingly, the United States isn't spared. At one time, the iodization of salt and the addition of iodine to bread seemed to solve the problem in the U.S. More recently, as a study in the *Journal of Clinical Endocrinology and Metabolism* in October 1998 shows, Americans have decreased their iodine intake. Nearly 12 percent of Americans studied had insufficient iodine in their urine. (The urine test is a reliable measurement of daily iodine intake.) This percentage compares with only 3 percent of people with insufficient iodine intake 20 years earlier.

Food manufacturers added iodine to salt and bread not for health reasons but because they needed it in the production process. As other substances have replaced iodine in the production process, the daily iodine intake of Americans has fallen. Although I advocate taking iodine in iodized salt in this book, I recommend limiting your salt intake to lower blood pressure in my book *High Blood Pressure For Dummies* (Wiley). Reduction in salt intake has become standard practice in the last few decades to combat the growing prevalence of high blood pressure and is another reason for the fall in total iodine in our diets.

Measuring iodine deficiency

In order to determine whether iodine deficiency is present in large populations, developing simple tools to measure a lack of iodine became necessary. One simple technique is a measurement of iodine in the urine. In areas where iodine isn't deficient, the iodine in the urine is 100 micrograms per day or more.

If a country or population undertakes an iodization program, the population takes a urine test before it receives iodine and at intervals afterward to see whether the program is working. (If it is, a much higher level of iodine appears in the urine after iodization begins.)

The second important measure of iodine deficiency is the frequency of goiters. A goiter is present if the lobes of the thyroid are larger than the end parts, or *terminal phalanges,* of the thumbs. Unfortunately, such a measurement of the thyroid is very hard to make in practice, especially in small children, where a measurement is most important. To overcome this difficulty, doctors use a portable ultrasound device (see Chapter 4), which produces a measurement that's highly accurate and reproducible.

Finally, measurement of thyroid hormones and TSH in the blood can evaluate the production of thyroid hormones.

Western Europe also used to be virtually free from iodine deficiency, but recent studies among Europeans have shown decreases in iodine intake as well.

Facing the Consequences of Iodine Lack

If your body lacks iodine, it can't produce sufficient thyroid hormone. Iodine deficiency has severe consequences at every stage of life. This section discusses the price your body pays in bad health and abnormal function at every stage of life, beginning with the pregnant woman and her fetus.

Doctors divide iodine deficiency into four categories: *none* when iodine intake is greater than 150 micrograms (ug) per day, *mild* between 75 to 149 ug per day, *moderate* between 30 to 74 ug per day, and *severe* when less than 30 ug per day. The occurrence of goiters in a population increases as the intake falls, from less than 5 percent of the population with goiters when no deficiency exists to greater than 30 percent when iodine is severely reduced.

From pregnancy to adulthood

The entire body's formation is dependent on adequate T4. If sufficient hormone isn't available, congenital anomalies may occur. The infant may not survive much past birth. If it does, it may not live more than a few years.

As you can see in the following sections, the costs of iodine deficiency disorder are enormous both for the individual and for society. A village filled with people like those I describe here wouldn't be able to govern itself, provide an economic base to help better the condition of the people, or take the steps necessary to overcome the problem, including using iodine.

Pregnancy

Thyroid hormone, T4, has iodine in its basic structure. Even before pregnancy, a lack of T4 hormone has a harmful effect. Women who are hypothyroid have greater difficulties becoming pregnant, and they have more miscarriages and stillbirths than women with normal thyroid function. The recommendation for iodine intake for pregnant women is 200 ug per day.

A fetus doesn't begin to make thyroid hormone until the 24th week of pregnancy. Until then, it's dependent on the mother's T4. During this time, the fetal brain is developing, and the entire chain of events that produces a normal brain requires T4 at every stage. If this hormone is lacking, the consequences are severe.

If a fetus is deficient in T4, its brain triggers an increase in the amount of the enzyme that converts T4 to T3 within the brain. This form of the enzyme isn't in other tissues, so the brain may experience protection from hypothyroidism while the rest of the body doesn't.

In this nuclear age, realizing that a thyroid gland that isn't making enough thyroid hormone will take up large amounts of iodine from whatever source it can is important. In a nuclear accident where radioactive iodine is released, a hypothyroid mother concentrates the iodine and passes it on to her growing fetus. If radioactive iodine doesn't completely destroy the fetal thyroid, that thyroid will at least be very prone to developing thyroid cancer.

Infancy

A new baby deprived of iodine will have a goiter and show signs of hypothyroidism. Depending on the severity of the lack, the baby may be a cretin, which I explain later in this chapter in "Defining the problem: Endemic cretinism." The brain of a newborn continues to develop up to age 2, so providing iodine starting immediately after birth may prevent retardation. A baby lacking in iodine also shows increased susceptibility to radioactive iodine (or any iodine). Infants should take at least 110 ug of iodine up to six months of age and 130 ug from 7 to 12 months of age per day.

Childhood

Iodine-deficient children often have goiters. They show reduced intelligence and poor motor function, and they may be deaf. Like infants, these children have a tendency to accumulate iodine from any source and are at greater risk in the case of a nuclear accident. Children should consume 90 to 120 ug of iodine daily.

Adulthood

After the iodine-deficient child grows up, a goiter is often present in an iodine-deficient adult, though not always. He or she is intellectually retarded and may have movement difficulties. This person's thyroid gland is highly susceptible to radioactivity. Adults should eat at least 100 to150 ug of iodine every day.

Changes brought on by iodine deficiency

Your body goes through a series of changes as your iodine level falls:

1. **Your serum T4 level falls.**

2. **Your pituitary releases more thyroid-stimulating hormone (TSH).**

3. **TSH causes the thyroid to enlarge.**

4. **The production of T3 increases within the thyroid relative to T4, because T3 is 100 times more biologically active than T4 and requires only three iodine atoms rather than four.**

5. **Your body produces a goiter that's smooth at first but nodular later.**

6. **You become hypothyroid.**

Defining the problem: Endemic cretinism

Shabmir is a 46-year-old woman living in Pakistan. Since she can remember, she has had a huge growth on the front of her neck that the doctors tell her is a goiter. She isn't alone, because more than 70 percent of the villagers around her suffer from the same condition.

Shabmir attended the local school but seems to have no aptitude for learning. Because of the unsightly growth on her neck, she has been discriminated against by those who don't have the same problem (perhaps because they come from an area with sufficient iodine in the food). The goiter is so large that she has difficulty moving her head and neck, which makes it hard for her to earn a living. She didn't marry until she found another person who had a severe goiter.

For years, Shabmir was unable to become pregnant. When she did, the baby was stillborn. She hasn't been pregnant again.

She appears swollen and lethargic. She has very little interest in her neighbors or her surroundings, and she tends to sleep a lot.

Shabmir's story is typical of the way that iodine deficiency disease affects the lives of millions of people. It's a worldwide plague that can render whole populations unable to function. The shame is that this condition is completely preventable!

In this section, I show you the different ways that iodine deficiency disease appears in people. The manifestations of iodine deficiency disease that I describe here are far worse than the hypothyroidism commonly found in the United States (see Chapter 5), because the hypothyroidism in iodine deficiency states begins when babies are conceived. Their mothers were already hypothyroid. Unless and until providing sufficient iodine breaks the chain of iodine deficiency, the disease will continue to disrupt the lives of a quarter of the world's population.

Endemic cretinism is the term used to describe the group of signs and symptoms in severe iodine deficiency disease. The Pan American Health Organization has defined endemic cretinism. It consists of several features:

✔ **An association with endemic goiter and severe iodine deficiency.**
Endemic goiter means that more than 5 percent of children in a population age 6 to 12 have enlarged thyroid glands.

✔ **Mental deficiency.** Patients also show one of the following:

- **Nervous cretinism:** Predominantly nervous system symptoms (like defects of hearing and speech) as well as defects when they stand and walk

- **Myxedematous cretinism:** Symptoms of hypothyroidism and stunted growth

Where iodine has been adequately replaced, cretinism doesn't occur.

Figure 12-1 shows a typical goiter on a person living in an area of endemic cretinism.

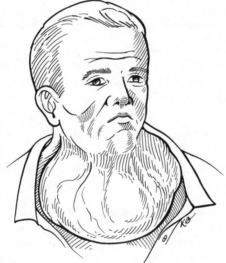

Figure 12-1:
A typical goiter for a person living in an area of endemic cretinism.

Goiter: The body's defense

The thyroid and the rest of the body do what they can to prevent hypothyroidism. The body's first response is a fall in the production of T4. When this drop occurs, the pituitary gland doesn't sense sufficient T3 in the brain, and it responds by secreting more TSH (see Chapter 2). The thyroid reacts by getting larger, thus forming a goiter, and by making more of the active hormone T3 (relative to the amount of T4). At the same time, the body converts more T4 into T3 away from the thyroid.

If a person's intake of iodine is severely limited, T3 production starts to fall. The consequence is severe hypothyroidism, which is particularly damaging in the brain.

Neurologic cretinism

Scientists believe that neurologic cretinism results from a lack of thyroid hormone from the mother during the third to the sixth month of pregnancy. The severe iodine lack means that the growing fetus is unable to contribute thyroid hormone either. During this time period, the brain should be achieving the ability to hear as well as perform important motor functions, so neurologic cretinism affects hearing and motor abilities most.

Neurologic cretinism has three major characteristics:

✔ Mental deficiency or retardation, although memory and social functions are unaffected.

✔ Deafness and often loss of speech.

✔ Stiffness of the arms and legs and an increase in the reflexes (both sets of symptoms opposite to those in hypothyroidism). The result is that a person with neurologic cretinism has a shuffling gait or may not be able to walk at all.

Neurologic cretins may not be hypothyroid later in life. If they receive sufficient iodine, they can have a thyroid that makes sufficient thyroid hormone. But the damage done by the lack of thyroid hormone during development of the brain is irreversible.

Myxedematous cretinism

People with myxedematous cretinism aren't as mentally retarded as those with neurologic cretinism. They don't tend to be deaf or mute as a result of their cretinism. Instead, they demonstrate the signs and symptoms of severe hypothyroidism from birth, including the following:

✔ Very dry, scaly, and thickened skin

✔ Retarded growth

✔ Thin hair, eyelashes, and eyebrows

✔ Puffy features

✔ Delayed sexual maturation

People with myxedematous cretinism don't have enlarged thyroids, but scar tissue often replaces their thyroids. As a result, their uptake of radioactive iodine is reduced despite having very high TSH levels. The levels of T4 and T3 hormones are very low. Many individuals have a combination of neurologic and myxedematous cretinism.

Just why such a difference exists between neurologic and myxedematous cretinism isn't clear. The difference may have to do with social forces in various cultures. In the Andes, where neurologic cretins are more widely present, a tradition of taking extraordinary care of these very handicapped individuals endures. This tradition of caring may not be present in places where neurologic cretins are more sparse; in these places, they haven't received the kind of care required and therefore have died. Or the environments of some areas may be too severe for neurologic cretins to survive in.

A study done by Dr. Stephen Boyages and published in the *Journal of Clinical Endocrinology and Metabolism* in 1988 sheds some light on this subject. Dr. Boyages studied a group of cretins in Qinghai Province in China and found both neurological and myxedematous cretins along with a mixed group. The length of time that they were hypothyroid after birth explained the difference between the types of cretins, the myxedematous cretins having suffered for a longer time than the neurologic cretins. The neurologic cretins, after suffering mental retardation from a lack of thyroid hormone during brain development, experienced normal thyroid function after birth by getting enough iodine for the production of normal amounts of thyroid hormone. Myxedematous cretins had thyroid destruction, while neurologic cretins had normal thyroid function. The conclusion of the researchers was that myxedematous and neurologic cretinism are actually the same disorder, only modified by the amount of hypothyroidism after birth.

Looking at the geographic distribution

Endemic cretinism is present in the mountainous regions of the world, as I explain earlier in the chapter. It's most common in the Andes and the Himalayas. It was present in the Alps until iodine replacement began several decades ago, but areas in the Alps still exist where people don't get sufficient iodine. It's present in mountainous regions of China, the Pacific, and the Middle East, as well as in lowlands away from the ocean where heavy rains wash iodine out of the soil. It's present in central Africa, in central Brazil, and even in Holland.

- ✔ **Africa:** In Africa, endemic cretinism is present in Cameroon, the Central African Republic, Nigeria, Uganda, Rwanda, the Sudan, Tanzania, Zaire, and Zimbabwe.

- ✔ **Australia:** Australia has iodine deficiency in its mountainous regions, especially Tasmania.

- ✔ **Europe:** Iodine deficiency disease remains a significant problem in numerous countries, including Austria, Belgium, Bulgaria, the Commonwealth of Independent States (including Russia), Croatia, Germany, Greece, Holland, Hungary, Ireland, Portugal, Romania, Spain, and Turkey.

✔ **Latin and South America:** In Latin and South America, large populations lack iodine in Bolivia, Brazil, Chile, Ecuador, Mexico, Peru, and Venezuela — mostly in the Andes Mountains and the mountains of Mexico.

✔ **South Asia:** In South Asia, iodine deficiency disease is common in Bangladesh, India, Nepal, Tibet, and Pakistan.

✔ **Southeast Asia:** In Southeast Asia, large populations of people with goiters exist in Myanmar, Vietnam, Thailand, and New Guinea.

Contributing factors

Lack of iodine is, without a doubt, the main factor in endemic cretinism, but other issues definitely play a role in different areas of the world.

Dietary factors

Dietary factors other than iodine consumption are a major aspect of iodine deficiency disease. A number of foods contribute to the problem:

✔ **Cassava:** In some areas of iodine deficiency disease, the normal diet includes substances that are harmful to the thyroid. In Africa, for example, cassava is a major part of the diet. Cassava contains cyanide, which you can destroy only by properly preparing the food. If not, the cyanide converts to thiocyanate in the body. Thiocyanate competes with iodine for uptake by the thyroid, thus decreasing even further the tiny amount of iodine that gets into the thyroid. (If someone consumes sufficient iodine, it overcomes any block from thiocyanate.)

✔ **Soybeans:** Soybeans also interfere with thyroid function, preventing the production of thyroid hormone in the thyroid gland (see Chapter 10). Again, sufficient iodine can overcome the block and permit normal production of thyroid hormone, but when iodine is scarce, the extra loss of thyroid hormone can make a huge difference.

✔ **Broccoli and cauliflower:** A third group of foods that may contribute to endemic cretinism is the Brassica group of vegetables, which includes foods such as broccoli and cauliflower. Hypothyroidism is more common in areas where these vegetables make up a large part of the diet and the diet is deficient in iodine.

✔ **Others:** Other foods that impair thyroid hormone production and are significant sources of food calories in certain areas of the world are bamboo shoots, sweet potatoes, corn, and lima beans.

Lack of selenium

Another important contributing factor in the development of iodine deficiency disease is the absence of selenium in the diet in certain areas, especially in China, Siberia, Korea, Tibet, and central Africa — places where iodine deficiency is already present. *Selenium* is a mineral that the body needs in order to create the enzyme that turns T4 into the more potent T3.

Selenium may play a role in reducing the number of goiters associated with iodine deficiency. The enzyme in the thyroid that selenium helps to produce also has the function of disposing of hydrogen peroxide, a side product of thyroid hormone production. A buildup of hydrogen peroxide may destroy thyroid cells, leading to a small thyroid. But the small thyroid is still not healthy, despite the lack of a goiter.

When both selenium and iodine are absent from the diet, a disease called *Kashin–Beck disease* develops. This disease can lead to short stature as a result of the destruction of the growth plates of bones, the *cartilage.* The damage is different than that in the short stature associated with myxedematous cretinism, which I describe later in the chapter. Scientists previously thought that Kashin–Beck disease resulted from selenium deficiency alone, but the combination of deficiencies makes the disease even worse.

Managing the Problem of Iodine Deficiency

You may think that managing the problem of iodine deficiency disease — preventing all goiters, cretinism, thyroid-related retardation, and hypothyroidism — should be easy. The trick is just to get everyone to eat a sufficient amount of iodine. The daily requirement is less than a pinhead of iodine. An individual requires only a teaspoon of iodine over a lifetime. But consuming enough iodine is much easier said than done. And sufficient iodine consumption must occur prior to the conception of a baby to prevent cretinism.

A sprinkle of salt

As far as food sources of iodine, the highest content is present in fish and, to a lesser extent, milk, eggs, and meat. Fruits and vegetables contain very little iodine. Using iodine-rich foods to solve the problem isn't likely to be globally successful, though, because diets and tastes differ throughout the world, and the logistics of transporting sufficient daily amounts of fish, milk, eggs, or meat to everyone in the world are overwhelming.

Because virtually every culture in the world uses salt, which is cheap and simple to iodize, iodized salt has been the standard way of overcoming the problem of iodine deficiency disease. The amount of salt needed to carry the daily requirement of 200 to 300 micrograms of iodine is very small and easily consumed.

In many countries, salt iodization has worked well, but some of its success has been less than glowing. Numerous international meetings have set goals and dates to eliminate iodine deficiency by. Charitable organizations, particularly the Kiwanis Clubs, have made the elimination of iodine deficiency disease a major goal. Some areas have achieved the goal of elimination of iodine deficiency, but in many other areas, the problem continues to exist.

One major organization, the International Council for the Control of Iodine Deficiency Disorders (ICCIDD), serves as the central organization for coordination of these efforts. This organization has created the *global iodized salt logo,* which appears on packages of salt that have been properly iodized (see Figure 12-2).

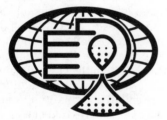

Figure 12-2: The global iodized salt logo.

The history of efforts to overcome iodine deficiency disease in Bangladesh serves as an excellent illustration of the problems of eliminating iodine deficiency disease. The UNICEF statistical summary for Bangladesh says that only 55 percent of households consume iodized salt, despite international efforts to rid the nation of iodine deficiency.

Bangladesh is subject to annual flooding with monsoon rains that have effectively washed all iodine out of the soil. The iodine has washed into the Bay of Bengal, which means that the fish caught there contain plenty of iodine. However, most of the population of the country lives in rural areas far from the supply of iodine. More than 50 million people in Bangladesh have goiters.

The Law of Iodination in Bangladesh has made it illegal since 1984 to sell salt in Bangladesh without iodizing it. However, no penalties were established until 1992. The cost of iodized salt in Bangladesh is 25 cents per kilogram, and noniodized salt is 14 cents per kilogram. The poorest families buy the cheaper salt.

The cost of iodizing salt is only 5 cents per person per year. Iodization is a simple process that can take place in a salt factory. But tests of iodine in salt show that as many as half the factories in Bangladesh are producing salt with insufficient iodine. In a country with a population the size of Bangladesh, this represents inadequate iodine intake for millions of people.

Some of the so-called iodized salt isn't iodized at all in Bangladesh so that the provider can make an extra profit. Bangladesh sometimes imports salt from other countries, which is mislabeled as iodized and sells for a cheaper price than Bangladesh iodized salt. The country borders on Myanmar (formerly Burma) and India, which don't enforce iodization as strictly as Bangladesh. So smuggling contributes to iodine deficiency disease in Bangladesh as well.

One step in the right direction is the development of a simple kit by UNICEF that can detect whether salt contains iodine. A drop of liquid solution added to salt turns the salt blue if iodine is present. UNICEF distributes these kits to school children, who test their salt at home.

Another example of a successful iodization program is the situation in Tasmania, Australia. A paper in the *Journal of Clinical Endocrinology and Metabolism* described the situation in June 2002. The authors tell us that before 1950 a great deal of goiter in Tasmania led to the detection of iodine deficiency. At that time, children began to receive potassium iodide pills; iodine was also added to bread and was present in a disinfectant used for cattle. The problem seemed to disappear, but then the government stepped in and established an upper limit of iodine in milk, while the addition of iodine to bread ceased. As a result, many children in this study were in the moderate group of iodine deficient people and had thyroid enlargement. The children of Tasmania are again getting supplements to insure that they have sufficient iodine in their diets.

You can see that a successful iodization program involves much more than passing a law and setting up salt iodization programs in salt factories. A mountain of barriers can block such a simple solution.

An injection of oil

A highly effective way of managing iodine deficiency disorder is to inject iodized oil, called *lipiodol,* into the muscle of iodine deficient people. A single injection provides enough iodine to last four years or longer. People can also take lipiodol by mouth, although it lasts only a little more than a year when consumed orally. Iodine given through lipiodol has resulted in significant shrinkage of goiters in just a few months. However, giving iodine injections also has its problems.

Iodine deficiency is present in rural areas, where giving sterile injections isn't always possible. Qualified people aren't always available to give the injections. Sufficient supplies of sterile needles and the iodized oil must be available. Also, in this age of AIDS, many people are reluctant to accept an injection. The oral form of lipiodol, of course, solves all these problems.

A slice of bread or cup of water

Other ways of managing iodine deficiency that have proven effective in some areas include the iodization of bread and the addition of iodine to the water supply. The problem with the iodization of bread is that bread consumption varies widely, and so this method works only in limited areas. Adding iodine to water doesn't work in areas with no public water supply, as is the case in most areas of the world where iodine deficiency disease is most prevalent.

Delineating the Drawbacks of Iodization

One major problem of iodization programs is the occurrence of hyperthyroidism when a person whose thyroid is under hyperstimulation with TSH receives a lot of iodine. Hyperthyroidism happens with iodine injections and even with iodized salt that contains excessive iodine. The tools for managing hyperthyroidism (see Chapter 6) in a rural environment may not be readily available, especially if a large number of cases exist. This is another issue that is most important in the less developed nations of the world.

People commonly take a number of drugs that provide iodine in fairly large amounts. Among the most important are the following:

- ✔ Amiodarone with 75 mg of iodine per tablet
- ✔ Calcium iodide with 26 mg of iodine per milliliter (ml)
- ✔ Iodine-containing vitamins with .15 mg per tablet
- ✔ Kelp with .15 mg per tablet
- ✔ Lugol's solution containing 6.3 mg per drop
- ✔ Supersaturated potassium iodide solution with 38 mg per drop
- ✔ Tincture of iodine with 40 mg/ml
- ✔ Radiology contrast agents
  - Telepaque with 333 mg per tablet
  - Ipodate with 308 mg per capsule
  - Visipaque with up to 320 mg/ml
- ✔ Vioform with 12 mg/gram

The preceding drugs and other sources of high levels of iodine can cause either hypothyroidism or hyperthyroidism, depending on the clinical state of the patient. Patients who become hypothyroid may have no underlying disease. Hypothyroidism occurs in newborns, infants, and adults who take large amounts of iodine, which blocks production of thyroid hormone.

A group of people with some thyroid condition already present develop hypothyroidism when they take iodine in large amounts. Some of the patients in this category include the following:

✔ Patients with chronic thyroiditis (see Chapter 5)

✔ Patients with controlled Graves' disease (see Chapter 6)

✔ Patients with subclinical hypothyroidism (see Chapter 5)

✔ Patients with subacute thyroiditis (see Chapter 11)

✔ Patients on lithium

On the other side are patients who become hyperthyroid as a result of too much iodine. The people in this category include the following:

✔ Patients with nontoxic nodular goiter (see Chapter 9)

✔ Patients with one nodule that's autonomous, or not under the control of TSH

✔ Patients with nontoxic diffuse goiter, a large thyroid with normal function

✔ Patients without any thyroid disorder who live where mild iodine sufficiency exists

Chapter 13

Surgery of the Thyroid

· ·

In This Chapter

▶ Determining whether you need surgery

▶ Picking the surgeon

▶ Preparing for surgery

▶ Understanding the procedure

▶ Managing after surgery

· ·

*I*f you need to have a thyroid operation, the good news is that the thyroid is in a very convenient location — a few millimeters under the skin of the neck — so surgeons easily find it. Except in rare circumstances in which the gland is matted down and can't be freed up, thyroid surgery isn't difficult in the hands of a skilled surgeon. Complications are few and infrequent, and the result is usually very satisfactory. If you're about to have surgery, you need to know a few things to make the experience as benign as possible. Revealing those things is the purpose of this chapter. You probably won't be able to perform thyroid surgery after reading it, but you will have a good idea of what to expect so that you won't get any surprises.

Deciding If Surgery Is Necessary

Orlo Blunt is a 45-year-old man who has a solitary thyroid nodule — a lump on the thyroid. His doctor performs a fine needle biopsy, which shows a *follicular lesion,* tissue that looks like normal thyroid follicles (the circles of cells that make thyroid hormone). The pathologist is uncertain whether the nodule is cancerous. Orlo's doctor refers him to Dr. Allen, a thyroid surgeon with extensive experience, for thyroid surgery. After examining Orlo, Dr. Allen tells him that he needs a *lobectomy* (removal of one lobe of the thyroid). During the surgery, a pathologist examines the tissue that the surgeon removes. If the lobectomy shows that Orlo has follicular cancer, Dr. Allen will do a total *thyroidectomy* — he will remove the entire thyroid.

Orlo undergoes blood studies before the surgery, including thyroid function tests, which come back normal. Orlo doesn't eat the morning of surgery, which is supposed to start at 7 a.m., but due to various glitches, the operation begins at 9 a.m. Dr. Allen puts him under general anesthesia. The operation goes smoothly. The lesion proves to be a follicular *carcinoma* (cancer), so Dr. Allen performs a total thyroidectomy. Dr. Allen feels no nodes on the side of the thyroid but removes nodes in the central neck to look for cancer there. The pathologist determines that these nodes aren't cancerous.

After the surgery, Orlo feels some soreness in his neck but isn't hoarse. A clear plastic bandage covers the incision on his neck. Orlo has a chest X-ray and bone scan to make certain that cancer hasn't spread to those areas. These tests come back negative, indicating no cancer spread.

Several weeks after surgery, Orlo receives a dose of radioactive iodine (see Chapter 6) to destroy any remaining thyroid tissue. For the next several years, Orlo sees his doctor every six months with no evidence of recurrence.

A number of reasons may bring you to the thyroid surgeon. Orlo's situation is one of the most serious — thyroid cancer (see Chapter 8). But surgery is the best way to handle several other thyroid situations as well.

- ✔ If you're hyperthyroid, antithyroid pills don't successfully treat your condition (or you're allergic to them), and you don't want to have treatment with radioactive iodine, surgery is your only other choice (see Chapter 6).

- ✔ If you're pregnant and develop hyperthyroidism (see Chapter 17), and you're unable to take the antithyroid pills because of allergies, surgery is your only option. (You can't receive radioactive iodine during pregnancy.)

- ✔ If you have a large thyroid that's causing local symptoms in your neck, such as trouble swallowing or breathing, or if the goiter is especially unattractive, (see Chapter 5) surgery is necessary, though you may also try radioactive iodine.

Finding Your Surgeon

Usually, your doctor picks your surgeon for you and you agree, assuming that your doctor has your best interest at heart. In most cases, your doctor does have your best interest at heart, so this is a good method to follow. But sometimes other factors determine the doctor's choice as well. Perhaps the surgeon is an old friend and colleague your doctor has been working with for years. Or perhaps your doctor wants to keep your case within the confines of a particular hospital. (Occasionally, your insurance mandates that you can go to only certain surgeons.)

The three most important criteria for a surgeon are experience, experience, and experience. If a surgeon does an operation once a month, that isn't experience. If he or she does it several times a week, that's experience. But how do you find a surgeon with the kind of experience you need? I devote an entire chapter (Chapter 3) to the subject of finding a doctor to treat your thyroid condition. And much of the research I suggest that you do there is applicable to finding an experienced thyroid surgeon, including checking out the following organizations on the Web:

- American Association of Endocrine Surgeons (`http://endocrine surgery.org`)
- American Association of Clinical Endocrinologists (`www.aace.com`)

Another good resource is `www.thyroid.org`.

Simply because a doctor is an endocrine surgeon doesn't mean that he or she specializes in thyroid surgery. Many endocrine organs — the pancreas, the adrenals, the ovaries, and so forth — require a surgery that's entirely different from thyroid surgery. Be sure you find a *thyroid* surgeon.

Don't go to a surgeon unless you're certain that you're ready for surgery. The job of the surgeon is to cut, and he or she probably won't try to talk you out of having surgery. You and your thyroid specialist should agree on the need for surgery before you arrive in the surgeon's office.

After you find a potential surgeon, your responsibility to your neck isn't over. You need to ask the surgeon some hard questions before you give him or her the privilege of cutting into you. The most important questions are the following:

- How often do you perform this surgery? (The answer should be more than three times a month, at least.)
- Have you had any deaths in the last five years while doing this surgery? (The answer had better be "no.")
- Have your patients had any serious and permanent complications from your surgery? (Keep reading for information about specific complications.)

If you're happy with the surgeon's answers to these questions, go ahead and sign up.

Making Final Preparations Before Surgery

In the weeks before you head in for surgery, you may have to juggle some medications, depending on your condition.

- ✔ If you're having an operation for hyperthyroidism, you'll probably take antithyroid pills for four to six weeks prior to surgery to get your thyroid function to be normal, which a free T4 test shows. (If you can't take antithyroid pills because of an allergy, obviously you skip this step.) You often get iodine for ten days before surgery to reduce the size and blood vessels of the thyroid. Your doctor may also place you on *propranolol,* a beta blocker, to control symptoms such as a rapid heartbeat or shakiness.

- ✔ If you have hypothyroidism, you need to take thyroid hormone replacement pills prior to surgery so that your thyroid function is normal. Anesthesia is risky if a patient is very hypothyroid.

- ✔ If you're taking aspirin or other medications like coumadin that thin the blood (and therefore prolong bleeding), stop taking them a week before surgery.

A few days prior to surgery, you have blood tests to confirm that your organs, such as your liver and kidneys, are performing satisfactorily. The doctor also wants to confirm that you don't have anemia, although you won't lose much blood during thyroid surgery.

You should eat nothing after supper the night before surgery. The anxiety, the trauma of surgery, and the anesthesia all make you more prone to vomit, and you don't want to have anything in your stomach in case you do.

What Happens During Surgery

You generally come to the hospital on the morning of surgery. A staff member wheels you into the operating room, where the anesthesiologist gives you general anesthesia. (Rarely, local anesthesia is used.) Two hours later, you awaken minus some or all your thyroid. (But thyroid surgery isn't the greatest way to lose weight.)

Making the initial incisions

The anesthesia may be local (an injection in the area of the surgery that doesn't put you to sleep) or general (a medication that causes you to sleep through the operation). Most patients prefer the latter. After all the preparations of cleaning and covering the area of the operation, the surgeon makes an incision about 3 inches (8 centimeters) long horizontally over the area of the thyroid. The surgeon minimizes the scar by carefully placing the incision over the normal skin fold (the place where your skin folds when you bend your head forward) and by making the smallest possible incision. If the surgeon has to remove lymph nodes (as can be the case with thyroid cancer), the surgeon may carry the incision up in the direction of the ear at one or both ends of the incision. The incision cuts through the fat underneath the skin and a thin muscle called the *platysma*. The surgeon pulls the skin and the muscle overlying the thyroid back to reveal the thyroid gland.

The surgeon then sees what he or she will be dealing with in the next hour or so. The thyroid is shaped like a butterfly, with an *isthmus* (a narrow strip) of thyroid tissue connecting the two "wings" of the butterfly (check out the illustration in Chapter 2). Above the isthmus, the surgeon may see a projection of thyroid tissue called the *pyramidal lobe.* Surgeons usually remove the pyramidal lobe during any partial thyroid operation so that it won't regrow as a large bump on the front of the neck when the gland grows to restore thyroid hormone production.

The surgeon knows that the thyroid is firmly fixed to the trachea and larynx in back, so any operation has to free it up before the surgeon can remove the thyroid tissue. He or she sees two *superior thyroid arteries* entering the thyroid from above and two *inferior thyroid arteries* entering the thyroid from below. A fifth artery sometimes enters the thyroid in its central portion from below. The surgeon may have to tie and cut one or all of these arteries, depending on how much of the thyroid he or she is removing.

The surgeon must also deal with the thyroid veins. The *middle thyroid veins* connect to the thyroid from the side. The surgeon must tie and cut them. The surgeon also ties and cuts the veins connecting to the top of the thyroid, called the *superior thyroid veins,* if the plan is to remove the entire lobe.

Dealing with surgical obstacles

Between three and six parathyroid glands, as well as the recurrent laryngeal nerves (one on each side), are found on the back of the thyroid, and the surgeon must carefully preserve them if possible. In any thyroid surgery, the main obstacles to easy surgery are the parathyroid glands and the recurrent laryngeal nerves.

Parathyroid glands

The *parathyroid glands* sit on the back of the thyroid and share blood supply with it. There are usually four of these tiny glands, but there may be more or less, and surgeons find them in many locations. They weigh only 30 to 40 milligrams each and may be accidentally removed, damaged, or lose their blood supply during surgery because they're so tiny.

The parathyroids are responsible for managing the calcium level in the blood. If they aren't functioning, the calcium level falls. Sometimes the trauma of surgery causes the parathyroids to shut off temporarily, but they recover in a few days.

When you have a total thyroidectomy, preserving the parathyroid glands often isn't possible. In this case, the surgeon cuts them into small pieces and injects them back into a muscle, for example in the shoulder, where they seem to function just fine.

If a patient has symptoms of low calcium after surgery, oral calcium supplements can usually manage the problem. The symptoms that may occur include:

- ✔ Feelings of numbness, tingling, and prickling along the extremities, as well as loss of sensation in those areas
- ✔ Increased irritability
- ✔ Fatigue
- ✔ Mood swings
- ✔ Hoarseness
- ✔ Muscle cramps

Rarely, a person needs intravenous calcium. If, by chance, the parathyroids don't recover their function after surgery, the patient takes vitamin D and calcium for life — a rare occurrence associated with only 1 in 300 surgeries of the thyroid.

Recurrent laryngeal nerves

The two recurrent laryngeal nerves, one behind each thyroid lobe, can be major obstacles to the surgeon. Each nerve controls the vocal cord on its side. Both nerves lie close to the thyroid; a surgeon can easily cut them accidentally or include them in a knot that's tying off a blood vessel. If the diagnosis is thyroid cancer, one or both of the recurrent laryngeal nerves may already be included in the cancer, and the patient may have to sacrifice them at the time of surgery.

The trauma of surgery may temporarily damage recurrent laryngeal nerves. If so, the patient has a hoarse voice for a few days after surgery. If surgery damages both nerves, the situation is more serious, and the patient may need a *tracheostomy* (an opening from the neck into the breathing tube) to breathe. The damage and the hoarseness may be permanent. Damage to a recurrent laryngeal nerve should be very rare. In good hands, it doesn't happen more often than once every 250 operations on the thyroid.

The superior laryngeal nerve may suffer an injury during surgery as well. Damage to this nerve produces milder symptoms than those of recurrent laryngeal loss. Loss of this nerve produces voice fatigue and a decrease in the range of the voice.

Determining the extent of surgery

The purpose of the surgery determines what happens next. If the surgeon is removing a hot nodule (see Chapter 7), the surgeon locates any blood supply to it, cuts and ties off the blood supply, and removes the nodule. If hyperthyroidism is the reason for surgery, the surgeon performs a *subtotal thyroidectomy,* leaving a few grams of the part of the thyroid nearest the trachea to avoid damaging the parathyroid glands.

A debate rages about how much thyroid to remove when a cancer is present in the thyroid. Most of the debate concerns small thyroid cancers — the ones that measure less than 1.5 centimeters (0.6 inches) in diameter. The survival rate for this size of cancer seems to be just as good whether you have a total thyroidectomy or less than a total thyroidectomy. Less than a total thyroidectomy leaves thyroid tissue in the area of the recurrent laryngeal nerve in order to avoid damaging it.

A *total thyroidectomy* is an attempt to remove all visible thyroid tissue. It's an extensive surgery that's more difficult than partial removal of the thyroid. A total thyroidectomy results in more frequent damage to parathyroids and nerves. Therefore, many surgeons do a *subtotal thyroidectomy,* leaving a small piece of one lobe of the thyroid intact, when the tumor has a diameter less than 1.5 centimeters.

Other surgeons elect to do a total thyroidectomy on all thyroid cancer patients. They offer fairly convincing arguments:

- The morbidity and mortality rate of this surgery in their hands is very low.

- Thyroid cancer is often *bilateral* — it affects both lobes of the thyroid. If radiation is the cause of cancer, the cancer is almost always bilateral.

- Scanning for evidence of new tumors and treating any new tumors is much easier when no thyroid gland remains to take up radioactive iodine.

- After surgery, levels of thyroglobulin in the blood fall to zero. Therefore, if blood tests later show that a patient's thyroglobulin levels are rising, that's a strong indicator that a tumor is recurring.

If cancer brings you to the surgeon, a very important part of your history is whether you've had radiation therapy to your neck. If you have, then a total thyroidectomy is the correct operation because cancers tend to be in both lobes in this situation. Most surgeons remove the entire thyroid even if the tissue that was suspicious turns out to be free of cancer, because cancer in the rest of the thyroid is so likely.

After the surgeon removes all or part of the thyroid, the question arises whether to remove lymph nodes, especially if none are enlarged. Many surgeons remove nodes over the trachea because cancer often spreads there first. They biopsy nodes to the side of the thyroid if they're enlarged, and they remove most of those nodes if the tissue has cancer — a procedure called a *modified radical neck dissection.* A more extensive form of this surgery is called an *unmodified radical neck dissection,* which involves removing muscles and other tissues. No study shows that this extensive surgery improves mortality; it leaves the patient disfigured for no reason.

Studies show that if a surgeon injects a dye into the thyroid, it goes to the chain of lymph nodes on the trachea behind the isthmus. The surgeon knows that this chain is where to look first for the spread of cancer.

The following outlines surgical treatment approaches particular to each of the types of thyroid cancer (which I discuss in Chapter 8):

- ✔ **Papillary or follicular cancer:** After surgery, doctors put patients with papillary or follicular carcinoma on suppressive doses of thyroid hormone for life. A suppressive dose is a dose that keeps the TSH between 0.1 and 0.5. This is a value below the normal range, which means that the patient has slightly too much thyroid hormone in her system, but the dose seems to prevent growth of new thyroid tissue without causing damage to the patient.

- ✔ **Medullary cancer:** A tumor of the medullary type (see Chapter 8) is managed with a total thyroidectomy and the removal of the central nodes around the trachea; a surgeon removes lateral nodes to the side of the thyroid only if they're visibly enlarged. Medullary tumors often secrete hormones that cause diarrhea or stimulate the adrenal gland, so removing as much tissue as possible prevents or reverses these complications.

  A medullary tumor may be part of a hereditary condition known as *multiple endocrine neoplasia* (MEN). MEN patients have tumors of their adrenal glands and occasionally their parathyroids. Some experts recommend removal of the thyroid before age 5, because the likelihood of cancer is so great. If an adrenal tumor is present, a surgeon should remove it first, because surgery on the thyroid may be dangerous when a malignant adrenal is making large amounts of adrenal hormones as surgery is occurring.

Dealing with a tumor in the thorax

Sometimes most of the cancerous tumor is located in the thorax, under the sternum, the breast bone. The surgeon can usually bring the thyroid up through the neck and remove it, in the process of the standard surgical procedure I outline in the "What Happens During Surgery" section. Occasionally the thyroid surgeon has to go into the chest by splitting the sternum if the mass is especially large and the surgeon can't remove it through the neck, if the blood supply to the thyroid in the chest is especially great in the chest, or if the large mass is a cancer.

✔ **Undifferentiated cancer:** The surgeon attempts to remove as much cancer and thyroid as possible if the tumor is the undifferentiated type. By the time surgery occurs, these tumors usually have spread, and doctors can do little. But surgery can slow the inevitable local spread of this aggressive type of tumor.

If a surgeon has any concern about bleeding after surgery, or if the surgeon has removed so much tissue that a large space is left in the neck, the surgeon leaves a drain in the wound. A drain is necessary only rarely, and the surgeon usually removes it after a day or two in any case. The drain helps prevent fluid accumulation and results in a better cosmetic outcome.

Considering a New Approach

Recently, surgeons have been trying a less invasive approach to thyroid surgery called *endoscopic thyroid surgery*. Surgeons perform this surgery when a diagnosis of cancer is uncertain and a nodule needs to be removed. The surgeon inserts a tiny tube in the neck, and a stream of carbon dioxide gas opens up the area. The surgeon uses high magnification to see the area in excellent anatomical detail. Another tube inserted into the area has a cutting edge that allows for removal of the nodule. The result is a less unsightly scar and a quicker return to activity for most patients, although the amount of pain that patients feel is about the same as those who have a conventional operation.

Endoscopic thyroid surgery may take a little longer than an open operation. If the surgeon finds cancer during the endoscopic surgery, the surgeon usually opens the neck to proceed with an open, total thyroidectomy. However, endoscopic thyroid surgery is promising as a way to avoid large scars and shorten the time between surgery and returning to work. As surgeons gain more experience with this method, it may start to replace the open operation.

Recuperating After the Operation

You'll have a permanent scar after surgery, but it may not be very visible. Most people leave the hospital the same day of the surgery if no complications develop, which is usually the case. But as I note later in this section, the possibility of hemorrhage is rare but present. You must stay in the hospital for 24 hours after surgery to deal with this complication. Don't let the hospital staff kick you out early.

Getting back on your feet

A week is usually necessary to recover from thyroid surgery. During that time, you feel some neck stiffness and tenderness. Your throat is sore, and your voice is hoarse. You have a cough for a few days and feel some pain when you swallow, but pain killer medicine usually manages it. The scar becomes hard initially and then softens over the next month. An occasional patient forms a very thick scar called a *keloid,* which will be permanent because attempts to remove keloids with plastic surgery often result in new keloid formation.

The only postoperative restriction is that you shouldn't submerge yourself in water for the first day or two (no swimming). You can drive a car as soon as your head can turn without difficulty. You can resume most of your usual activities after a week, building up to them slowly. Many people are back at work in two weeks. The surgeon often wants to see you again about three weeks to check on your results.

Any patient who has had extensive removal of the thyroid needs to take thyroid hormone replacement for life. If the operation is for thyroid cancer, you receive enough thyroid hormone to mildly suppress your thyroid-stimulating hormone.

Dealing with complications

In the hands of an experienced thyroid surgeon, complications should be rare and insignificant. Death is a very rare occurrence after thyroid surgery. Seven problems exist that you may need to manage after surgery:

  ✔ **Hypothyroidism** is normal after removal of most of the thyroid, and doctors treat it by giving the proper amount of thyroid hormone. Usually T4 is all that's needed. If the surgery is for benign disease, then the patient receives enough T4 to make the TSH normal. If the surgery is for cancer, the patient receives T4 in a sufficient amount to suppress the TSH, as I describe in the preceding section, "Getting back on your feet."

✓ **Thyroid storm** occurs when the patient who is having surgery for hyperthyroidism isn't prepared properly with antithyroid drugs and propranolol before surgery (see Chapter 6 for more on this condition). Thyroid storm should never occur when the patient is made ready for surgery properly.

✓ **Wound infection** occurs in less than 1 percent of thyroid surgeries, and antibiotics and drainage treat it.

✓ **Wound hemorrhage** is also rare. It occurs in less than 1 percent of operations. It begins with swelling of the neck in the first 12 hours after surgery. Often, the patient has some bandage placed over the site of the operation. If the bandage is too tight and bleeding occurs, the bleeding can compress the trachea and cause breathing difficulties. Sometimes the patient has to have the wound opened at the bedside in an emergency.

✓ **Injury to the recurrent laryngeal nerve** is often temporary. The voice becoming hoarse or husky allows doctors to discover it. This injury is the result of one side of the vocal cord being paralyzed. The situation is much worse if recurrent laryngeal nerves on both sides of the thyroid are injured. Then the patient may be unable to breathe and has to have a tracheostomy.

✓ **Hypoparathyroidism** sometimes occurs for a brief time after surgery, but the glands recover. Permanent hypoparathyroidism is a very rare event when experienced surgeons are doing the operation. A low serum calcium plus the symptoms I describe in the "Parathyroid glands" section such as a feeling of numbness in the extremities, mood swings, hoarseness and muscle cramps allow doctors to easily diagnose it.

✓ **Tracheomalacia** is a softening of the trachea due to pressure from a large goiter. Every time the patient breathes in, the trachea narrows and may even collapse. Sometimes a tracheostomy is necessary to allow a person to breathe.

Part III

Reviewing Special Considerations in Thyroid Health

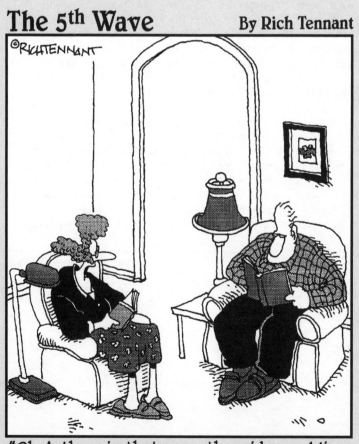

The 5th Wave   By Rich Tennant

"Oh Arthur, is that your thyroid grumbling again? Why don't you use your salt lick?"

In this part . . .

These chapters clue you into some special situations that can affect your thyroid, such as medications you take for other conditions. You discover the genetic link to thyroid diseases and what scientists are doing to try to prevent their transmission from one generation to the next. I also synthesize the latest findings in thyroid treatment to help you stay informed and up to date.

Certain groups of people are affected differently from the rest of us by thyroid disease. These include pregnant women, children, and elderly people. Their special needs are taken up in this part. Plus, there is plenty you can do to keep your thyroid happy and making those essential hormones in the right quantities. The last chapter in this part discusses some ways you can manage your body so that thyroid function takes place in a healthy environment.

Chapter 14

The Genetic Link to Thyroid Disease

• •

In This Chapter

▶ Grasping the basics of genetics

▶ Discovering how your genes impact your thyroid

▶ Planning for the prevention of hereditary thyroid disease

• •

Throughout this book, I introduce you to several members of the Dummy family: Sarah, Stacy, Karen, and Tami. The reason these five women, who come from the same prestigious family, all suffer from thyroid conditions is that thyroid diseases often run in families. Many (though not all) thyroid diseases are hereditary.

In this chapter, I discuss the various hereditary thyroid diseases and how they're passed from one generation to the next. The progress that scientists have made in the last decade alone in understanding the inheritance of thyroid disease is nothing short of amazing. But all this new information has made the subject pretty complicated.

I try to clear up some of the complications of *genetics,* the science of heredity, in this chapter, but I'll be honest: This subject isn't for the fainthearted. If you're interested in knowing how genetics program your body to experience a certain disease, this chapter definitely tickles your intellect. If you're reading this book solely to determine how to treat your present thyroid condition, you may want to head over to the chapter that details your specific condition instead.

But even if the term *genetics* strikes fear in your heart, you may want to jump to the end of the chapter (the section called "Viewing the Future of Managing Hereditary Thyroid Disease") to discover some of the exciting ways that scientists are attempting to prevent people from inheriting thyroid disease and many other genetic diseases in the future.

Taking Genetics 101

To understand how genetic disease affects the thyroid, you need a basic understanding of genetics. This section provides the background that you need. This book isn't about genetics, so I've made this section as brief as possible while still giving you the essentials.

Pouring over pea plants

Gregor Mendel, an Austrian monk, is the starting point for all the great discoveries in genetics, although he never got credit for his pioneering efforts in his lifetime. Mendel studied pea plants, looking at the ways that various characteristics of the plants were inherited, such as height, the texture of the seeds, the plumpness of the pods, and so forth.

Mendel knew that pea plants form new seeds when the *pollen* (which functions the same as sperm) in the male part of the plant called the *anther* manages to attach to the *stigma,* the female part, and get down to the *ovary* (the egg), which the pollen fertilizes. The result is a seed, which grows into a plant.

Mendel carefully controlled the fertilization of his pea plants so that he knew which plant provided the pollen and which plant provided the ovary. He took, for example, the pollen of short pea plants that had never produced anything but short pea plants, and used that pollen to fertilize the ovaries of tall pea plants that had never produced anything but tall pea plants. Then he took the pollen from tall pea plants and fertilized the ovaries of short pea plants. Much to his surprise, the result in both cases was always tall pea plants (he expected the short and tall plants to combine to form a medium-sized plant).

Mendel then crossed the tall offspring from this first fertilization (called the *first cross*) with each other. The offspring of the second cross weren't all tall: Three-fourths were tall, and one-fourth was short. When Mendel crossed the short plants from the second cross with other short plants from the second cross, the result was plants that were always short. But if he crossed short and tall plants from the second cross, the new plants were usually, but not always, tall. The same pattern held true for the other characteristics that Mendel studied.

On the basis of these studies, Mendel made the following observations of the pea plant:

- A feature of the pollen and the egg determines whether a plant is tall or short. (This feature is now called a *gene;* Mendel didn't use this term.)
- When the gene (what he called an *atom of inheritance*) from the tall plant combines with the gene from the short plant, the genes don't mix to form an average-sized plant.

✔ If a plant has two characteristics for the same gene, such as tallness and shortness, one tends to appear more often than the other when they're crossed. (The gene that produces the trait that appears more often is the *dominant* gene, and the gene producing the trait that appears less often is the *recessive* gene.)

✔ Two different genes can exist for a trait. (Two genes that determine the same trait are called *alleles.*)

✔ Genes follow the principle of *independent assortment:* Plants inherit each trait separately from all other traits. When plants are crossed that have two different traits, such as height and texture of the seed, these traits are passed to the offspring independently of one another. For example, a tall plant doesn't always have a smooth seed or always have a wrinkled seed.

Mendel's work received little attention when he announced it in 1865, but scientists rediscovered it in 1900. He got posthumous credit for his discoveries (for what that was worth).

Talking the genetics talk

Using Mendel's research, scientists later began to create the new language of genetics so that you and I couldn't possibly understand what they were talking about. I'm going to test my interpretation skills here to walk you through the maze they've created.

If a person (or a plant, dog, or chimpanzee) has two copies of the same allele, he or she is said to be *homozygous* for that gene. If he or she has one of each allele, the person is *heterozygous* for that gene. (We now know that, within an entire population, more than two different alleles can exist for each gene. However, any given person, animal, or plant has only two alleles for each gene because a single individual has only two copies, while others in the population may have two different copies.)

The appearance of the trait controlled by a gene is called the *phenotype,* while the genes that make up that phenotype are called the *genotype.* For instance, two tall pea plants may have the same appearance (phenotype), while their genotype may be different. One plant may have only tall genes and is tall, while the other has a tall gene and a short gene and is still tall — because tallness is the dominant gene.

A quick quiz: Based on your in-depth knowledge of genetics, can two short pea plants have different genotypes? The answer is no, because shortness is the recessive gene. If you throw a tallness gene into the mix, the plant is tall. Therefore, all short pea plants must have only the genes for shortness.

Observing the great divide

At the same time that the world was ignoring Mendel's work, great things were happening under the microscope. Scientists were seeing that tissues are made up of cells and that new cells come from the division of old cells. As two new cells form, the old cell produces two copies of everything so that each new cell has exactly what the old cell had. *Mitosis* is the whole process by which one cell becomes two.

One particular area of the cell, which looks like a cell within the cell, was especially intriguing to scientists. This area is called the *nucleus* of the cell. As two new cells are being formed, some substances in the nucleus double and separate so that each new cell gets a complete set of these substances, called *chromosomes*.

Over the years, scientists discovered that each plant and animal has a set of chromosomes, but the numbers of chromosomes may differ between species. For instance, humans have 23 pairs, or 46, chromosomes, while chimpanzees have 24 pairs, or 48, chromosomes. (But chimpanzee chromosomes look more like human chromosomes than ape chromosomes, so don't be thinking that you're so smart.)

Examining the division of egg cells and sperm cells (the so-called *germ cells*), scientists discovered that each of these cells contains only half the normal number of chromosomes. In humans, for example, each egg cell and each sperm cell has one set of 23 chromosomes (while other human cells have 46 chromosomes). When these cells divide to form more sperm or egg cells through a process called *meiosis,* the result is again 23 chromosomes per cell. When the egg and the sperm join together in fertilization, the combination, called a *zygote,* has the normal number of 46 (23 pairs) chromosomes.

When a zygote forms, one set of its chromosomes comes from the female, and one set of chromosomes comes from the male; these sets pair up two by two. The members of each chromosome pair are called *homologous* chromosomes.

As is always the case, the rule that all chromosome pairs have identical sets of genes has an exception. But like the French say, *vive le difference.* Loosely translated, that means "thank goodness for this particular set of chromosomes." I'm referring to the sex chromosomes that determine whether you're a boy or a girl. All other pairs of chromosomes have matched genes; if a gene exists for a given characteristic on one of the chromosomes of the pair, the other chromosome has a gene for that same characteristic. A female has two matched sex chromosomes (called *X chromosomes*), and a male has two different sex chromosomes (called an *X chromosome* and a *Y chromosome*).

Mapping traits with genes and chromosomes

Any given plant, animal, or human has far more traits than its number of chromosomes. Recognizing this fact, scientists realized that each chromosome must contain many genes.

Each chromosome is passed down to its *daughter cells* — the cells created when a cell divides. Therefore, some genes (and the traits they create) get passed down together from generation to generation. (They don't follow the principle of independent assortment.) Genes on the same chromosome are *linked.*

Even though some genes are linked, they sometimes do get inherited independently, just as Mendel predicted, which happens because *crossing over* takes place. What is crossing over? During the process of meiosis, which produces sperm and egg cells, as the sets of chromosomes line up close together, genes on one chromosome can cross over to the other while their alleles cross over in the other direction. In this way, *recombinant* chromosomes are formed — new combinations that help to make your offspring different from you.

The discovery of crossing over meant that scientists could start to *map* chromosomes. That is, scientists could determine which genes are on which chromosomes and where, because the closer two genes are, the less likely they're separated by a cross-over. The farther genes are from one another, the more likely they are to separate.

Another way that a new trait replaces an old one is when a *mutation* takes place. In a mutation, a new gene replaces as old one as a result of faulty copying of the chromosome or an outside influence, such as radiation, chemicals, or the sun. Usually mutation isn't noticed, either because the gene is recessive or because the mutation may kill the individual so that it isn't reproduced. Once in a while, a mutation is good for the animal or plant in which it occurs, producing a useful trait.

Getting down to the DNA

Genes consist of long, long, long chains of *nucleic acids.* Nucleic acids have three components: a sugar called *deoxyribose,* a *phosphate* attached at one end of the sugar, and a *base,* which may be adenine, cytosine, guanine, or thymine, attached to the sugar at another point. The genes contain *deoxyribonucleic acid,* or DNA.

Within the DNA, the number of adenine molecules is always equal to the number of thymine molecules, while the amount of cytosine equals that of guanine. In 1952, biochemists James D. Watson and Francis H. C. Crick showed that this equality is because each gene contains two chains of nucleic acids. The adenine on one chain is always paired with the thymine on the other, while cytosine on one chain is always paired with guanine on the other. Other researchers had shown that DNA has a helical structure, so Watson and Crick called the structure a *double helix* — a shape that looks like a spiral staircase.

One of the best outcomes of the identification of the double helix was that scientists understood how the genes copy themselves, or *replicate*. The helix can break apart into two strands. The two individual strands then each act as a template so that a new strand forms on each in the only way it can, by connecting to the only nucleic acid it can combine with — namely, a nucleic acid containing adenine connects to a nucleic acid containing thymine, and a nucleic acid containing cytosine connects with a nucleic acid containing guanine. The result is two new double helixes.

The DNA has to somehow control the creation of the animal or plant and the ongoing processes that allow it to live. The DNA does so by producing *ribonucleic acid,* or RNA. RNA comprises nucleic acids just like DNA. But the sugar in RNA is ribose, and the bases are adenine, cytosine, and guanine, with uricil replacing thymine.

In the same way that the double helix can break apart to reproduce itself, it can break apart and construct a complementary RNA molecule. This process is called *transcription.* The RNA remains a single strand, not a double helix. The RNA is called *messenger RNA* because it carries the message from the DNA to the next level of control, the *enzyme.* An enzyme is a protein that acts as a facilitator for a chemical reaction — for example, the breakdown of a complex carbohydrate like glycogen (the storage form of glucose — the body's source of immediate energy) into small glucose molecules that the body can instantly use.

The messenger RNA accomplishes its task by acting as a template in its turn for the production of the enzyme or protein in the process of *translation.* Proteins consist of amino acids. Every three bases in the messenger RNA, called a *triplet,* causes one particular amino acid to line up opposite them. Each group of three is a *codon,* because it codes for a specific amino acid. By making up artificial messenger RNA that contained the same codon again and again, determining which amino acid each codon selected became possible.

With 4 different bases in sets of 3, the maximum number of codons is 64, but only 20 amino acids exist. Different codons select the same amino acid, and some codons act as the code for the end of a protein without selecting an amino acid.

Just to complicate the issue a little further, the amino acids don't actually line up opposite the codons but are carried at one end of another RNA molecule, called *transfer RNA*. At its other end, transfer RNA has the bases that are complementary to the codon. So the transfer RNA lines up neatly against the messenger RNA, while the amino acids line up next to one another at the other end. A series of other steps that you don't need to know to understand hereditary thyroid disease bind the amino acids into a protein that may be an enzyme or a muscle or whatever.

Genes also contain large segments of bases that don't code anything and, in fact, have to be cut out from their complementary RNA before the RNA can produce a protein. These sequences are called *introns,* and scientists don't know what their function is.

Determining whether to be a liver or a heart

A fertilized egg reproduces itself by the process of mitosis, creating two identical cells. But how can each identical cell transform itself into a thyroid cell or a liver cell or even a brain cell?

The gene uses a number of techniques to turn gene action on and off. Short sequences of bases called *promoters* precede the active gene. When various factors bind to a promoter, it turns on the action of the gene to begin transcription. Other sequences of elements called *enhancers* increase the activity of the gene further, while *silencers* tend to shut down the activity of the gene. The process of transcription from DNA to messenger RNA comes to a halt when certain sequences of bases are reached.

Because all cells contain the same genetic information, a thyroid cell differs from a brain cell as a result of the particular genes that are *expressed* (active) in each cell. Many different factors determine whether a gene is expressed. Promoters and enhancers increase their activity in response to various hormones or growth factors that may be present in one cell but not another.

The expression of a gene may be controlled at the level of the gene itself, or it may be controlled after transcription has taken place so that the messenger RNA never makes the protein.

In these and in many other ways scientists have yet to discover, cells use only the genes they need to function within their environment.

Probing the Origins of Genetic Thyroid Diseases

Now that you have a basic understanding of genetics, you can apply your knowledge to thyroid diseases that are transmitted through inheritance. A child inherits a thyroid disease in one of three basic ways:

- ✔ A single gene from a parent transmits a dominant or recessive trait to the child. This method goes back to Mendel and his peas.

- ✔ The child inherits all of the many genes involved in the inheritance of a disease.

- ✔ An entire chromosome is abnormal. For example, if a female ends up with only one X chromosome, that lack can produce a condition known as *Turner's syndrome,* which often includes a thyroid disorder.

Inheriting a disease through a single gene

People inherit many diseases through a single gene, often as a result of a gene mutation, in one of three ways:

- ✔ **As a recessive gene:** Both parents must supply the same gene in order for the disease to appear.

- ✔ **As a dominant gene:** Only one parent supplies the gene necessary to cause the disease.

- ✔ **With the X chromosome in a recessive form:** A male gets the disease (because he has only one X chromosome), but a female is spared unless both her X chromosomes have the gene.

You can find the entire list of diseases transmitted by single-gene inheritance at www.ncbi.nlm.nih.gov/entrez/query.fcgi?db=OMIM, the home-page of Online Mendelian Inheritance in Man (OMIM), a huge database compiled by Dr. Victor McKusick at Johns Hopkins University and others. If you search the term "thyroid" from the homepage, 554 different thyroid diseases appear (at the time of this writing). A full description accompanies each one, with citations of all the research that has been done to define the defect and a complete bibliography at the end of each description.

Inherited thyroid diseases can affect every step in thyroid hormone production, transportation, and action. The ones I list in the following sections are only 14 of the 554 currently listed in the OMIM database. Scientists are discovering new conditions all the time. These 14 are the best understood.

Recessive inheritance

Many conditions where the body doesn't make thyroid hormone properly fall into the category of recessive inheritance. Two "bad" genes are necessary to develop one of these conditions. If you have just one bad gene, you're a carrier of the disease, but you don't experience it yourself. The phenotype (the way this gene makes itself known) is usually a large thyroid that doesn't produce sufficient thyroid hormone. Note that several of the conditions appear to be the same because the final result of the condition is absence of thyroid hormone, but each condition involves a defect in a different step in the production of thyroid hormone. Among the conditions inherited this way are the following:

- **A defect in the creation of the enzyme that produces thyroid hormone:** (see Chapter 4): Patients with this condition are hypothyroid (see Chapter 5) and have goiters.

- **Thyroid hormone unresponsiveness:** If you inherit a bad gene instead of the gene that makes the receptor protein for thyroid hormone, your end organs aren't responsive to the thyroid hormone your body produces. This condition causes patients to be deaf and have goiters. With this condition, the T3, T4, and TSH levels are all elevated (see Chapter 4).

- **Pendred syndrome:** Patients with this disease are deaf and have goiters, but their thyroid function is normal. The disease also causes mental retardation and an increased tendency to develop thyroid cancer. The defect is in the production of thyroid hormone, but at some point it improves so that hypothyroidism isn't present later on.

- **Thyroid transcription–factor defect:** Patients have goiters and decreased levels of thyroglobulin. If you remember that *transcription* is the term for the production of messenger RNA from DNA, you understand that this defect arises from a failure to produce the enzyme necessary to make thyroid hormone.

- **Defect in thyroid production:** This disease is different from thyroid transcription–factor defect. Patients are hypothyroid, have goiters, and experience mental retardation. Lab tests show a defect in the formation of thyroid hormone. Normally, two molecules of tyrosine with iodine attached couple to form thyroid hormone, but this process fails in this particular inherited condition.

Dominant inheritance

Many inherited thyroid conditions pass from parents to children through dominant inheritance: One "bad" gene produces the disease. These diseases tend to be more common than those inherited by recessive genes. Examples of diseases inherited this way are as follows:

- **Thyroid hormone–receptor defects:** A number of receptor defects are possible. With one of these conditions, your body is resistant to the action of thyroid hormones. At the same time, you experience mild hyperthyroidism. Patients with this condition have short stature, learning disabilities, deafness, and goiters. Lab tests show high levels of T3, T4, and TSH. These conditions are rare, resulting from a mutation in the gene responsible for the thyroid receptor. Another type of receptor defect produces a child with severe cretinism of the neurologic form (see Chapter 12).

✔ **Papillary thyroid carcinoma** (see Chapter 8). This type of cancer usually occurs at an earlier age than thyroid cancer that's not inherited.

✔ **Thyroid hormone resistance** (also found in a recessive form). Patients with this condition have a goiter and begin to speak at a later than expected age but have normal thyroid function. Lab tests show that T3 and T4 levels are high, but the TSH level is normal.

✔ **Multiple endocrine neoplasia, type II:** This condition causes tumors on multiple organs, including the thyroid (see Chapter 8), the adrenal gland, and the parathyroid glands. Lab tests show increased levels of epinephrine and calcitonin in the blood.

✔ **Medullary carcinoma of the thyroid, familial:** Patients with this condition have medullary cancer (see Chapter 8).

X-linked inheritance

X-linked inheritance presents fewer examples of thyroid disease because men have only one X chromosome, and women have two, compared to 44 other chromosomes that can produce a disease by recessive or dominant inheritance. If a disease passed on by the X chromosome is recessive, both parents must give the gene to a daughter in order for the disease to appear. But a son gets the disease if only one parent passes along the gene. Because Y chromosomes are only present in males, Y-linked inheritance is only found in males, and it's rare because the Y chromosome is so small. Some examples of diseases inherited this way include

✔ **Immunodeficiency and polyendocrinopathy:** A baby with this condition has unmanageable diarrhea, diabetes, and thyroid autoimmune disease and usually dies very young.

✔ **Thyroid-binding globulin abnormality:** This condition produces retardation. Lab tests show that patients with this disease have decreased thyroid-binding globulin (see Chapter 3).

✔ **Multinodular goiter:** The thyroid is larger than normal and multinodular (see Chapter 9).

Inheriting a disease through multiple genes

The major thyroid disease inherited as a result of abnormalities of multiple genes is *autoimmune thyroiditis*. This disease is much more common in women than in men, so you may assume that the inheritance is linked to the X chromosome somehow. But if this is the case, scientists don't know the method by which the X chromosome passes the disease along. One idea is that the female sex hormone influences the occurrence of this disease, but scientists don't understand just how this may happen.

Autoimmune thyroiditis is easy to diagnose because lab tests show that a person has autoantibodies (see Chapter 5) that damage the thyroid. Many genes are involved in the production of autoantibodies. The substance (such as thyroid tissue) that provokes antibodies is called an *antigen*. The antigen is broken into small pieces that proteins called *major histocompatibility molecules* bind to cells. This combination of cells and antigens leads to the activation of another cell called the *T cell*. The T cell helps yet another cell, the *B cell,* recognize the antigen and produce antibodies against it. All these steps involve multiple genes.

The major histocompatibility region of the chromosomes is on the short arm of chromosome six. It is a set of genes that determines which antigens are found on white blood cells. These antigens are the *human leukocyte antigens* (HLA). Scientists can identify the antigens chemically. In this way, scientists have shown that in whites, HLA-B8 and HLA-DR3 are the antigens associated with Graves' disease (see Chapter 6), while in Koreans, the DR5 and DR8 are most common. In Japanese, the antigen most associated with Graves' disease is DR5, and in Chinese, the DR9. All of this knowledge is important because doctors can test for these antigens in relatives of affected individuals. If the antigens are present, they're more likely to get the disease.

Autoimmune thyroid disease really comprises three different conditions:

- ✔ **Graves' disease:** This disease consists of hyperthyroidism, eye disease, and skin disease (see Chapter 6).

- ✔ **Chronic thyroiditis:** This condition consists of goiter in a person with normal thyroid function or hypothyroidism (see Chapter 5).

- ✔ **Myxedema:** This condition is severe hypothyroidism.

When scientists examine the thyroid glands of patients with the preceding conditions, the appearance is amazingly similar despite the completely different clinical outcome. In addition, as the Dummy family shows throughout this book, different members of the same family can have one or the other of these conditions. And the same person can have one or the other of these conditions at different times. Which type of antibody a person's body is producing determines which condition is present. If an antibody that stimulates the thyroid is predominant, then Graves' disease is present. If antibodies that block thyroid-stimulating hormone are predominant, then chronic thyroiditis or myxedema is present.

The greater occurrence of other autoimmune conditions in people with autoimmune thyroiditis strengthens their autoimmune basis for this disease. These other autoimmune conditions include the following:

- ✔ **Myasthenia gravis:** A disease of muscle weakness that activity worsens and rest improves, resulting from an autoimmune attack at the place where nerves and muscles come together.

- ✔ **Pernicious anemia:** A reduction in red blood cells caused by a lack of *intrinsic factor,* a substance made in the parietal cells of the stomach that's essential for absorbing vitamin B12 into the body. An autoimmune attack destroys the parietal cells.

- ✔ **Vitiligo:** A loss of pigmentation of the skin caused by autoimmune destruction of *melanocytes,* the cells that produce pigmentation.

- ✔ **Type 1 diabetes mellitus:** (See my book *Diabetes For Dummies,* 2nd Edition [Wiley].) A disease caused by excessive levels of glucose in the blood as a result of an autoimmune attack on the pancreas, which makes insulin, the chemical that controls the blood glucose.

- ✔ **Addison's disease:** Failure of the adrenal gland to produce hydrocortisone as a result of an autoimmune attack on the hydrocortisone-producing adrenal cells.

- ✔ **Alopecia areata:** Patchy loss of hair in any part of the body, caused by an autoimmune attack on hair follicles.

- ✔ **Ovarian failure:** Loss of function of the ovaries, resulting in infertility on account of an autoimmune attack on the ovarian follicles, the structures that nurture the eggs.

- ✔ **Testicular failure:** Loss of fertility as a result of autoimmune attack on the sperm in the testicles.

- ✔ **Pituitary failure:** Loss of function of the pituitary gland with failure to make the hormones that stimulate other glands, including the thyroid, the adrenal gland, and the ovaries and testicles, as a result of autoimmune attack on pituitary cells.

- ✔ **Rheumatoid arthritis:** Systemic lupus erythematosis and Sjorgren's syndrome, all examples of autoimmune attacks on the joints of the body.

Antigens in autoimmune thyroiditis

A number of antigens are present in autoimmune thyroiditis against which antibodies are formed, but three antigens are most important.

✔ **Thyroglobulin** is the substance within the thyroid that contains thyroid hormones T4 and T3. Not just one kind of thyroglobulin exists, but different kinds in different people. Thyroglobulin is also present in tissue in the eye. Some of the eye disease of Graves' disease may be due to the reaction of antibodies against thyroglobulin in the eyes.

✔ **TSH receptor,** the second antigen, is the substance on the thyroid cell to which TSH binds in order to stimulate the thyroid. Antibodies to TSH receptor bind to it and cause hyperthyroidism by acting like TSH.

✔ **Thyroid peroxidase,** which used to be called antimicrosomal antigen, is the third important antigen. As its previous name implies, scientists found it in a part of the thyroid cell called the microsome. Its antibody is the most easily measured thyroid antibody and is most often positive in autoimmune thyroiditis.

Whew! That's really quite a list. But don't worry. The chances that you'll get any of the preceding conditions in combination with your autoimmune thyroid disease are quite small, though greater than if you don't have the thyroid condition.

Thyroid autoantibodies are also present in several other clinical conditions, but whether they're the cause of these conditions or represent a marker for a disturbance in autoimmunity that's to blame isn't clear. These clinical conditions are as follows:

✔ Increased risk of miscarriage in women attempting to become pregnant by in-vitro fertilization

✔ Breast cancer

✔ Depression in middle-aged women

Another disease that's found more often in people with certain human leukocyte antigens is postpartum thyroiditis (see Chapter 11). In whites, the antigens are HLA, DR3, DR4, or DR5, while in Chinese, the antigen is DR9. The antigens are not certain for other ethnic groups.

Inheriting a chromosome abnormality

During the creation of a zygote, as new cells are being formed, a mistake can occur in the division of the chromosomes into the two new cells — one cell ends up with an extra chromosome, and the other ends up with one less chromosome. The most well-known conditions associated with this kind of chromosome mistake are Turner's syndrome and Down's syndrome. Both conditions are associated with hypothyroidism, but Down's syndrome is also associated with hyperthyroidism on occasion.

Down's syndrome results when the new cells have an extra chromosome — they have three copies of the 21st chromosome instead of two. People with this condition have a typical physical appearance with characteristic facial features that are recognizable at birth. Children with Down's syndrome have palms that have a single crease, and their muscles lack tone. Reduced intelligence and other abnormalities are part of this syndrome.

Turner's syndrome results when an X chromosome is left behind so that a female is born with a single sex chromosome. The woman has distinctive facial features, including low-set ears, folds of skin in the inner corner of the eye, and drooping eyelids. The woman also may have diabetes mellitus, cataracts, rheumatoid arthritis, and cardiac abnormalities in addition to chronic thyroiditis.

Viewing the Future of Managing Hereditary Thyroid Disease

Up to now, scientists haven't been successful in their attempts to remove a "bad" gene from a human and replace it with a healthy gene — a process known as *genetic engineering*. The problem is that they don't yet know how to insert the new gene successfully. If scientists can determine how to do so, they can open the door to preventing diseases that people inherit through a single gene.

Genetic engineering

If a recessive gene causes a disease, replacing that gene with its dominant form in sufficient amounts should be enough to cure the condition. Usually in a recessive-gene disorder, the disease occurs because that particular gene isn't functioning at all, so providing even a small level of function may cure the condition.

The disorders that may most easily respond to genetic engineering are disorders of the blood system, because doctors and scientists may easily remove blood. A new gene can be spliced into the cells and the blood reintroduced to the patient. The first trial of gene therapy, performed in 1990, was for a disorder that resulted in severe loss of immunity so that the patient was very susceptible to any infection, as well as a cancer. Scientists were able to introduce the necessary gene into the blood cells of the patient by connecting the gene to a virus, which infected the cells and added the gene to their DNA. The cells were grown to increase their number and reinserted. Unfortunately, the trial didn't work, probably because the efficiency of splicing the gene into the cells was low.

Other genetic disorders for which trials of gene therapy have taken place include

- ✔ **Familial hypercholesterolemia:** Excessive production of cholesterol leads to early death by heart attack.

- ✔ **Cystic fibrosis:** Lack of a certain gene leads to excessive production of a thick mucous in the lungs, resulting in chronic lung infection.

- ✔ **Duchenne muscular dystrophy:** Severe muscle deterioration leads to the individual dying by the third decade of life.

A trial of gene replacement in all three of these conditions has been unsuccessful.

Another novel way of managing diseases caused by defective genes is to find a gene that's active during fetal life (but becomes dormant later on) and that can replace the activity of the defective gene if it can be made to express itself. A prime candidate for this treatment is sickle cell disease. In this disease, abnormal hemoglobin (hemoglobin is the chemical in red cells that carries oxygen to the tissues of the body) leads to the early loss of red blood cells, which become sickled (crescent shaped) in appearance and can block blood flow to tissues, causing great pain. A gene active during fetal life produces fetal hemoglobin, which doesn't sickle. If this gene can be turned on during adult life, it can replace the defective hemoglobin made by the patient. Scientists are looking for the drug that may be able to turn this gene on.

Cancer treatment has seen a lot of activity in the area of gene therapy. Gene therapy can treat cancer of the thyroid in a number of ways, including the following:

- ✔ Inserting a gene that increases the sensitivity of the cancer to a drug, or inserting a poison into cells that are injected directly into the tumor.

- ✔ Inserting a gene that increases the activity of the patient's immune system.

✔ Inserting a new gene into blood cells to restore tumor-suppressor activity. This treatment works because some tumors arise when the activity of tumor suppressors (chemicals in the body that suppress the growth of tumors) declines.

✔ Using a virus to introduce a gene into a thyroid cancer cell. The virus causes the DNA to change so that the cell takes up radioactive iodine, which can kill the cell. (This approach is the newest cancer treatment and is outlined in a paper in *Thyroid* in June 2004.)

All these treatments have seen some success, but no one has yet been cured of cancer with gene therapy.

Scientists are also attempting to increase a tumor's immune response by modifying the tumor so that it provokes body cells against it. Scientists perform this technique by inserting genes into the tumor that cause it to produce new antigens that the body can fight against. Tumors like malignant melanoma and colon cancer have been the target of this type of therapy. A similar technique involves inserting a gene directly into a tumor that activates a cancer-killing agent, which is subsequently injected. These techniques have led to some decrease in tumor size but, so far, no cures of cancer. Interestingly, gene therapy isn't limited to tumors brought on by faulty genes but can be directed at any tumor, genetic or not.

Exploring the ethics of germline gene therapy

You can see that the range of techniques for using genetic engineering to cure disease is enormous. Scientists are discovering new methods of delivering healthy genes to replace disease-conferring genes as you read this book. This approach would certainly be the simplest and most successful way of treating the diseases provoked by inheritance of a single dominant gene. However, this type of treatment would cure only the particular individual without affecting the transmission of the disease to his offspring. To eliminate the disease from future generations, genetic engineering has to take place in the sperm and/or the egg, the *germline* of the individual.

Germline gene therapy raises tremendous ethical questions. If we have the tools for eliminating the recessively inherited Pendred syndrome by replacing a Pendred gene with a normal gene, don't we also have the tools for changing skin color, height, or any other body characteristic in future generations? An entire field of genetics concerns *ELSI,* the ethical, legal, and social implications of genetic science.

So far, germline gene therapy has actually been successful in some animals, but hasn't been done on humans for several reasons:

✔ The methods used so far are very imprecise, so the final product is uncertain, including the possible introduction of harmful genes.

✔ Many people fear that germline gene therapy may lead to germline enhancement, an attempt to produce a "superior" human being.

✔ Whether germline gene therapy is even needed is uncertain, because a harmful recessive trait requires mating with another human with the same trait to express itself, while dominant traits are present in only half of a germline. Identifying the sperm or egg with the normal gene and using that gene in fertilization makes more sense than trying to modify the sperm or egg with the abnormal gene. Scientists should perform genetic testing of the germline if they are to eliminate these diseases.

Clearly, genetics is the current frontier in medical science. Genetics promises to prevent or cure many of the diseases that plague humans, including hereditary thyroid disease and nonhereditary tumors. But the road to those cures and preventions is full of cracks and bumps that assure a very uneven ride.

Chapter 15

The Thyroid and Your Mental Health

*T*he term *myxedema madness* may not be familiar to you, but it was popular when it was introduced in 1949 and for many years thereafter. *Myxedema* refers to low thyroid function, or hypothyroidism. The term *myxedema madness* resulted in the unfortunate association that all people with low thyroid function were somehow mad. My goal in this chapter is to clear up this misconception.

The abnormal production of thyroid hormones, which I explain in Chapter 3, can cause changes in the mood of a patient, and these changes can be severe in rare instances. But for most patients, simply treating their overactive or underactive thyroid allows them to live psychologically and physically normal lives.

In this chapter, I share what doctors currently understand about how changes in the production of thyroid hormones (both overproduction and underproduction) affect your personality. You discover how often personality or mood disorders are associated with thyroid abnormalities and why thyroid hormones play a role in the treatment of depression, even when no thyroid problem exists. Because the emphasis in this chapter is on the psychology of thyroid abnormalities, I don't discuss physical signs and symptoms here; those discussions occur elsewhere in the book, especially in Chapters 5 and 6.

The Underactive Thyroid and Your Mood

Sarah Dummy is a 44-year-old woman who hasn't been herself for several months. Her husband, Milton, notices that she is much less talkative than before. She often forgets to pick up the food that they need at the supermarket or to stop at the dry cleaner's to pick up clothes she dropped off.

Milton wants to discuss a vacation with Sarah, but she doesn't seem to care. Sarah is usually the one responsible for making plans with their friends, but she hasn't made any for months. Everything she does seems to take more time than it used to, like preparing dinner or getting ready to go to bed. When she finally gets in bed, she isn't particularly interested in having sex anymore. The most serious change is that Sarah, usually a happy person, seems sad a lot of the time.

Worried about these changes, Milton encourages Sarah to see Dr. Rubin, who examines her and sends her for some lab tests. A few days later, Dr. Rubin tells Sarah that she has hypothyroidism — her thyroid gland isn't making enough thyroid hormone. He gives her a prescription for replacement thyroid hormone, and about a month later Sarah is well on her way to becoming her old self. Milton is happy because he has clean underwear again.

Sarah is an excellent example of the changes in personality that occur when the body doesn't produce enough thyroid hormone. Depending on the level of the deficiency, the changes are more or less severe and include the following:

- Decreased talking
- Memory loss, especially for recent events at first, and for remote events later on
- General loss of interest
- Inability to concentrate
- Withdrawal from society
- A general slowing of movement and thought
- Depression, generally mild but sometimes severe (see the "Fighting Depression" section, later in the chapter)
- Loss of interest in sex
- In severe cases, a kind of ironic sense of humor

Patients and doctors can easily confuse many of the preceding complaints, which are nonspecific and poorly defined, with depression. For this reason, both patients and doctors can easily miss their significance.

No one or group of the preceding mental changes means that you definitely have low thyroid function, but they certainly suggest that you need testing to find out.

If your doctor determines that lack of thyroid hormone is the cause of your symptoms, then the right dose of hormone replacement should reverse them. If it doesn't, then you and your doctor need to look elsewhere for the cause, which may be underlying depression. See Chapter 5 for a thorough discussion of hypothyroidism.

Any person over the age of 60 who has a psychosis and reduced mental ability should receive testing for possible thyroid disease.

And keep in mind the following additional hypothyroid–mental illness related issues:

✔ Occasionally, a patient who has schizophrenia has hypothyroidism. Giving thyroid pills may not completely cure the patient, because some changes may be irreversible.

✔ If a patient with manic-depressive psychosis caused by hypothyroidism receives lithium, the lithium may make the problem worse because it causes hypothyroidism as well.

The most severe mental symptoms — historical notes

Years ago — I'm talking about more than 50 years ago — doctors saw patients with much more severe and longstanding cases of hypothyroidism and hyperthyroidism than we see today.

At one time, doctors saw many more hypothyroid individuals with decreased accuracy of perception that led to visual and other hallucinations. Still later, bizarre behavior appeared. Patients showed increasing drowsiness, difficulty in arousal, sleeping for long periods, and finally coma followed by death if they didn't receive treatment for their hypothyroidism.

Doctors found hyperthyroid patients with huge thyroid glands who were visibly shaky and nervous, unable to sit still for more than a few moments, resembling mania. Such severe hyperthyroidism very rarely happens now, because doctors usually diagnose the condition earlier, but rare cases of severe, prolonged hyperthyroidism may result in hallucinations, both in vision and hearing. In fact, a severely hyperthyroid patient first caused me to become very interested in thyroid disease. She had a large goiter, and I saw her in the medical psychiatric ward during my training days at Bellevue Hospital Medical Center at New York University School of Medicine.

But doctors rarely see patients suffering from such severe symptoms today, and the medical literature and descriptions of such cases relies on the observations of people living in a very different society fifty or more years ago.

Overactivity of the Thyroid and Your Mind

Sarah Dummy's sister, Margaret, who is five years younger, began showing some big personality changes a few years ago. Previously a fairly even-tempered person, she now becomes easily excited and loses her temper after fairly mild provocation. Her small children never know when their mother is going to yell at them. She sometimes has a crying spell but, if asked, can't give a reason why.

At other times, Margaret is extremely happy, but she can't explain the reason for that either. When she tries to do a task, she often loses interest rapidly and gets distracted. She can't sit still for very long and seems to be always moving. Her memory of recent events is poor.

Margaret and her husband, Fred, go to see Dr. Rubin about her condition after a few months of absolute chaos in their home. During an examination, Dr. Rubin discovers a number of physical findings, including a rapid pulse, a large thyroid gland, and a fine tremor of Margaret's fingers. He confirms his findings with lab tests (see Chapter 4). Two days later, he tells the concerned pair that Margaret is suffering from hyperthyroidism — her body is producing too much thyroid hormone. He begins treatment with medication, and in three weeks a definite change begins to occur. After six weeks, Margaret is just about back to normal. Margaret and Fred take the kids to Lollipop Land to make up for all the yelling.

Margaret is an excellent example of the psychological changes that occur when the body produces excessive levels of thyroid hormone. Some of these changes are

- ✔ Increased excitability and agitation
- ✔ Anxiety
- ✔ Impaired concentration
- ✔ Insomnia
- ✔ An emotional roller coaster of moods
- ✔ Outbursts of anger for no reason
- ✔ Crying spells
- ✔ A tendency to get easily distracted

Psychiatric illness is present in about 10 percent of patients with hyperthyroidism.

Other conditions seem to be indicators of hyperthyroidism but turn out not to be when doctors perform thyroid function tests. They include

- ✔ **An anxiety state or neurosis:** A compulsion to do something continuously like washing the hands, cleaning the windows, or making certain sounds or an extreme and unrealistic fear are examples.

- ✔ **Panic attacks:** Panic attacks are associated with rapid heart rates that mimic hyperthyroidism.

- ✔ **Thyrotoxicosis factitia:** This is a condition of false hyperthyroidism brought on by secret ingestion of thyroid hormone, usually by nurses. This is a psychiatric disorder.

- ✔ **Mania:** Characterized by extreme excitability and excessive activity.

When hyperthyroidism affects elderly people (who I define as anyone older than I am), the condition may actually look like hypothyroidism. An elderly patient with hyperthyroidism may feel sad and depressed, apathetic, and withdrawn from society. I explain how thyroid problems affect the elderly in Chapter 19.

The treatments for hyperthyroidism, which I describe in Chapter 6, are very effective in reversing all the mental and physical symptoms, particularly in younger people who often get the disease. If the mental symptoms are present long enough, however, curing the hyperthyroidism may not cure the manic state.

Stress is sometimes blamed for bringing on hyperthyroidism, but little objective evidence supports this claim. Hyperthyroidism may precede stress. Most people who live through severe stress don't develop hyperthyroidism. However, some evidence suggests that patients with established hyperthyroidism may do better if they're able to handle stresses that come along while they're receiving treatment and afterward. If they're able to handle the stress, then relapse is less likely.

Fighting Depression

Depression may be a symptom of a lack of thyroid hormone. On the other hand, thyroid hormone may help in the treatment of depression, even when tests indicate that the patient has enough thyroid hormone. The following sections explain the role that thyroid hormone plays in depression.

Determining if the thyroid is the cause

Depression is a prominent symptom of thyroid disease, especially hypothyroidism. Therefore, when someone receives a diagnosis of depression, determining whether a thyroid disease is the cause is important.

Studies show that most depressed people don't have hypothyroidism. However, the condition may be present in a mild form in as many as 20 percent of depressed people, more often in women than in men. If a person receives a diagnosis of hypothyroidism, a doctor should determine whether the patient is taking a drug for treatment of depression that may actually be causing hypothyroidism (see Chapter 10). Two such drugs are lithium and carbamazepine.

If a drug is responsible for hypothyroidism, a person has two options. The patient can stop taking the drug, in which case its contribution to the depression disappears, but the patient may still be depressed for other reasons. Alternately, the patient can receive thyroid hormone as treatment if the doctor feels that the drug is helping the depression a great deal and no substitute exists.

If you're receiving treatment for depression and haven't had thyroid function tests, ask your doctor to perform them.

Using thyroid hormone to treat depression

Many doctors believe that replacement thyroid hormone has a role in the treatment of depression, even when no thyroid abnormality is present.

Given by itself, thyroid hormone doesn't seem to reverse depression in a patient who doesn't have a thyroid disease. However, when a patient takes the thyroid hormone *triiodothyronine* (see Chapter 3) together with antidepressants, it can improve the effectiveness of the treatment. This is especially true when a patient is taking a class of drugs called *tricyclic antidepressants,* which have brand names like Elavil, Tofranil, Etrafon, Norpramin, and Sinequan. The thyroid hormone is particularly effective in turning people who don't respond to tricyclic antidepressants into responders. It also increases the effectiveness of those drugs when they do work.

When used to help treat depression in patients who don't have thyroid disease, the patient can stop taking the thyroid hormone after a few weeks or months, and the positive effect persists.

TSH, autoantibodies, and depression

Thyroid abnormalities are often associated with other chemical changes in the blood besides too much or too little thyroid hormone. A patient with hypothyroidism, for example, may have too much thyroid-stimulating hormone (TSH) or high levels of thyroid autoantibodies, both of which I explain in Chapter 3. Could these other chemical changes promote depression in some patients?

Doctors haven't yet found a correlation between levels of TSH and thyroid autoantibodies and depression. Patients may sometimes have high autoantibodies while their thyroid function is normal, in which case they don't experience thyroid-related depression. The level of TSH in the blood doesn't seem to impact depression either.

Current research indicates that the level of the thyroid hormones themselves affects mood, and the levels of TSH and thyroid autoantibodies don't.

Chapter 16

What's New in Thyroid Treatment?

. . . .

In This Chapter

▶ Managing hypothyroidism

▶ Zeroing in on the right dose of hormone

▶ Treating hyperthyroidism

▶ Shrinking nodules and goiters

▶ Understanding antithyroid drugs

▶ Dealing with thyrotoxic periodic paralysis

▶ Overcoming thyroid cancer

▶ Correcting iodine deficiency

. . . .

In November 2005, I visited PubMed, an online search page of the National Library of Medicine (www.pubmed.gov), and did a search for "thyroid disease." The result was more than 9,500 citations to studies done by thousands of scientists that were published in medical journals since the first edition of this book. (Thousands more studies were offered for publication but didn't get into the journals for one reason or another.) This research represents the cutting edge of medicine. But how do you stay on the cutting edge without slipping and getting sliced up? One of the reasons you bought this book is so I can do the work of sifting through the research for you.

In this chapter, you find a selection of the most important discoveries in thyroid medicine during the last couple years. Some discoveries are single studies of a subject that a similar study can revise or even overturn. You have to keep an open mind when new (and not necessarily validated) material presents itself in the future.

Knowing something about the observer is equally important as knowing what someone is observing. For instance, one of the studies about whether thyroid nodules shrink when a doctor gives a patient thyroid hormone points out that two different observers differ by as much as 50 percent in their observation of the size of the same thyroid nodule. So any change less than 50 percent can be observer "error" as much as it can be true change.

Furthermore, some observers have a self-interest in what they're observing. Unfortunately, the drug or equipment companies pay for most studies of new drugs and techniques that require special equipment. Is it likely that these companies will continue to fund researchers who constantly come up with negative findings? The best studies are those that aren't connected to specific companies, but knowing which studies don't have such connections is sometimes hard. So don't be surprised if today's magic cure-all turns out to be tomorrow's source of major side effects.

Even with no observer bias, results that are excellent when a drug is tested on a few hundred or thousand people may be very different when hundreds of thousands of people begin to use the drug.

As I write this chapter, researchers are studying just about every aspect of thyroid disease, with articles in every medical journal andnew findings that are getting ready to join the thousands of studies before them. Being up to the minute in a book isn't possible given the constraints of a publishing deadline and the amount of information coming out. If you have a particular problem that concerns you or a loved one, don't hesitate to use the enormous amount of free resources at your disposal. Go to the PubMed Web site (www.pubmed.gov), or check out your local bookstore and hospital library. And be sure to utilize the references you find in Appendix B of this book.

Treating Subclinical Hypothyroidism

One of the great debates in thyroid management is what to do about *subclinical hypothyroidism,* condition in which the patient's TSH level is slightly elevated (say to 6 or 7), the free T4 level is normal, and the patient has some nonspecific symptoms that can be the result of hypothyroidism or something else. Doctors have been studying these patients, looking for signs of low thyroid function or a response to thyroid medication, because they aren't sure whether treatment is necessary.

One study from Italy, published in the *Journal of Clinical Endocrinology and Metabolism* in March 2001, looked at the function of the heart in 20 people with subclinical hypothyroidism, all of whom showed some abnormality in heart activity. Half of the study participants were given thyroid treatment, and the other half were given a placebo. The study found that people given the thyroid-treatment drug showed an improvement in heart function, while those given a placebo showed no change. The study concluded that people with subclinical hypothyroidism have measurable abnormalities that thyroid treatment improves.

Another study from Germany, published in *Thyroid* in August 2000, looked at heart disease and heart attacks in patients with subclinical hypothyroidism. The author of the study found that these patients sustained a definite increase in heart disease and heart attacks over patients without the condition. Various tests of normal heart function, such as changes in heart rate with exercise, indicated that those functions were impaired in people with subclinical hypothyroidism. The most at-risk people were women over age 50 who smoked and had TSH levels greater than ten. Giving the study patients thyroid medication improved these functions and also improved the levels of fats in the blood. The author of this study felt that these changes justified the use of thyroid treatment in subclinical hypothyroidism. He noted, however, that giving a patient thyroid-replacement hormone tends to speed up the heart rate and may worsen chest pain, which doctors must consider when treating someone with this condition.

A more recent study in the *Annals of Family Medicine* in July 2004 provides further evidence that patients with subclinical hypothyroidism probably don't need treatment. The authors of the study looked at people who didn't have a diagnosis of hypothyroidism and weren't taking thyroid pills. They found that a subgroup of those people had subclinical hypothyroidism, which they defined as a TSH between 6.7 and 14.9 with a normal thyroxine (T4). The authors looked at the fat levels of these patients and found that although they had slightly more total cholesterol, their levels of HDL cholesterol (good cholesterol) and LDL cholesterol (bad cholesterol) as well as triglyceride were no different from people with normal TSH levels. Even the levels of total cholesterol weren't different in the two groups when adjusted for age and sex. The authors' conclusion was that subclinical hypothyroidism doesn't need to be treated, as least as far as treating to benefit fat levels in the body. They raised the possibility that other abnormalities may benefit from treatment.

This remains a very controversial topic. At this time, my bias is to treat subclinical hypothyroidism since on balance the evidence suggests that these patients suffer heart abnormalities that are improved by thyroid hormone treatment.

If you have subclinical hypothyroidism, you and your doctor should look carefully for subtle evidence of low thyroid function and treat the condition with thyroid-replacement hormone if you find such evidence. Then determining whether thyroid hormone makes a difference in those subtle findings becomes important.

Finding the Right Dose of Hormone

A question that keeps coming up among doctors who treat hypothyroidism is "What is the correct dose of thyroid medication?" Some physicians believe that lowering a patient's level of thyroid-stimulating hormone (TSH) to under five is sufficient to eliminate signs and symptoms of low thyroid function, but many patients are still symptomatic at that level. In a study published in the *Medical Journal of Australia* in February 2001, the authors show that lowering the TSH to between ⅓ and 2 may be beneficial.

Recent examinations have taken place of the question of whether combined T4 and T3 is better treatment for hypothyroidism than T4 alone. A report in the *Journal of Clinical Endocrinology and Metabolism* in May 2005 evaluated all the carefully controlled studies comparing treatment with T4 and T3 to T4 alone. Nine studies met the authors' of the report's criteria, which was that the studies were double-blind (neither the patient nor the doctor knew what the patient was getting). Only one study found that the patients given both hormones had improved mood, quality of life, and psychological measurements compared with T4 alone. Later studies didn't confirm this study. The authors conclude that no evidence supports that combined T4 and T3 have advantages over T4 alone in treating hypothyroidism.

If you're being treated for hypothyroidism and still have symptoms when your TSH level is between three and five, ask your doctor to treat you to lower that level. I believe that doing so will improve your health.

Dealing with Hyperthyroidism

Despite the availability of several treatments for hyperthyroidism (see Chapter 6), specialists aren't satisfied with any of them. Each treatment is associated with either frequent failure or undesirable side effects like hypothyroidism. The search for better therapy continues.

A study published in January 2001 in the *Journal of Clinical Endocrinology and Metabolism* emphasizes the importance of measuring calcium levels of patients with thyroid conditions, especially hyperthyroidism. This German study shows that after thyroid surgery, *hypoparathyroidism* — the loss of parathyroid function — frequently occurs and leads to low calcium levels. (A high calcium level, on the other hand, may be caused by *hyperparathyroidism* — excess parathyroid function. In this study, excess parathyroid function was also relatively common in association with thyroid disease.)

Both decreased and increased parathyroid function occur at a higher rate in patients with hyperthyroidism than in people who don't have thyroid disease. If you have hyperthyroidism, be sure to have your calcium level checked regularly.

Connecting hyperthyroidism and the heart

People with hyperthyroidism have an increase in heart disease and death. The main types of heart disease are heart failure and blood clots from the heart. Thyroid hormone has many effects on the heart, including the following:

- Increased heart rate
- Increased force of the heart
- Increased flow of blood from the heart
- Increased consumption of oxygen by the heart muscle

- Enlarged heart
- Decreased diastolic blood pressure
- Decreased blood-vessel resistance

Because of the preceding effects, especially in patients who have other heart problems, diagnosing and treating hyperthyroidism as early as possible is important. These abnormalities lead to a number of symptoms and signs. The most important are as follows:

- Feeling that the heart is beating rapidly
- Intolerance to exercise
- Shortness of breath on exertion
- Rapid heart rate
- Atrial fibrillation (a very irregular rhythm of the heart)

In the elderly, atrial fibrillation may be the only sign of hyperthyroidism. An elderly person with atrial fibrillation should always be tested for hyperthyroidism.

Blood clots are a major complication of atrial fibrillation and should be prevented by *anticoagulation,* administration of a drug that prevents clots.

Subclinical hyperthyroidism, where the T4 is normal but the TSH is low, is also associated with heart problems, including a rapid heart rate, reduced tolerance to exercise, and atrial fibrillation. Subclinlical hyperthyroid patients, especially those over 60 with other heart problems, need to receive treatment to make the TSH normal. But atrial fibrillation, if present, won't always return to a normal heart rhythm after treatment.

Amiodarone, as I note in Chapter 12, can also induce hyperthyroidism, increasing the blood-iodine level 40 times. If the patient was previously deficient in iodine, the result may be hyperthyroidism. As a result of its other properties, amiodarone can conceal hyperthyroidism. Amiodarone also stays in the body long after it's stopped, so hyperthyroidism can occur months later.

The best treatment for amiodarone-induced hyperthyroidism is to stop the amiodarone. Other treatments may be more helpful for maintaining a normal heart rhythm and can replace the amiodarone. Scientists are investigating other compounds that work as well as amiodarone but don't contain iodine.

Exploring hyperthyroid eye disease

Severe hyperthyroid eye disease, though rare, can lead to blindness. Just exactly why hyperthyroid eye disease occurs isn't clear, but researchers generally believe that it has a basis as an autoimmune disorder (see Chapter 4).

One suggestion is that thyroglobulin enters the muscles of the eyes, and antibodies react against it. A study from Italy in the journal *Thyroid* in 2001 showed that thyroglobulin can, indeed, be found in the muscle tissue of the eyes. The study demonstrated that the thyroglobulin originated in the thyroid gland, which confirms that the autoimmune reaction in the thyroid is very similar to the autoimmune reaction in the eyes. The findings of the study help bolster the argument in favor of using anti-immunity therapy for hyperthyroid eye disease, as I discuss in Chapter 6.

Hyperthyroid eye disease has a very negative impact on quality of life, even when it's moderate, which is usually the case. Severe eye disease occurs less than 5 percent of the time, but treatment works in only two-thirds of patients. The eye disease goes through three phases:

- **First phase:** High activity with redness of the eye, pain, tearing, and sensitivity to light.
- **Second phase:** Stabilization of the signs and symptoms.
- **Final phase:** Improvement of the eye disease, which becomes inactive.

The duration of these phases varies, but the eye disease burns out within a couple of years. Steroids are helpful during the first active phase.

Steroids given intravenously are more effective than steroids by mouth for thyroid eye disease. Steroids can be injected right into the muscles around the eye and are effective there. Doctors give IV steroids in very high amounts, which can cause liver damage. IV steroids are effective about 90 percent of the time, while liver damage occurs only 1 percent of the time.

If steroids aren't successful, then doctors perform orbital radiation therapy. This therapy is successful about 60 percent of the time. Using both steroids and orbital radiation at the same time is even better than either alone.

Recent studies of other therapies, including drugs called somatostatin analogs and antioxidants, haven't shown that these therapies are effective. Antioxidants may be useful for mild eye disease but not moderate or severe forms.

Three factors are definitely important in the progression of hyperthyroid eye disease, and should be managed as strongly as possible:

- **Cigarette smoking:** Cigarette smoking not only promotes the development of eye disease but blocks the effectiveness of steroid and orbital–radiation therapy treatments. Quitting smoking is probably the most important preventive measure in this disease.
- **Active thyroid dysfunction:** Active thyroid dysfunction, whether hyperthyroidism or hypothyroidism, promotes the progression of eye disease. Both conditions need to be corrected as soon as possible.
- **Radiation therapy:** This hyperthyroidism treatment causes progression of the eye disease as well. A course of steroids can prevent this progression.

Assessing Goiters and Nodules

Goiters and nodules remain a very common problem in thyroid medicine. Newer studies are changing how doctors manage patients with these conditions. Ultrasound studies pick up nodules in the necks of as many as 67 percent of people who don't have a nodule by physical examination.

Differentiating benign from malignant nodules

The fine-needle biopsy remains the best way to diagnose a thyroid nodule, but it's much more effective when guided by ultrasound, especially when the nodule is very small (less than 1.5 centimeters in size). The fine-needle biopsy guided by ultrasound permits a correct diagnosis of cancer 60 percent of the time compared to 40 percent when not guided by ultrasound.

It's not possible to make a definite diagnosis about 10 percent of the time with fine-needle biopsy. Of these 10 percent, only 15 percent turn out to be cancers. The problem is how to pick out that 15 percent that will need surgery; the other 85 percent can be followed medically. Two chemical markers have recently shown some promise in telling the difference. Doctors can assess both of these chemical markers in the clinical laboratory. They may become generally available if they prove their success in further studies. The two chemical markers are as follows:

- **Human bone marrow endothelial cell-1:** This chemical is an antibody that seems to be specific for thyroid malignancy. When cells are exposed to this antibody attached to a substance that causes staining, strongly positive staining occurs for the papillary and follicular cancers, but little or no staining for benign tissues.

- **Galectin-3:** Galectin-3 is found in tissues of patients with thyroid cancer but not in those with nonmalignant thyroid tissue. Cancerous tissues stain positive for galectin-3, and those that aren't don't stain. Ninety-five percent of tumors stain positive. Very few malignant thyroid glands don't have this marker.

Doctors can watch and restudy small thyroid nodules less than 1.5 centimeters (0.6 inches) that high-resolution ultrasound discovers. Most of the nodules are "incidentalomas," with no clinical significance. The decision as to whether they should be biopsied is still controversial. My opinion is that careful monitoring with high-resolution ultrasound is sufficient because most of the nodules, even if they turn out to be microcancers, don't change in size over five years.

Recent studies have taken up the question of whether to measure calcitonin routinely to diagnose medullary thyroid cancer. This cancer makes up only

5 percent of thyroid cancers. Calculations suggest that screening routinely costs $20,000 to pick up one malignancy. If the level of the calcitonin isn't high enough to make a definite diagnosis, the cost for more testing is even greater. Therefore doctors don't recommend it.

Performing surgery after ethanol injections

One of the newer techniques for eliminating nodules in the thyroid is the injection of ethanol directly into the nodules (see Chapter 7). When this technique was brand new, it raised the question of whether surgeons would face complications if they had to operate on patients who had ethanol injections. For example, a surgeon may need to operate if the ethanol fails to eliminate a nodule, if a doctor suspects that a nodule is malignant, or if a nodule is compressing the trachea. A 2000 study in the periodical *Thyroid* reported that surgeons didn't encounter any special surgical problems while operating on the thyroids of 13 people who had received injections.

One suggestion for improving this technique of injecting ethanol directly into the nodules is to remove the fluid with a second puncture in an attempt to reduce pain. In a study reported in the *American Journal of Neuroradiology* in September 2005, the authors wrote that the second puncture greatly prolonged the procedure, wasn't appreciated by the patients, and didn't result in reduced pain or more frequent success in destroying the nodule. The authors recommended against it.

Another study in the *Endocrine Journal* in August 2005 evaluated the long-term effects of ethanol injections in three types of nodules: benign cystic nodules (which contain fluid), toxic nodules (which make the patient hyperthyroid), and solitary nodules (which aren't overactive). The authors of the study found that they were successful in partially or completely eliminating cystic nodules and solitary nodules but were successful in treating toxic nodules only 1 in 24 times, so this technique may not work for a toxic nodule.

Serious complications of ethanol injections are extremely rare. As more and more physicians become skilled in using them, ethanol injections may become the treatment of choice for cystic nodules and nontoxic solitary thyroid nodules.

The best assurance that ethanol injections don't cause problems down the road is to do your research and make certain that the person giving you an injection is highly skilled and experienced. You should always receive ethanol injections under ultrasound observation.

Shrinking goiters and nodules

Doctors have used thyroid hormone for decades to treat goiters; the hope has always been that the hormone will help to shrink the goiter. Most recent studies have shown that goiters respond little if at all to thyroid hormone.

In a study published in 2001 in the *Journal of Clinical Endocrinology and Metabolism* from the Netherlands, the authors compared thyroid hormone to radioactive iodine in the treatment of goiters. They used ultrasound to measure goiter size, and they measured the thyroid function of all test patients.

The researchers found that patients who received radioactive iodine had, on average, a 44 percent reduction in goiter size, while those patients who took thyroid hormone had a reduction of 1 percent. Only 1 of 29 patients didn't respond to radioactive iodine, while 16 of 28 had no response to thyroid hormone. Almost half the patients who got radioactive iodine developed hypothyroidism, while 10 of 28 taking thyroid hormone had symptoms of hyperthyroidism. In addition, those patients on thyroid hormone developed increased bone turnover and a loss of bone mineral density. The conclusion of this study is that radioactive iodine is more effective and better tolerated than thyroid hormone in the treatment of goiters.

If you have a goiter and want to get rid of it, you're much better off with radioactive iodine than thyroid hormone. The days of using thyroid hormone for this condition may be numbered.

On the other hand, benign thyroid nodules respond to thyroid hormone by shrinking, according to studies that looked at large numbers of studies of this question. One of the problems in interpreting whether shrinkage occurs is the difference between different observers. In a study done in Germany and reported in *Thyroid* in October 2005, three different observers evaluated the size of the nodules in a group of patients. A variability of 49 percent existed between observers of the same thyroid nodule. This variability means that any change less than 50 percent is as likely to be due to the observer as to actual shrinkage. This study brings into question all those reports that thyroid hormone shrinks nodules when the shrinkage noted is less than 50 percent.

Unless a change of 50 percent or greater occurs, saying a true change in the size of at thyroid nodule has occurred isn't possible. Until we have a definitive answer to the question of whether thyroid hormone can shrink benign thyroid nodules, using thyroid hormone in an attempt to shrink benign nodules is worthwhile.

Using Antithyroid Drugs Properly

The two antithyroid drugs available in the United States, propylthiouricil (PTU) and methimazole (tapazole), are thought to have slightly different actions, but their clinical effectiveness is about the same. PTU not only blocks the formation of the thyroid hormones within the thyroid but also blocks the conversion of T4 into T3. Methimazole has the former but not the latter activity. In clinical practice, patients do just as well with either drug.

Studies show that these drugs block the autoimmune reaction from taking place and restore the body to its more normal state. This effect makes them more useful in treatment than surgery or radioactive iodine (RAI), both of which may worsen the autoimmunity. However, the rate at which the hyperthyroidism returns is up to 50 percent, while surgery and RAI usually accomplish a permanent cure.

No change you can measure tells you whether a patient will eventually remain normal or have a return of hyperthyroidism. Neither the size of the thyroid, the level of thyroid hormone, nor the level of antibodies can predict the eventual outcome.

PTU and methimazole can cause some serious side effects, the principal one being *agranulocytosis* — failure of production of white blood cells, which usually occurs within the first 90 days of treatment. Switching from one drug to the other may not help because the drugs have similar properties, so that a reaction to one may occur with the other (a *cross-reaction*). Cross-reacting occurs in about 1 in 300 patients.

If you have a sore throat or fever when taking an antithyroid drug, stop taking it and notify your physician. Sudden onset of high fever, chills, and severe weakness is especially worrisome. A drug called granulocyte colony-stimulating factor may help to reverse this serious problem. Minor side effects include rashes, pain in the joints, a slight reduction in white blood cells, and stomach upset in about 5 percent of the people who take these drugs.

In pregnancy, PTU is the preferred drug because women have reported abnormalities of the fetus with methimazole. Both drugs cross the placenta and should be used at the smallest possible dose to protect the fetus. Doctors find both drugs in the mother's breast milk but in very tiny amounts. Babies of women taking these drugs aren't physically or mentally abnormal.

Handling Thyrotoxic Periodic Paralysis

Thyrotoxic periodic paralysis is a disorder that occurs when a patient, especially an Asian patient, has hyperthyroidism of any cause, including Graves' disease, toxic nodular goiter, excessive thyroxine use, or a solitary toxic thyroid nodule. Some new information has been discovered about periodic paralysis in the last few years. Thyrotoxic periodic paralysis has the following characteristics:

- ✔ Thyrotoxic periodic paralysis occurs between the ages of 20 and 40.

- ✔ Thyrotoxic periodic paralysis is much more common in men (20:1) compared to women, despite the greater frequency of all types of hyperthyroidism in women.

- ✔ Two percent of Asians but 0.2 percent of Caucasians suffer from it.

- ✔ Patients have muscle aches, cramps, and muscle stiffness before an attack.

- ✔ The attack consists of severe weakness, sometimes progressing to paralysis.

- ✔ Serum potassium levels during an attack are below the normal range but not always.

- ✔ Hard exercise or eating a lot of carbohydrates can bring on an attack.

- ✔ Patients may not know they have hyperthyroidism.

- ✔ Spontaneous improvement occurs within hours to two days, but abnormal heart rhythms and respiratory failure may kill the patient.

- ✔ Between attacks, patients are free of symptoms.

The condition results from a sudden shift of potassium from the bloodstream into cells. Exactly why this shift happens isn't clear. The total potassium in the body of these patients is normal, so immediate treatment is directed to restore the potassium in the bloodstream without overloading the patient. When this treatment is done, rapid improvement takes place. The danger is that the potassium in the cells will be released, leading to the patient having too much potassium in the blood — which happens in up to 70 percent of patients given potassium, unless the dose is kept fairly low. Lower doses work just as well and avoid excess potassium.

Permanent treatment consists of bringing the hyperthyroidism under control with antithyroid drugs, radioactive iodine, or surgery. Propranolol also works to reverse the movement of potassium. Giving potassium between attacks doesn't work.

While waiting for definitive treatment, patients should avoid precipitating activities, such as

- ✔ Heavy exercise
- ✔ Trauma
- ✔ Cold exposure
- ✔ Infection
- ✔ Emotional stress

Thyrotoxic periodic paralysis isn't hard to treat. The key is recognizing the condition, especially when the patient has previously had hyperthyroidism.

Taking New Approaches to Thyroid Cancer

Not surprisingly, much of the research concerning advances in thyroid disease centers around thyroid cancer. The following sections provide you with some of the more provocative and important studies of the last year or two. Undoubtedly, many more studies are to come.

Understanding the impact of radioactive iodine exposure

More than 15 years after the nuclear disaster in Chernobyl, researchers still follow up with the children who were exposed to excessive radioactive iodine. In the *World Journal of Surgery* in 2000, a group of Russian scientists published the results of surgery on 330 children who had thyroid cancer after Chernobyl. The cancers tended to develop rapidly after exposure, were more aggressive than typical thyroid cancers, and spread early to distant sites in the body. The patients were treated by *total thyroidectomy* (removal of the entire thyroid), followed by radioactive iodine treatment and suppression of TSH. The authors of the study emphasize that doctors will find many more cases of thyroid cancer among the children of Chernobyl, who need to be monitored over the next several decades.

Are any environmental factors protective in the situation of radioactive-iodine exposure? A study in *Environmental Health* in 2000 looked at people in Germany who were exposed to radioactive iodine. The study confirmed that drinking coffee and eating cruciferous vegetables like broccoli reduce the risk of developing cancer in people exposed to radioactive iodine. If a patient had a goiter prior to the exposure, or if he consumed decaffeinated coffee instead of caffeinated, he was at increased risk for malignant or benign tumors.

These researchers also found that tomato consumption was a risk factor for malignant disease. They suggest that off-season tomatoes coming from areas where the farmers are careless about the use of chemicals may promote the development of thyroid cancer.

There are a number of recent reports of the children exposed to radioactive iodine at Chernobyl. The best was in May 2005 in the *Journal of the National Cancer Institute.* The authors reported several new and important findings:

✔ Diets deficient in iodine increase the chance of radiation-induced thyroid cancer occurring.

✔ The more radiation exposure, the more thyroid cancer.

✔ Boys and girls have the same risk of developing thyroid cancer.

✔ Use of dietary supplements rich in iodine reduces the chance of getting thyroid cancer.

✔ Children who were iodine deficient but were given iodine supplements after exposure to radioactive iodine were one-third as likely to get thyroid cancer as those not given iodine after exposure.

The effect of iodine supplements may be good news for populations where no iodine deficiency exists. This could not be studied in Russia because all exposed areas were iodine deficient. But if there is sufficient iodine in the diet, the occurrence of thyroid cancer after exposure may be low, and giving iodine even weeks to months after exposure may reduce the instances of thyroid cancer even more.

Blocking estrogen to slow tumor growth

One source of bewilderment about thyroid cancer is that it occurs more often in women than in men. One study suggests that the reason may lie with the fact that women make estrogen as their primary sex hormone, and estrogen may stimulate thyroid tumor-cell growth. The authors of a study in the March 2001 *Journal of Clinical Endocrinology and Metabolism* describe an experiment in which estrogen was shown to stimulate tumor cells and, to a lesser extent, benign cells. (Estrogen activates a metabolic pathway that leads to much greater growth activity in both malignant and benign cells.) When patients received a drug that blocks estrogen action, the tumor cells were no longer stimulated.

Predicting thyroid cancer

Is it possible to predict the future occurrence of thyroid cancer? The authors of a study from Iceland present an analysis of blood taken many years before the diagnosis of thyroid cancer was made in 164 patients. Their study was published in *Acta Oncologica* in 2000. The authors report that levels of *thyroglobulin,* the chemical that resides in the thyroid and that doctors monitor when following thyroid-cancer patients, can also be found in much elevated levels up to 15 years before the diagnosis of thyroid cancer is made. In contrast, the authors found no difference in the blood levels of TSH or thyroid hormone in the thyroid-cancer patients compared to patients who never had thyroid cancer.

Detecting residual thyroid cancer

Another important recent advance is in the ability to detect thyroid cancer that remains after surgery. Thyroglobulin plays a major role in detecting remaining cancer. Another important tool that doctors often use is the whole–body radioactive iodine scan, which can locate active thyroid tissue. The limitation of the scan is that it can't locate thyroid tissue that isn't making thyroid hormone. Sometimes a thyroglobulin level is high, indicating that active thyroid tissue is present, but the body scan is negative.

A newer type of scan called a *PET scan* is able to localize thyroid tissue that isn't functioning well as thyroid tissue but is very metabolically active. A study in *Advances in Internal Medicine* in 2001 reviews the successful use of the PET scan for this purpose. The study points out that the need still exists for new agents that attack these tumor tissues when they don't concentrate radioactive iodine.

If you've had thyroid cancer and discover a new growth that doesn't concentrate radioactive iodine on a thyroid scan, ask your doctor about the possibility of having a PET scan.

Following up on thyroid-cancer treatment

Does the thyroid-cancer patient need to be followed for life, or does the patient reach a point at which she can be considered cured of the disease? The authors of a study in *Annales Chirurgiae* in 2000 attempt to answer this question.

The study's authors contend that studying patients for seven months after thyroid surgery is necessary. At that time, patients can be divided into groups:

- ✔ **Group I:** Patients with microcancers
- ✔ **Group II:** Patients with no lymph-node involvement or metastases and normal thyroglobulin
  - • **A:** Younger than age 45
  - • **B:** Age 45 or older
- ✔ **Group III:** Patients with cancer with lymph-node involvement but a normal thyroglobulin level
- ✔ **Group IV:** Patients who have extension of the cancer beyond local lymph nodes or an elevated thyroglobulin level

Table 16-1 shows the survival rates for these groups.

Table 16-1	Survival Rates for Thyroid-Cancer Patients	
Length of Time after Surgery	*10 Years*	*15 Years*
Group I	100%	100%
Group II A	100%	100%
Group II B	96%	92%
Group III	100%	100%
Group IV	86%	73%

The latest time of a recurrence in groups I and II A was at 12 years. For groups II B, III, and IV, tumors were discovered as late as 16 years after treatment. The study emphasizes that patients must have thyroglobulin tests and whole-body scanning every five years. Doctors need to follow patients in groups I and II A for up to 15 years; they should follow other patients for 20 years before saying with certainty that the disease is eliminated. If a recurrence happens, then the doctor needs to follow the patient another ten years with no more cancer before declaring that she is cancer-free.

Knowing what to expect from medullary thyroid cancer

Medullary thyroid cancer (MTC) is different from thyroid cell cancers like follicular or papillary cancer (see Chapter 8). MTC arises from the C-cells in the thyroid, and doctors can't detect it with radioactive iodine.

A study from Finland in the *Annales Chiarurgiae Gynecologica* in 2000 provides helpful information about the prognosis of medullary thyroid cancer. The authors divided their cases into hereditary (inherited) MTC and sporadic (not inherited) MTC. They found that sporadic MTC is a much deadlier disease than hereditary MTC.

Both groups were treated with total thyroidectomy and lymph-node dissection. The group with sporadic MTC had a ten-year survival rate of 57.9 percent. Within the group of patients with sporadic MTC, those who had recurrent cancer in their lymph nodes that doctors found and removed had a survival rate of only 51.4 percent at ten years. More important predictors of survival than lymph nodes were distant metastases and local spread of the cancer in the neck.

Using recombinant TSH with thyroid-cancer patients

Recombinant TSH is a valuable tool both for the detection and treatment of residual thyroid cancer. Before recombinant TSH, in order to be tested for residual cancer with a total body scan, patients had to be taken off thyroid-replacement hormone for four weeks or longer to allow their tissues to become hypothyroid. Going off hormone replacement greatly enhances the uptake of radioactive iodine, allowing for a more accurate scan of thyroid tissue.

Doctors have always been concerned that this time off the thyroid hormone allows cancer to grow more rapidly. For this reason, they use recombinant TSH to stimulate uptake and identify cancer recurrences without needing patients to stop taking thyroid hormone.

A group in Massachusetts, writing in the *Journal of Clinical Endocrinology and Metabolism* in 2001, explored the dosages of recombinant TSH required for optimal effect. The group looked at patients' thyroglobulin levels as well as TSH, T4, and T3. The group found that a dose of 0.3 milligrams of recombinant TSH produced the maximal increase in thyroglobulin and radioactive-iodine uptake. Going higher than 0.3 milligrams didn't increase the effect of treatment.

Another group from New York showed in the *European Journal of Endocrinology* in 2001 that using recombinant TSH was just as good as taking patients off thyroid medication in stimulating thyroglobulin secretion and radioactive-iodine uptake. The group concluded that, in terms of diagnostic accuracy, preparing patients for a scan with recombinant TSH is equivalent to taking patients off thyroid hormone.

Finally, doctors can use recombinant TSH to stimulate thyroid cancer to take up radioactive iodine in order to destroy it. In a study published in 2001 in the *European Journal of Endocrinology,* scientists used recombinant TSH to increase uptake. They noted that the recombinant TSH was free of side effects other than mild nausea. The results were excellent. The thyroid-cancer treatment was as effective as with patients who were taken off thyroid hormone therapy prior to treatment. By using recombinant TSH, patients avoid the discomfort of being without thyroid hormone for weeks and avoid becoming hypothyroid.

Checking testicular function after radiation therapy

Scientists don't know whether radiation therapy to ablate remaining thyroid tissue after surgery for thyroid cancer or for treatment of recurring cancer leads to damage to the production of sperm. The authors of a study in the

Annals of Andrology in May–June 2005 showed a reduction in sperm production and evidence of damage to the testes, especially after more than one treatment with radioactive iodine. Levels of a hormone called FSH rose after radiation treatment and declined over time, indicating that the testicles were damaged but recovered. Patients who got several radiation treatments didn't show this recovery.

If you require several treatments with large-dose radioactive iodine, protect your future as a father by banking sperm before you receive the treatments.

Testing calcium levels after cancer surgery

In the process of removing the thyroid gland because of thyroid cancer, patients inevitably experience some trauma to the parathyroid glands that lie on the back of the thyroid lobes. Most of the time, these glands recover, but sometimes the trauma results in permanent hypoparathyroidism, which causes a patient to have low calcium levels.

In a study published in the *Journal of the European Society of Surgery and Oncology* in 2000, researchers wanted to establish how long cancer patients take to recover their normal calcium levels. The researchers also wanted to determine how often treatment is necessary. The study showed that if a patient had just one lobe of the thyroid removed, even though two of the parathyroid glands weren't touched, the patient experienced a 10-percent drop in the level of calcium. Thirty-four percent of patients with this type of surgery required some calcium treatment because the level fell too low. Their calcium levels returned to normal within one week after surgery and remained normal.

When patients had both sides of the thyroid operated on, as expected, the operation had more effect on the parathyroids and the calcium. Calcium levels decreased 15 percent on average; some patients experienced severely low levels early in their recovery. The calcium decline was greater if the number of preserved parathyroid glands was fewer. Fifteen percent of these patients needed calcium treatment for 2 to 7 days, 26 percent for 8 to 180 days, and 9 percent for longer than a year. Only 1 patient of 82 required permanent treatment for low calcium after a single thyroid surgery on both sides. One of four patients who had several thyroid surgeries needed permanent calcium treatment.

Understanding familial papillary thyroid cancer

In the last few years, specialists have recognized an inherited familial form of papillary thyroid cancer. The familial form differs from sporadic thyroid cancer in a number of ways:

✔ The age of onset is younger (age 38 rather than age 45 to 50).

✔ Females are only twice as likely to get it.

✔ Many locations in the thyroid tend to be involved.

✔ Benign nodules are present more often.

✔ The cancer recurs a little more often.

At present, identifying carriers of the abnormal gene who don't have symptoms isn't possible. Removal of the thyroid in advance of the development of thyroid cancer isn't recommended because carriers can't be found, and the tumor grows very slowly.

Tackling Iodine-Deficiency Disease

When you consider the numbers of people affected by iodine-deficiency disease (see Chapter 12), you may think that most of the articles on thyroid disease concern themselves with this topic. But iodine-deficiency disease isn't a common problem in the United States, so American scientists, who make up the majority of the world's investigators, don't tend to write about it. Still, plenty is going on in this area. This section describes the more important recent studies on iodine-deficiency disease.

Recognizing the importance of selenium

Selenium is an element that plays a role in thyroid-hormone production because it's part of an enzyme responsible for converting T4 into T3. Until now, researchers and doctors have generally believed that selenium deficiency alone doesn't cause hypothyroidism; only when an iodine deficiency exists does selenium deficiency contribute to the disease. However, a study from the journal *Biological Trace Element Research* in 2000 contradicts this belief. The study's authors describe three girls who had hypothyroidism due to lack of selenium alone. When given replacement selenium, all returned to normal thyroid function. This study is the first description of hypothyroidism due to lack of selenium alone.

Writing in *Endocrine Reviews* in September 2005, the authors provided further information about the importance of selenium in the thyroid and other endocrine tissues. In the thyroid, selenium protects thyroid cells from damage from hydrogen peroxide produced when the body makes thyroid hormone. Selenium is also present in higher amounts in endocrine tissues compared to other tissues. When selenium deficiency exists in the rest of the body, selenium is maintained in normal amounts in the thyroid and these other endocrine tissues. Although tiny quantities of selenium are necessary, selenium plays an important role in the body.

Selenium received further approval in a paper in the *Journal of Endocrinology* in March 2005. Selenium in an enzyme controls the amount of the T3 by removing iodine from the hormone. Men who are deficient in selenium have low sperm production and poor sperm quality, leading to infertility. Selenium also helps to reduce blood glucose and prevents the negative effects of diabetes on the heart and the kidneys.

Although selenium deficiency reduces the response of iodine-deficient patients to lipiodol (a type of iodized oil; see the following section for more), overall it doesn't prevent iodine from restoring thyroid function.

Using iodized oil for goiters

Doctors commonly use iodized oil injection to treat iodine deficiency and prevent goiter formation in areas of the world where iodine deficiency persists (see Chapter 12). The authors of a study in *Medicine* in 2001 wanted to consider any potential problems associated with lipiodol, a type of iodized oil. When lipiodol was given to a person who already had a multinodular goiter, that person sometimes became hyperthyroid. The hyperthyroidism tended to be mild and didn't last long. If the patient was a pregnant woman, the iodine sometimes entered the bloodstream of the fetus but didn't affect the fetus. The study confirms that using iodized oil for the replacement of iodine is a safe, cheap, and effective way to treat iodine deficiency.

Iodine deficiency and hypothyroidism also contribute to hearing difficulties in children. A study in the *Journal of Endocrinological Investigation* in July 2005 showed that supplementation of iodine with iodized oil can greatly reduce the hearing loss that these children suffer. That the supplementation be continuous is important. Ten years of giving iodine improved hearing almost to normal in a large group of iodine-deficient children.

Doctors usually give lipiodol by injection, which requires all kinds of precautions and equipment that may not be available in rural areas where it's needed most. The authors of a study in the *Journal of Endocrinological Investigation* in 2003 showed that oral lipiodol once a year gives prolonged protection from iodine deficiency just as effectively as intramuscular lipiodol, as shown by increased urinary iodine. Intramuscular lipiodol lasts for two to three years in the body, while oral lipiodol must be renewed once a year. But the ease of administration and lack of a need for special equipment may make oral lipiodol the preferred route of administration.

In some areas of the world, people aren't only iodine deficient but iron deficient as well. A Swiss group studied whether iodine supplementation would be successful despite iron deficiency. The group reported in the *American Journal of Clinical Nutrition* in July 2000 that iodine would eliminate goiters in children who were iron deficient. Restoring iron stores is necessary before using iodine.

Iodized oil does have some side effects associated with it. Iodized oil causes a rash in a small percentage of people who get it, but the rash doesn't last long. Iodized oil can bring on hyperthyroidism in some patients, but the incidence is less than 1 percent. The hyperthyroidism is mild and doesn't last long but may require the use of antithyroid medication for a period of time. Iodized oil can also bring on hypothyroidism, again with a very low incidence of less than 1 percent, which is treated with thyroid hormone.

Increasing the intelligence of babies born to hypothyroid mothers

Babies born to hypothyroid mothers tend to have low intelligence. In a study done in Taiwan and published in the *Journal of the Formosa Medical Association* in 2001, researchers looked at the level of intelligence of 62 babies of hypothyroid mothers and sought an early screening to avoid retardation. They found that the level of T4 at the time of diagnosis was a good predictor of the future intelligence of the baby. By measuring T4 at birth and giving thyroid-replacement hormone, the researchers improved the outlook of these babies in terms of their intelligence.

The screening of babies with TSH tests doesn't always discover newborn hypothyroidism, especially when the baby has very low birth weight. In a study in the *Journal of Pediatrics* in November 2003, the authors found that some babies with very low birth weight, especially those with heart disease, had normal TSH values at birth but elevated values when tested weeks or months later. The authors recommended TSH tests for all babies with very low birth weight.

In another paper, this time in the journal *Clinical Biochemistry* in September 2004, the authors looked at the TSH at different times after birth. TSH taken within the first 24 hours wasn't reliable for making a diagnosis of hypothyroidism. The best time to do a TSH test is at 48 hours after birth. If it is taken earlier, the cutoff value for an abnormal TSH has to be set too high, and some truly hypothyroid babies will be missed.

Chapter 17

The Thyroid and Pregnancy

*I*n the last ten years, doctors have learned a lot about how the thyroid functions during pregnancy. This new level of understanding makes a tremendous difference in your ability to have a healthy baby, even if you have a thyroid disorder. If you and your doctor keep up with the latest information available, thyroid disease shouldn't seriously impact your ability to have a healthy baby.

This chapter is about the wonderful state of pregnancy, with particular reference to how it changes thyroid function and how abnormalities of thyroid function affect the pregnancy. As I explain in earlier chapters, thyroid disease is very common among women. Many women come into a pregnancy with a thyroid condition, whether they know it or not. Others develop a thyroid condition during pregnancy. For the health of both the mother and the fetus, detecting the condition and treating it appropriately are important. This chapter explains how you and your doctor should monitor your thyroid function during pregnancy and describes some of the consequences that could occur from not managing a thyroid condition.

The Normal Thyroid During Pregnancy

Three important changes occur in a woman's body during pregnancy, leading to a much greater need for iodine:

- ✔ Early in pregnancy, the flow of blood to a woman's kidneys increases, resulting in more clearing of iodine and a greater loss of iodine through the urine.

- ✔ Because the fetus can't make thyroid hormone at first, it takes thyroid hormone from the mother through the placenta.

- ✔ The growing fetus starts to make its own thyroid hormone after a while and needs iodine to do so.

At the same time, as a result of increases in hormones, particularly estrogen, the mother makes much more thyroxine-binding globulin — a protein that transports thyroid hormone through the blood — than she used to. (In fact, the concentration doubles.) She also makes a form of thyroxine-binding globulin that leaves the circulation much more slowly. This substance takes up a lot of the thyroid hormone that the mother's body is making, which leads to an even greater need for iodine to make more.

The daily requirement for iodine in pregnancy is at least 250 micrograms per day, a figure recommended at a meeting of the World Health Organization in 2005. In much of the United States, Canada, and Western Europe, this requirement is generally met. However, in other parts of the world, getting this increased amount of iodine can be a problem (check out Chapter 12 for more on iodine deficiency).

The increased need for iodine has important consequences for pregnant women in iodine-deficient areas:

- ✔ If the woman is depending on iodized salt for her iodine needs and has to be salt-restricted, she may quickly become iodine deficient.

- ✔ Some areas thought to be iodine sufficient are discovered to be low in iodine when the greater needs of pregnancy must be taken into account, even in areas of the United States.

- ✔ Different areas of the same country may differ greatly in the amount of iodine in the diet.

Iodine levels must be constantly monitored in areas where iodine is deficient, even though supplemental iodine is being given.

If you're hypothyroid and take thyroid hormone pills, understanding all these changes is important. To maintain normal thyroid function, you probably need to increase your dose of thyroid-hormone replacement early in pregnancy, based on your level of thyroid-stimulating hormone (TSH).

While all these changes are happening, the placenta — the tissue that connects the fetus to the mother — is making a lot of a hormone called *human chorionic gonadotrophin* (HCG). HCG has some parts that look very much like TSH. It reaches the mother's thyroid and starts to stimulate it into making more thyroid hormone, just as TSH does. As a result, the mother's level of free T4 rises, causing a fall in the amount of TSH her body produces. If she is having twins, her HCG level can be especially high and can persist for weeks. As I show you in the section "Hyperthyroidism in Pregnancy," later in this chapter, the result may be a form of hyperthyroidism.

A condition called *hyperemesis gravidarum* occurs early in pregnancy. The symptoms are severe nausea, vomiting, and dehydration, which may require hospitalization. Doctors believe that the temporary increase in thyroid hormone stimulated by HCG along with the significant increase of estrogen that results from the same HCG stimulation cause this condition. Morning sickness may be a milder form of the same condition. The amount of vomiting is directly proportional to the level of HCG and T4 and inversely proportional to the level of TSH.

These changes in levels of thyroid hormone and TSH mean that the usual way of defining normal thyroid function, a normal free T4 and a normal TSH, doesn't apply in pregnancy. TSH is actually below the lower level of the normal range in one-fifth of healthy pregnant women. So far, no ranges for normal for these tests during pregnancy have been established, but doctors agree that a temporary rise in free T4 occurs in the first trimester and a decrease to normal from that level in the second and third trimesters.

The need for more thyroid hormone as well as the increased stimulation of the thyroid gland by the HCG causes the thyroid to enlarge, especially in areas where iodine is deficient. A goiter is one consequence of the pregnancy. The thyroid may enlarge symmetrically, or it may form nodules. The enlarged gland and the nodules don't necessarily shrink away when the pregnancy ends, which may be one explanation for the great increase in thyroid disease in women compared to men.

One of the confusing aspects of pregnancy with respect to thyroid disease is that many signs and symptoms of a normal pregnancy are similar to the findings in hyperthyroidism. These signs and symptoms include

- A rapid heart rate
- Intolerance to heat
- Tiredness
- Anxiety
- Trouble sleeping
- Sweating

Your weight is the biggest clue as to whether hyperthyroidism is an issue. Most pregnant women gain weight throughout their pregnancy (although some women lose a few pounds initially if they experience vomiting). A hyperthyroid woman often doesn't gain weight and sometimes loses weight during pregnancy.

Pregnancy and Hypothyroidism

The fact that a mother's body doesn't reject a fetus as a foreign intruder just as it would reject any foreign invasion is a miracle. (Even a few foreign cells injected inside your body wouldn't last long.) The fact that the mother's body doesn't reject the fetus is evidence that a general decline in immunity takes place during pregnancy.

As a result, women who have autoimmune diseases prior to pregnancy often discover that they improve during a pregnancy, with their condition returning to its original state again after delivery. This is true for women with either hypothyroidism or hyperthyroidism that results from an autoimmune condition — the most common cause of both hypothyroidism and hyperthyroidism in the United States and Europe (see Chapters 5 and 6). If levels of antibodies are measured, they are found to fall throughout the pregnancy. Along with this is a general fall in the inflammation that is found in most autoimmune diseases.

After the pregnancy, a woman may experience a rebound in levels of autoantibodies, and the diseases that they represent may worsen.

Decreased fertility

If a woman has hypothyroidism that goes untreated, she will probably have a difficult time becoming pregnant because the hypothyroidism decreases her fertility. In a study of infertile women in Finland published in *Gynecological Endocrinology* in 2000, 5 percent were hypothyroid. If the hypothyroid woman does become pregnant, the risk of a miscarriage is much higher than if she didn't have a thyroid condition.

Antithyroid antibodies, which are present in women with autoimmune thyroid disease, are associated with an increased risk of miscarriage. They may not be the cause of the miscarriage, but they are present much more often in women who miscarry than in the general population of women.

If you suffer one or more miscarriages, be sure to have your doctor check your thyroid function.

If you're hypothyroid and aren't receiving thyroid-hormone replacement, you may suffer from a number of obstetric complications if you become pregnant. Complications may include high blood pressure, problems with the placental connection to the fetus, and problems with delivery. You can avoid all these complications with proper treatment of the thyroid.

Iodine deficiency

A mother with an iodine deficiency during pregnancy can't make sufficient thyroid hormone for herself and her fetus. (The fetus gets the thyroid hormone it needs from its mother up until the 20th week of the pregnancy.) As a result, the mother is chronically stimulated by TSH to make more thyroid hormone, and she develops a goiter.

A goiter doesn't develop in the mother during a normal pregnancy. If a mother develops a goiter, she is experiencing iodine deficiency, hypothyroidism, or hyperthyroidism.

The mother's goiter may not fully shrink after delivery, when her iodine needs are reduced. This may partly explain the much greater incidence of thyroid enlargement in women when compared with men.

Iodine deficiency also strongly affects the fetus. It may develop a goiter as well, and it may suffer from abnormal brain development (see Chapter 12). A goiter in the fetus can result in problems during delivery.

Laboratory tests show that iodine-deficient pregnant women have

- ✔ Reduced T4 and, if severe, reduced T3 hormone levels
- ✔ Increased TSH
- ✔ Increased ratios of T3 to T4, because the thyroid begins to prefer making T3
- ✔ Increased thyroglobulin

Autoimmune hypothyroidism

Autoimmune thyroid disease is much more common in iodine-rich countries than in iodine-deficient countries. Most cases of hypothyroidism in pregnancy result from this disease. Autoimmune hypothyroidism probably affects between 2 percent and 4 percent of pregnant women at some time during their pregnancy. Pregnant women with type 1 diabetes have an even higher incidence of chronic autoimmune thyroiditis and hypothyroidism.

Understanding the risks to the mother and fetus

If lab tests show that a woman has thyroid autoantibodies — even if her doctor doesn't diagnose her as hypothyroid because her thyroid function tests are normal — she is at an increased risk for a miscarriage. Doctors aren't clear why this is so. One suggestion is that these women really have mild hypothyroidism despite the normal test results. Another is that the autoantibodies are just a marker for other autoimmune diseases that may be responsible for the miscarriage. A third hypothesis is that miscarriage in these autoimmune mothers is meant to prevent the transmission of autoimmune diseases to the next generation.

The thyroid autoantibodies can be transmitted to the fetus through the placenta, causing hypothyroidism in the fetus. Usually if the mother is hypothyroid and is receiving adequate treatment with thyroid hormone, enough thyroid hormone gets to the fetus to prevent hypothyroidism. If the baby is born with hypothyroidism, the pediatrician places the baby on thyroid-hormone replacement until the autoantibodies are cleared from the baby's circulation, usually in three or four months. The baby doesn't need treatment after that.

Knowing when to treat the mother

At what point do women who have autoimmune hypothyroidism in pregnancy need treatment? If a mother's TSH level is greater than 4, treatment is appropriate. She needs to have thyroid function tests during every trimester of pregnancy to confirm that she is receiving the right amount of thyroid medication.

If the mother's TSH level is between 2 and 4 and she tests positive for thyroid autoantibodies, her doctor should probably treat her and should check the fetus for goiter or other signs of a thyroid abnormality. Fortunately, recent studies show that if the mother has very mild hypothyroidism in early pregnancy, the hypothyroidism has no negative effect on the newborn's hearing or physical activity.

Several obstetrical complications are associated with a mother who is hypothyroid. These complications include

- ✔ Anemia, when a woman has decreased red blood cells
- ✔ Bleeding after delivery
- ✔ Preeclampsia, where a woman has high blood pressure, headache, weight gain, and blurred vision
- ✔ Rupture of the placenta

Making the thyroid hormone levels normal can prevent the preceding complications.

Although autoimmune hypothyroidism generally improves during pregnancy, after the baby is born, the mother's hypothyroidism may become worse, and her T4 level may decrease further. Her doctor should check her TSH every six to eight weeks after delivery.

The experts make no general recommendation for screening for hypothyroidism in pregnancy despite the high incidence and the severe consequences if maternal hypothyroidism is present. Women who are at high risk should certainly be tested. Make sure you're tested if any of the following apply to you:

✔ Members of your family have chronic thyroiditis or hypothyroidism.

✔ You already take thyroid hormone.

✔ You have type 1 diabetes mellitus or another autoimmune disease.

✔ You have diminished thyroid reserve as a result of surgery or a history of neck irradiation.

If you have hypothyroidism during pregnancy, have thyroid function tests done about two months after delivery to verify that you're taking the right dose of thyroid hormone.

Treatment of newly diagnosed hypothyroidism in pregnancy is with levothyroxine. In an effort to make the mother normal rapidly, doctors often give a large dose for several days followed by the usual dose. Women have to undergo retesting in six weeks to make sure the dose is correct.

Certain drugs that women commonly take during pregnancy, such as iron, sucralfate, and aluminum hydroxide (see Chapter 10), can block the absorption of thyroid hormone. Pregnant women should take these drugs several hours before or after taking the thyroid hormone.

Hyperthyroidism in Pregnancy

Hyperthyroidism occurring in pregnancy is much less common than hypothyroidism. It occurs in about 2 in 1,000 pregnancies. If doctors don't recognize it, the baby will be premature at birth and have a low birth weight, not to mention possible hyperthyroidism.

Hyperthyroid women who wish to become pregnant should make sure that their disease is under control before they do so. It is important that women have normal thyroid function when they conceive their baby. The miscarriage rate for babies conceived by a hyperthyroid mother is greater than normal, just like the situation I describe in the preceding section for hypothyroidism.

Women who have previously received treatment for Graves' disease and are now normal, with or without thyroid medication, also have to be aware that hyperthyroidism can still occur in their baby during the pregnancy. If the treatment was antithyroid drugs, the risk is much less. But if surgery or radioactive iodine were the treatments, the mother may still have thyroid-stimulating autoantibodies that she passes to the baby. Doctors can measure these autoantibodies in the mother's blood. If they're not present, then hyperthyroidism in the baby is unlikely.

Some women with Graves' disease who are already pregnant but don't realize it receive radioactive iodine in treatment. Most radiation therapists ask the woman if she may possibly be pregnant. Occasionally she is unaware of a pregnancy and denies it. Whether damage to the fetal thyroid results depends on the stage of the pregnancy.

The following considerations determine whether radioactive iodine mistakenly given to the pregnant woman will cause damage to the fetal thyroid:

✔ The fetal thyroid begins to concentrate iodine after the 10th to the 12th week of gestation.

✔ The fetal thyroid takes in iodine more avidly than the maternal thyroid.

✔ Fetal tissues are more radio sensitive than maternal tissues.

✔ Radioactive iodine given to a pregnant woman up to the tenth week isn't an indication for termination of the pregnancy.

At birth, sampling the umbilical cord blood for thyroid hormone levels should determine the possibility of fetal hyperthyroidism. Such babies have a higher incidence of malformations, which doctors have to carefully look for.

Doctors once believed that most hyperthyroidism in pregnancy was due exclusively to Graves' disease. Recently doctors have become aware of another cause for hyperthyroidism in pregnancy that's actually more frequent than Graves' disease — a condition called *gestational transient thyrotoxicosis*. I discuss both conditions in this section.

Regardless of the cause, the symptoms of hyperthyroidism in pregnancy are those I mention earlier in this chapter: rapid heart rate, sweating, trouble sleeping, anxiety, heat intolerance, and fatigue. These symptoms are all fairly common for any pregnant woman. One way to determine whether the mother is hyperthyroid is that if she has Graves' disease, she usually won't gain a great deal of weight during pregnancy; she may even lose weight.

Lab tests show that a hyperthyroid mother has high levels of free T4 and low levels of TSH. In this situation, doing a total T4 test (see Chapter 4) isn't helpful at all, because the total T4 will always be elevated in view of the increase in thyroid-binding globulin in the mother's system.

Doctors need to control hyperthyroidism during pregnancy. If it's not controlled, some of the consequences may include

✔ Premature delivery

✔ Fetal malformations

✔ Low birth weight

✔ Hyperthyroidism in the infant

✔ High blood pressure and other problems in the mother

Graves' disease

Alice Dummy is a cousin of Stacy, Karen, Sarah, and Margaret — our friends from earlier chapters. She is married, but — conveniently for us — she kept her maiden name. She became pregnant about a month ago. She notices that her heart is beating very fast all the time and that she is feeling very warm. She has actually lost a few pounds. Her husband notices that her neck seems enlarged.

Alice and her husband go to their obstetrician, Dr. Ufbaum, who obtains thyroid blood tests to rule out hyperthyroidism. To her surprise, Dr. Ufbaum rules in the possibility of hyperthyroidism when she finds that the free T4 level in Alice's blood is elevated while the TSH level is suppressed. The doctor immediately refers Alice to her favorite endocrinologist, Dr. Rubin.

Dr. Rubin sends Alice for a blood test for thyroid-stimulating hormone–receptor-stimulating antibodies. The test result is very positive. He starts Alice on the antithyroid medication propylthiouricil. Within three weeks, Alice begins to feel better. By six weeks, she is gaining weight, and her heart slows noticeably. Alice can stop taking the propylthiouricil during the second half of her pregnancy, which proceeds normally. Dr. Rubin instructs Dr. Ufbaum to check carefully for hyperthyroidism in the fetus; fortunately, hyperthyroidism doesn't develop.

After the delivery, Alice again needs antithyroid medication, which she takes for a year. She does well.

Autoimmune hyperthyroidism is associated with antibodies that stimulate the TSH receptors on thyroid cells and trigger the production of more thyroid hormone. In some cases, the mother may have had Graves' disease prior to pregnancy and received successful treatment with radioactive iodine, surgery, or antithyroid drugs. She may have normal thyroid function, but she still has the antibodies that can be transferred through the placenta to the fetus, giving the fetus hyperthyroidism and a probable goiter.

Finding hyperthyroidism in the fetus

A number of signs indicate that the fetus has hyperthyroidism, most of which are determined by an ultrasound study of the developing fetus. They include

✔ Fetal goiter

✔ Very rapid fetal heart rate (over 160 beats per minute)

✔ Increased movement of the fetus

- ✔ Acceleration in the bone maturity of the fetus
- ✔ Fetal growth retardation

If you become pregnant after successful treatment for Graves' disease, your fetus can become hyperthyroid because you still have thyroid-stimulating antibodies that can pass through the placenta. It is important for your doctor to monitor the fetus for signs of hyperthyroidism and check you for TSH-receptor antibodies early in pregnancy . If your TSH receptor antibodies are elevated, but no signs of fetal hyperthyroidism appear, your doctor should check both again in six months.

Doctors give antithyroid drugs to the mother to treat hyperthyroidism in the fetus; the medication passes through the placenta to decrease the thyroid function of the fetus. The mother may need to also take thyroid hormone replacement, because the antithyroid drugs will reduce her thyroid function as well.

The fetus may also show hyperthyroidism at birth if the mother has Graves' disease that hasn't been well controlled or has a lot of TSH receptor–stimulating antibodies. A mother who has previously had a baby with neonatal hyperthyroidism is at especially high risk to have another baby with neonatal hyperthyroidism in a subsequent pregnancy.

Hyperthyroidism in the newborn may not appear until the antithyroid drugs, obtained through the placenta, clear out of the baby's system. The baby then has the usual signs of hyperthyroidism plus signs specific to a newborn, such as failure to thrive, increase in the yellow color of the skin (due to increased bilirubin), and increased irritability. After the mother's thyroid-stimulating antibodies are cleared from the baby's blood, the baby has normal thyroid function.

Treating the mother during pregnancy

As I mention earlier in the chapter, autoimmune hyperthyroidism tends to improve through the course of a pregnancy because of a general decline in the mother's autoimmunity. Other factors aiding the improvement of autoimmune hyperthyroidism include an increase in thyroxine-binding globulin, an increased loss of iodine in the urine, and an increase in TSH receptor–blocking antibodies as the TSH receptor–stimulating antibodies decline.

The usual treatment for Graves' disease during pregnancy is the use of antithyroid drugs. At one time, doctors preferred propylthiouricil because they thought that it didn't cross the placenta, while methimazole did. However, pregnant women use methimazole in Europe and Asia without any problem, so most specialists feel that using either one is fine.

The dose of antithyroid drug that doctors use is the least amount that can keep the free T4 in the upper part of the normal range (see Chapter 4). When this is done, the fetus receives the right amount of T4 from the mother.

A study of goiters in babies at birth found that 8 of 11 goiters were due to hypothyroidism in the baby, while 3 were due to hyperthyroidism. Of the eight hypothyroid babies, five of the goiters were a result of excessive amounts of antithyroid drugs that doctors gave to the mother during pregnancy. The results of this study emphasize how important it is to give the least amount of antithyroid drug that can make the mother normal.

A few circumstances require surgery rather than antithyroid drugs, including the following:

✔ The patient fails to take the antithyroid drug.

✔ The mother needs exceptionally high doses of medication — more than 300 milligrams of propylthiouricil or 20 milligrams of methimazole daily.

✔ A slow fetal heart rate indicates that the fetus may be hypothyroid due to the antithyroid drug the mother is taking.

✔ The mother has extremely severe hyperthyroid symptoms.

✔ The mother experiences side effects, like a fall in white blood cells, from the drug.

If a woman must have surgery, it's best done in the second trimester of the pregnancy, when it's least harmful to the fetus and the mother.

To prepare for surgery, doctors sometimes give the mother iodine. Iodine passes easily through the placenta to the fetus, where it can cause goiter and hypothyroidism. Iodine is also found in topical compounds and dyes used for better observation of the growing fetus. The use of iodine is necessary in these situations, but be aware of (and talk with your doctor about) the consequences of its use.

Checking mother and child after birth

The easiest way to check the thyroid status of a newborn is to check the levels of free T4 and TSH in the umbilical cord serum. Treatment depends on the findings.

After you deliver your baby, if your Graves' disease was under control during the pregnancy, you can expect a worsening of symptoms as the autoimmunity becomes severe again. Checking your thyroid function with blood tests after the delivery is important.

Postpartum Graves' disease isn't the same as postpartum thyroiditis (see Chapter 11). The treatment for these two conditions is entirely different. Postpartum thyroiditis is a condition associated with a low uptake of radioactive iodine and results when a damaged thyroid spills thyroid hormone (rather than from stimulation by TSH receptor–stimulating antibodies).

Thyroglobulin also spills into the blood in postpartum thyroiditis but not in postpartum Graves' disease.

Postpartum thyroiditis is associated with a finding of thyroid autoantibodies. Some specialists recommend that all pregnant women have tests for thyroid autoantibodies early in pregnancy, because about 50 percent of those with positive tests develop postpartum thyroiditis.

Breastfeeding with Graves' disease

For many years, doctors believed that mothers who were taking antithyroid drugs for Graves' disease shouldn't breastfeed because the drugs would enter the mothers' milk and pass to the babies. Recent studies have proved that this isn't the case.

One study shows no effect on breastfed infants when mothers take up to 750 milligrams of propylthiouricil (PTU) daily. In another study, no effect on breast-fed infants was found when the mothers were taking up to 20 milligrams of methimazole daily. (For more information on related studies, see Chapter 21.)

You can breastfeed safely if you're taking antithyroid drugs for hyperthy-roidism. Use the guidelines in the previous paragraph for the maximum dosage of drugs. Doctors should never give radioactive iodine for treatment to the mother with hyperthyroidism who is breastfeeding.

Gestational transient thyrotoxicosis

Holly Bright is a 27-year-old woman who has become pregnant for the first time. She has had a lot of morning sickness during the first several weeks of her pregnancy. She notices that she has lost some weight, but she believes that it's due to the morning sickness. However, in the last few days, she has had symptoms of a rapid heartbeat, fatigue, trouble sleeping, and a feeling of warmth all the time. She checks with her obstetrician, Dr. Ufbaum. As a result of her recent experience with Alice Dummy, Dr. Ufbaum is convinced that Holly has Graves' disease. Thyroid function tests seem to confirm this. She refers Holly to Dr. Rubin.

Dr. Rubin isn't as convinced. He notices that her thyroid isn't enlarged. He is concerned about the extent of the vomiting that Holly describes. He sends her to be tested for TSH receptor–stimulating autoantibodies. The result is negative. Dr. Rubin tells Holly that she probably has a condition called *gestational transient thyrotoxicosis*. He is able to reassure her that the condition will be brief. He gives her a low dose of propranolol, a drug that relieves her symptoms, along with a drug for her vomiting. Over the next few weeks, Holly returns to normal and has no further trouble with hyperthyroid symptoms. The thyroid function tests also return to normal.

Gestational transient thyrotoxicosis (GTT) is actually more common than Graves' disease in pregnancy, occurring as often as two to three times in 100 pregnancies. Fortunately, it's generally mild. But it's sometimes more serious, and doctors can confuse it with Graves' disease, leading to incorrect treatment.

The hormone human chorionic gonadotrophin (HCG), which I discuss in the section "The Normal Thyroid During Pregnancy," earlier in the chapter, causes GTT. HCG is at its highest level in the mother's circulation at around ten weeks of pregnancy, but it continues to be elevated above normal throughout. It may appear in a form that's cleared very slowly from the circulation of the mother. It can act as a stimulant on the thyroid, leading to increased free T4 and decreased TSH, which produces a diagnosis of hyperthyroidism. No TSH receptor–stimulating antibodies are found in GTT.

About half of GTT patients show the typical symptoms of hyperthyroidism. In addition, many patients experience a significant increase in vomiting associated with this condition, sometimes called *hyperemesis gravidarum,* as I mention previously. A goiter isn't usually present in patients with GTT.

Most patients need no more treatment than beta blockers like propranolol (see Chapter 6). Sometimes the mother has to be given fluids to replenish what she loses from vomiting. Occasionally, she needs to take antithyroid drugs for a short time, until levels of HCG begin to fall (usually after ten weeks of pregnancy). However, in twin pregnancies, HCG levels may be particularly high and sustained for a longer time period. Some studies don't show a difference in the level of HCG between pregnant women who vomit a lot and those who don't. This suggests that women who experience a lot of vomiting may be making a form of HCG that's especially stimulating to the thyroid.

The most severe vomiting associated with GTT occurs when the level of thyroid hormone, the level of HCG, and the level of estrogen in the pregnant mother are all at a maximum.

If you have symptoms of hyperthyroidism accompanied by vomiting early in pregnancy, your doctor should consider GTT as the diagnosis rather than Graves' disease. You can expect GTT to pass after several weeks, while Graves' disease requires treatment throughout the pregnancy in many cases.

Hydatidiform mole and choriocarcinoma

Occasionally, as a result of some abnormality of the mother's egg or in fertilization, the placenta forms a series of grapelike clusters called a *hydatidiform mole.* No viable fetus can result from this mole, but in about 10 percent of cases it can secrete large amounts of HCG and cause hyperthyroidism. The mother often experiences vaginal bleeding, and her uterus isn't the correct size for the stage of the pregnancy (it's usually too large).

Doctors often perform an ultrasound study in this situation, showing the mole very clearly. Because no viable fetus is present, the pregnancy is terminated.

Very rarely — about 2 percent of the time — the mole changes into a cancer called a *choriocarcinoma,* which also can make a large amount of HCG. Fortunately, this cancer is very treatable, and the patient may even be able to preserve the ability to have children.

New Thyroid Nodules in Pregnancy

Because pregnant women have frequent exams and their doctors follow them carefully, doctors sometimes discover thyroid nodules during pregnancy. In addition, pregnancy is a time of thyroid growth due to the need for increased iodine. Doctors find nodules in as many as 10 percent of pregnant women. Treatment depends on the tissue found in the nodule and the stage of the pregnancy.

The first step is to do a fine needle aspiration biopsy of the nodule (see Chapter 7). If the biopsy shows that a nodule is definitely cancer, and the patient hasn't yet reached her third trimester, she should have surgery of the thyroid at that time. The second trimester is the best time for this surgery, because it offers the least chance of interfering with the development of the baby or causing premature labor.

If the biopsy doesn't definitely show cancer, waiting until after the delivery, when a radioactive iodine scan is done (see Chapter 4), is safe. Keep in mind that after a woman has a radioactive scan, she can't breastfeed her baby. If the scan shows that the iodine uptake is high, the nodule probably isn't cancer. If the scan shows that the nodule remains cold, and the diagnosis remains uncertain, then the woman has surgery to obtain a final diagnosis and determine the appropriate treatment.

Some evidence exists that pregnancy and breastfeeding tend to stimulate the development of a new thyroid cancer if the woman is less than 45 years of age. No association exists between the number of births, the age of the mother during the first birth, or her age during the last birth and the incidence of thyroid cancer if the woman is over 45, according to one study.

Pregnancy doesn't make the cancer worse in terms of spread of the tumor or recurrence. A woman who has received treatment for thyroid cancer previously is permitted to become pregnant after the treatment. Even if she had received radioactive iodine, it doesn't put her or her baby at risk in a later pregnancy.

Chapter 18

Thyroid Conditions and Children

· ·

In This Chapter

▶ Understanding thyroid function in newborns and infants

▶ Screening for thyroid disease in babies

▶ Dealing with hypothyroidism and hyperthyroidism in kids

▶ Concentrating on goiters

▶ Treating thyroid nodules in the young

· ·

*N*ewborns and children who have thyroid abnormalities present special problems because their brains and bodies are developing at the same time that their thyroids aren't functioning properly. Thyroid hormones are a critical part of their development. The hormones must be available in the right amount at the right time in order for a child to have normal mental function and normal growth.

Children can experience all the kinds of thyroid diseases that are found in adults. This chapter discusses normal thyroid development and the impact of thyroid diseases on a developing human being. As a parent, you can do little to treat these conditions, but your early recognition of a problem, your understanding of the consequences if the problem isn't treated, and your continued support of your child through treatment and recovery can have a major impact on the way your child handles the challenges of thyroid disease.

Understanding the Onset and Development of Thyroid Function

The body produces thyroid hormones (T3 and T4) when *thyroid-stimulating hormone* (TSH) stimulates the thyroid to make them. TSH is released from the pituitary gland when the hypothalamus produces *thyrotrophin-releasing hormone* (TRH). (For an expanded discussion of thyroid hormones, see Chapter 2.) All these structures and their hormones are in place when a baby is born. Much recent research has established how this process comes about.

Focusing on the fetus

After just 15 weeks of development, the fetus shows function in its pituitary gland, and TRH is detectable. TSH and the other pituitary hormones start to appear between weeks 10 and 17. The thyroid is functioning by the 10th week, and its production of thyroid hormone becomes significant around the 20th week. The ability of thyroid hormone to shut off TSH production matures toward the end of the pregnancy and in the first two months after delivery.

The placenta acts as a barrier, preventing the mother's TSH from reaching the circulation of the fetus throughout the pregnancy. The placenta also contains an enzyme that breaks down the mother's thyroid hormones before they can reach the fetus. In breaking down the hormones, the enzyme releases iodine from the mother's hormones so the fetus can use the iodine to make thyroid hormone for itself. At the same time, the placenta is producing *human chorionic gonadotrophin (HCG),* a hormone that stimulates the thyroid (see Chapter 17).

As the pregnancy progresses, the enzyme in the placenta that breaks down the mother's thyroid hormones stops working as much, and other enzymes take over to convert T4 into the active hormone, T3. By not working so much, the placental enzyme no longer prevents the mother's T4 from getting to the fetus. This is very important, because the fetus needs the T4 for normal development, especially of its brain, at a time when it can't make much T4 for itself.

One enzyme, which converts T4 to T3, works in the liver, the kidneys, and the thyroid. Another enzyme works mainly in the pituitary gland. If the fetus isn't getting enough T4, the enzyme in the pituitary increases, and the other enzyme decreases so the fetal brain gets enough T3.

Keeping fetal T3 normal in the brain

Three chemicals in the fetus called enzymes affect the production of T3. The major enzyme, iodothyronine deiodinase 1 (D1), which converts T4 to T3 in the adult, is reduced in the fetus so blood levels of T3 are lower in the fetus than in the adult. The second enzyme, iodothronine deiodinase 2 (D2), which also converts T4 to T3, is found in the brain by seven weeks of gestation. The third enzyme, iodothyronine deiodinase 3 (D3), which converts T4 into inactive chemicals, is also found in the brain by seven weeks and protects the fetus from too much T4 from the mother. When T4 is too low, D2 increases its activity while D3 decreases it. Therefore, the brain always has enough T3, except in the most severe cases of lack of maternal T4.

Bringing a baby into the world

When the baby is born, leaving the warmth of the uterus for the colder temperatures of the outside world, the baby's pituitary releases a large amount of TSH. This increased flow of TSH stimulates the thyroid to release a large amount of T3 and T4, causing the temperature of the baby's body to rise. (The T4 concentration in the baby increases by 50 percent, and the T3 concentration increases three or four times.) This process is known as the *TSH surge*. The TSH surge peaks after only 30 minutes but continues to stimulate extra thyroid hormone for the next 24 hours. A large increase in the enzyme that converts T4 to T3 is also responsible for the great increase in T3. Babies also produce T4 at a much higher rate than adults.

A premature baby has similar hormone changes to a normal-term baby, but to a lesser extent. A premature baby doesn't have as much of a TSH surge and doesn't produce as much thyroid hormone. The T3 doesn't increase as much either, because the converting enzymes aren't yet as active. A premature baby can't defend its body temperature the way that a normal-term baby can.

As the baby grows, it stores more thyroid hormones in its thyroid along with thyroglobulin (see Chapter 2), and it produces more thyroid hormone. The thyroid gland grows so that the lobes are normally about the same size as the part of the baby's thumbs after the last joint (the *terminal phalanx*).

A lack of thyroid hormone during fetal growth has important consequences (see Chapter 12). Thyroid hormone is particularly important in the development of hearing, but many other body organs also need it for proper development. Some of the damage that results from lack of thyroid hormone includes the following:

✔ Immature bones

✔ Immature liver

✔ Reduced mental function

✔ Increased sleepiness

The brain is dependent on thyroid hormone for development for the first two to three years after birth. For every month that a hypothyroid newborn doesn't receive thyroid hormone, the baby suffers a loss of five IQ points.

During the first 20 years of life, the free T3 and free T4 slowly decline, as do the total T3 and total T4 (see Chapter 2 for an explanation of the difference between *free* and *total*). As estrogen levels begin to rise during puberty in the female, her body makes more thyroid-binding globulin, and she has more total T3 and total T4. The decrease in the free T3 and free T4 is probably because of a gradual decline in TSH.

Screening the Newborn

Noah Stern is the newborn son of Barry and Sally Stern. Sally finds that Noah feeds very poorly. He seems to be cold to the touch. Otherwise he appears fine.

According to law, Noah is screened for hypothyroidism a couple days after birth. The TSH level comes back elevated at 35. The pediatrician notifies the Sterns and asks them to bring Noah in for testing. A blood test confirms that his TSH is elevated, and the free T4 is low. The pediatrician diagnoses Noah with congenital hypothyroidism.

A thyroid scan is performed on Noah, which shows little active thyroid tissue. Noah is given thyroid hormone, and his feeding and his body temperature rapidly improve. Sally notices that Noah looks less puffy as well. The doctor measures thyroid functions frequently until Noah stabilizes. Noah grows and feeds normally. He doesn't appear to have any deficits in his intellectual development.

The major reason for screening for thyroid disease is to diagnose congenital hypothyroidism as early as possible. *Congenital hypothyroidism* means hypothyroidism that is present when the baby is born (see the next section, "Coping with Hypothyroidism in Children").

Because the consequences of not treating hypothyroidism in newborns are so great and the response to early treatment is so successful, screening for thyroid disease is essential in the newborn. In a study of 800 children who had congenital hypothyroidism before the era of screening began in 1974, the average IQ was 80, which is low. Some of these babies were noted to have signs of hypothyroidism and were tested. Children who testing confirmed to have hypothyroidism and who received any treatment experienced no lowering of the IQ. Within that group, some children didn't receive adequate treatment. Even these children had normal IQs, though somewhat lower than the fully treated children.

Screening is a simple process. A drop of blood is placed on filter paper. (This filter paper is the same type used for screening tests for other diseases as well.) Then the filter paper is tested for TSH (sometimes for total T4 instead). If the TSH is above 40, the baby has a regular blood test for TSH and free T4, and the doctor begins treating the baby with thyroid hormone while waiting for the result. If the TSH is between 20 and 39, the doctor performs blood tests but begins no treatment until the diagnosis is confirmed. The reason for this delay is that up to 75 percent of babies with a TSH at this level during screening test normal when they have a regular blood test.

A TSH surge occurs immediately after birth. Screening on the first day may result in a false positive test.

The screening test isn't perfect. Screening fails to diagnose children who have *secondary hypothyroidism,* which results from the body's failure to secrete TSH. Screening also won't identify children who have a normal TSH and a low T4 (which the screening doesn't measure) at birth, whose TSH becomes abnormal a week later. Premature babies, especially, may show this pattern. Babies who fail to secrete TSH often have failure of other hormones as well, which leads to many signs and symptoms that point to disease. It is the occurrence of these signs and symptoms that leads the doctor to do further testing.

Doctors can misdiagnose infants with low birth weight because these babies tend to be born with low levels of hormones that soon rise to normal.

Screening has shown that congenital hypothyroidism is more common than was previously thought, affecting about 1 in 3,750 babies. Doctors now do screening, by law, throughout the United States and in Western Europe, Japan, Australia, New Zealand, and Israel. A major campaign is under way to promote neonatal screening for thyroid disease throughout the world.

Not only does screening make excellent medical sense, but it makes excellent economic sense as well. A study in Denmark found that the future medical costs for the babies who were found to be positive at screening, had they not been discovered and treated, would have been 28 times the cost of screening all the babies in Denmark.

Coping with Hypothyroidism in Children

A number of conditions can cause hypothyroidism in the newborn and in the older child. You find out about these conditions in this section.

Specialists disagree as to whether pregnant mothers should be routinely tested for hypothyroidism to protect their babies from a hypothyroid environment. The incidence of hypothyroidism in the mothers is up to ten times as frequent as in the babies. Yet screening of the mothers very early in pregnancy isn't mandatory as it is for the babies, despite the great dependency of the fetus on the mother's T4, which is a strong argument for screening of all newly pregnant women. A study in the *New England Journal of Medicine* in August 1999 showed that babies experienced some slight loss of IQ if their mothers were hypothyroid and untreated during pregnancy.

My own bias is that every pregnant woman should be screened for hypothyroidism with a TSH test. For more on the thyroid and pregnancy, see Chapter 17.

Transient congenital hypothyroidism

Doctors diagnose some babies with hypothyroidism at birth because their TSH levels are found to be high, but these levels fall to normal shortly after birth. This condition is called *transient congenital hypothyroidism* because it doesn't last. One common cause of this condition is iodine deficiency in the mother.

This condition is especially prevalent in very low-birth-weight infants, who should be screened for thyroid disease not only at birth, but also at two and six weeks of age.

Because this condition is so common in premature infants, the question is whether premature babies need thyroid supplementation for a short time at birth. A study in the *Texas Medical Journal* in 2000 suggests that babies who have more than 27 weeks gestation at the time of birth don't need supplemental thyroid hormone at birth and that such treatment may actually harm them. Whereas babies who spend less than 27 weeks in the uterus may benefit from supplementation.

Sometimes, determining whether the hypothyroidism is transient or permanent isn't possible. In this case, the doctor treats the baby with thyroid hormone until the age of 4 and then stops treatment for a short time to see if the child can make her own thyroid hormone. This short pause in treatment doesn't damage the child's brain.

Congenital hypothyroidism

Babies who are born with hypothyroidism that doesn't correct itself shortly after birth have *congenital hypothyroidism.* This condition used to be a significant cause of mental retardation, but since neonatal thyroid screening began in the 1970s, doctors are able to prevent mental retardation from occurring.

Causes

Many causes lead to congenital hypothyroidism, but 80 percent of cases result from *thyroid dysgenesis* — a failure of the thyroid to grow or to end up in its proper place in the neck. The following are common causes of thyroid dysgenesis:

- ✔ No thyroid at all (a condition called *thyroid agenesis*)
- ✔ A small thyroid gland that can't make enough thyroid hormone (*thyroid hypoplasia*)
- ✔ A thyroid gland that grows in the wrong place, often at the base of the tongue (*ectopic thyroid*)

Some of the other far less frequent causes of congenital hypothyroidism include the following:

- ✔ The baby's thyroid doesn't respond to TSH.
- ✔ The mother is exposed to radioactive iodine that destroys the baby's thyroid.
- ✔ The hypothalamus doesn't release TRH (a condition called *hypothalamic hypothyroidism*).
- ✔ Some step of the synthesis of thyroid hormone is defective.

With the exception of maternal exposure to radioactive iodine, the conditions in the preceding list are all genetic diseases (see Chapter 14). In the United States, these diseases are rare among African Americans and more frequent among Hispanics.

Signs and symptoms

Many babies with congenital hypothyroidism have few signs or symptoms of hypothyroidism at birth. Screening discovers this condition (see "Screening the Newborn," earlier in the chapter). If the condition is severe, the baby shows some or all of the following signs:

- ✔ Low body temperature
- ✔ Slow heart rate
- ✔ Poor feeding
- ✔ Umbilical hernia (an outward protrusion of the umbilicus — the belly button — that may contain intestine)

Once doctors recognize and confirm the condition, treatment should begin immediately. Doing a thyroid scan just before treating the baby may help detect any functioning thyroid tissue, a lack of which indicates the need for lifelong treatment. Doctors may not see tissue or may find it in an unusual site. If no tissue is seen on the thyroid scan, a thyroid ultrasound shows whether tissue exists and whether it's unable to take up iodine, possibly due to a genetic abnormality. This information can be helpful in counseling the parents about hypothyroidism in future children.

Treatment

Babies with congenital hypothyroidism are usually given a relatively high dose of thyroxine (T4) hormone replacement for the first week to restore their thyroid hormone levels. The daily dose administered after that initial dose must be individualized.

Doctors should check the baby's thyroid function at 7, 14, and 28 days. In view of all the changes taking place in thyroid function soon after birth, the stabilization of thyroid function may take time. Once the tests are normal and stable, the tests are measured every three months until two years of age and then every year until the child shows normal and stable thyroid function three years in a row.

Doctors determine proper dosing of thyroid hormone not only by performing thyroid function tests but also by making sure that the baby is growing properly. Doctors check the height and weight of the baby regularly to verify the hormone dosage.

If thyroid hormone treatment is delayed more than four to eight weeks after birth, a child with congenital hypothyroidism will almost certainly have some decrease in intellectual function.

Acquired hypothyroidism

Children may acquire hypothyroidism at any time after birth. When hypothyroidism occurs in a child over the age of 2, it doesn't damage brain function, but it does greatly affect growth and development.

Causes

Children may develop hypothyroidism for all the same reasons that adults become hypothyroid. Iodine deficiency is, by far, the most common cause throughout the world. Where iodine is sufficient, autoimmune thyroiditis (see Chapter 5) is the leading cause. Less common reasons for acquired hypothyroidism include

- Drugs like iodine or lithium
- Irradiation — externally (for a tumor, for example) or internally, in treatment of hyperthyroidism with radioactive iodine
- Removal of the thyroid for any reason
- Abnormal production of thyroid hormone
- Resistance to thyroid hormone
- Central or secondary hypothyroidism due to a tumor in the pituitary or hypothalamus or a lack of production of TSH or TRH

Signs and symptoms

The signs and symptoms of acquired hypothyroidism in children are similar to the signs and symptoms found in adults, except that a growing, developing child experiences the consequences of poor growth. Constipation and dry skin are features of any hypothyroid person. The child, in addition, doesn't keep up with height and weight guidelines for growing children.

The child who becomes hypothyroid after he enters school starts to have trouble with schoolwork or keeping up with the physical activity of the other children. Lack of energy is a major complaint at this time.

Interestingly, some hypothyroid kids appear unusually muscular despite being weak. This is because they have swelling of their muscle fibers, called *pseudohypertrophy* of muscles.

The growth of the skeleton and the teeth is delayed. Other signs of acquired hypothyroidism include

✔ Enlarged thyroid (goiter), unless it has been removed

✔ Dry, cool skin that's puffy, pale, and yellowish

✔ Brittle nails and dry, brittle hair that tends to fall out excessively

✔ Swelling that doesn't retain an indentation, especially of the legs

✔ Hoarseness and slow speech with a thickened tongue

✔ An expressionless face

✔ A slow pulse

✔ Early sexual development (occasionally)

Early sexual development is thought to be the result of the large amount of TSH in these children's bodies. TSH has a structure that shares some features with *follicle-stimulating hormone* (FSH). The TSH activates cells that normally respond to FSH, so girls may have early vaginal bleeding, and boys may have large testicles for their age. The boys don't have a lot of male hormone, which is the result of stimulation by another hormone, *luteinizing hormone* (LH). TSH doesn't share features with LH. The girls, however, do have increased estrogen for their age because their ovaries can respond to the FSH-like properties of TSH; LH-like stimulation isn't necessary to accomplish increased estrogen production.

The adolescent who develops hypothyroidism has signs and symptoms that parallel the symptoms in a hypothyroid adult, with a few differences. If the child has begun puberty, puberty may stop unless the child receives thyroid hormone treatment. Also, a delay in the growth of permanent teeth may occur, and the child doesn't gain height as quickly as normal.

When central or secondary hypothyroidism (a lack of TRH or TSH; see Chapter 5) is the cause, the signs and symptoms of hypothyroidism tend to be milder. The main symptoms are due to the underlying cause, which may be a brain tumor, for example. The child complains of headaches or trouble with vision.

Laboratory confirmation

A TSH and free-T4 test confirm the diagnosis of hypothyroidism. In order to make a diagnosis of chronic (autoimmune) thyroiditis, doctors test the child for the presence of thyroid autoantibodies. X-rays that evaluate any growth abnormalities determine the child's bone age.

If central hypothyroidism is responsible, the free T4 and the TSH are low, as are the other hormones the pituitary gland makes. An X-ray of the pituitary is necessary to look for a tumor.

Treatment

The current treatment for hypothyroidism is thyroxine (T4) hormone replacement. However, recent studies suggest that giving both T3 and T4 replacement in the same proportions the normal thyroid makes may be more appropriate (see Chapter 5). This conclusion is based on studies in adults. Similar studies in children haven't been published.

In most cases, doctors change the dose of replacement hormone until the TSH is normal. However, if the cause is central hypothyroidism, doctors can't use the TSH as a guide because the pituitary isn't making any TSH.

In some cases, starting the child at a low dose of the replacement hormone and gradually increasing to the full therapeutic dose may be necessary. Some children show more symptoms when they suddenly go from no thyroid hormone to full replacement. They experience trouble sleeping, restlessness, and deterioration in their school performance. The rare patient has headaches due to increased pressure in the brain. Lowering the dose and gradually building it back up manages this situation.

If the child's growth has been delayed, she usually catches up when she takes thyroid hormone.

Giving too much thyroid hormone may cause early bone closure, resulting in stunted growth and a decrease in the mineral content of the bone.

Dealing with Hyperthyroidism in Children

Hyperthyroidism rarely occurs in babies and is less common in children and adolescents than in adults. Almost always, kids with hyperthyroidism have Graves' disease (see Chapter 6). When a newborn is hyperthyroid, usually the mother is also hyperthyroid (see Chapter 16), and the mother's thyroid-stimulating antibodies have passed to the fetus. When these antibodies are cleared from the fetus after is born, the hyperthyroidism subsides about 3 to 12 weeks after birth.

Signs and symptoms

When a mother with hyperthyroidism passes a large amount of thyroid-stimulating antibodies to the fetus through the placenta, the fetus develops hyperthyroidism. The signs of the hyperthyroidism in the fetus include

- Rapid heart rate
- Increased fetal movements
- Poor fetal body growth
- Abnormally rapid bone growth

After the baby is born, the baby shows a number of signs and symptoms of hyperthyroidism. They're the result of excessive metabolism in a baby who should be growing and developing normally. These signs and symptoms include

- Low birth weight and failure to gain weight
- Increased appetite
- Irritability
- Rapid heart rate
- Enlarged thyroid
- Prominent eyes

Hyperthyroidism is rare in children under the age of 5, and Graves' disease is usually the cause. Once in a while, the cause may be a functioning thyroid adenoma, a new growth of tissue on or within the thyroid that's making excessive amounts of thyroid hormone. Girls are more often affected than boys by thyroid adenomas. A family history of other autoimmune diseases may exist if the cause is Graves' disease.

In children under the age of 5, the signs and symptoms of hyperthyroidism are like those seen in adults (see Chapter 6). But the needs of a growing child who has reached school age temper these signs and symptoms. Unique signs at this age include the following:

- Poor school performance
- Trouble sleeping
- Poor athletic performance related to muscle weakness
- Tiredness
- More rapid growth in height but early closure of bone growth
- Irritability

Hyperthyroid children are hungry all the time but don't gain weight despite eating. They generally have mild eye disease. They have goiters and also have bowel movements more frequently than they should.

Hyperthyroidism in children before they reach puberty tends to be more severe than in children after puberty. They need longer treatment and go into remission less often than the older children, which is particularly true if the child is less than 5 years old.

Children with Graves' disease have a greater tendency to develop other autoimmune diseases (see Chapter 14), such as Addison's disease, type 1 diabetes mellitus, and so forth.

Laboratory confirmation

Obtaining a free T4 and a TSH level confirms the diagnosis of hyperthyroidism. If doctors suspect fetal hyperthyroidism, they can determine these levels from umbilical cord blood at birth. If hyperthyroidism is present, the free T4 is high and the TSH low. Rarely, if the hyperthyroidism is due to excessive TSH secretion from the pituitary, the TSH is high. In that case, the doctor should be on the lookout for a pituitary tumor. Doctors rarely do a thyroid scan and uptake unless they suspect that the child has subacute thyroiditis (see Chapter 11), which shows a low uptake, the opposite of Graves' disease.

Treatment

If your child has hyperthyroidism, you have many treatment options. The important point to remember is that your scrutiny doesn't end with treatment, because the recurrence of hyperthyroidism or the development of hypothyroidism can accompany all forms of treatment.

Be sure that you follow up with your child's condition regularly after treatment, because the disease process is ongoing. Regularly means every six months or yearly, as your doctor recommends.

If the fetus is hyperthyroid, the doctor gives antithyroid drugs to the mother. The drugs pass through the placenta to affect the fetus's thyroid hormone production. The goal is to have a fetal heart rate less than 140 beats per minute. Sometimes, the mother takes a beta blocker (such as propranolol) to control severe symptoms.

Antithyroid drugs are another treatment for hyperthyroidism in babies. Once the baby receives treatment, the baby rapidly improves. In a few months, the pediatrician withdraws the antithyroid drugs because the thyroid-stimulating antibodies that were passed from mother to baby disappear from the baby.

Radioactive iodine

At one time, doctors resisted using radioactive iodine to treat hyperthyroidism in children. However, doctors commonly use this treatment today because long-term studies have shown no negative effects upon the child. Specifically, radioactive iodine causes no increase in cancer, no loss of fertility, and has no negative effect on the offspring of children treated with radioactive iodine.

The problem with radioactive iodine is that most children become hypothyroid after some time. (The same is true of adults; see Chapter 6.) In addition, thyroid eye disease may get worse with radioactive iodine because of the release of a lot of antigen from the thyroid.

Antithyroid drugs

Antithyroid drugs, such as propylthiouricil (PTU) and methimazole, are the preferred treatment for hyperthyroidism in children. They take three to six weeks to work, but they control the disease in at least 85 percent of children. If the medication doesn't work, the child either has a very large goiter or doesn't take the medication as prescribed. In most cases, doctors continue the treatment for two to four years.

How does the doctor choose which of these drugs to use? PTU has the advantage of blocking the conversion of T4 to T3, whereas methimazole lasts longer after taking it. In practice, these differences don't seem to matter much. I tend to use methimazole only because I have more experience with it, not because I believe it's better.

If the disease recurs after the child stops taking the pills, the child usually has measurable amounts of TSH receptor–stimulating antibodies. Doctors do this test at the time they stop treatment to help to predict a recurrence. The drugs may fail to produce a permanent remission in up to half the patients treated, even though 85 percent can be controlled temporarily.

Just as in adults, antithyroid medications cause side effects in children. The most important is the halting of the production of white blood cells. The doctor should monitor white blood cells, and if the white blood cell count is less than 1,000, must stop the drug. If the doctor uses PTU initially, the child is not switched to methimazole and vice versa. The child receives a totally different treatment. Sometimes the white blood cell count falls a little, but it returns to normal after some weeks. Another important side effect is the development of a rash, which the doctor can treat without needing to stop the drug.

Surgery of the thyroid

Sometimes antithyroid drugs cause serious side effects, or the child doesn't take the pills correctly, and radioactive iodine isn't an option (usually because the parents are concerned about giving radioactivity to their child). In these cases, surgery is a safe and rapid form of treatment when done by a competent surgeon who has experience with children. If possible, the antithyroid drugs should secure normal thyroid function before the child undergoes surgery. The doctor gives the child iodine for two weeks prior to surgery to block the thyroid gland and reduce blood flow into it. The usual operation is a near total thyroidectomy (see Chapter 13).

Leaving enough thyroid tissue to retain thyroid function while eliminating hyperthyroidism may be possible, but the doctor must check the child at least every six months to a year to detect a recurrence or loss of thyroid function and the need for thyroid medication.

Diagnosing Goiters in Children

An enlarged thyroid gland (a goiter) is actually the most common thyroid abnormality doctors find in children. It occurs in about 5 percent of all children. A child with an enlarged thyroid usually has normal thyroid function.

The most common cause of thyroid enlargement in children is autoimmune thyroiditis (see Chapter 5). The second most common cause is a multinodular goiter (see Chapter 9).

Differentiating between these causes is important because autoimmune thyroiditis can lead to hypothyroidism (or sometimes hyperthyroidism), whereas a multinodular goiter doesn't. Thyroid autoantibody studies tell the difference, pointing to autoimmune thyroiditis if the results are positive. Testing the child's levels of free T4 and TSH verifies that her thyroid function is normal.

Children with autoimmune thyroiditis may have a negative thyroid antibody test the first time but develop the antibodies later. Therefore, doctors should perform testing more than once to find these children, especially if a family history of autoimmune thyroiditis exists.

These goiters sometimes get smaller and then larger again, sometimes growing at different rates in different parts of the thyroid, leading to a multinodular thyroid gland.

Doctors apply treatment if the large thyroid is pressing on nearby structures like the esophagus and trachea or is disfiguring. The treatment is either surgery or radioactive iodine. Doctors check the thyroid every six months for a few visits and then yearly.

If the goiter is painful, the diagnosis is more likely subacute or acute thyroiditis (see Chapter 11). These diseases cause similar signs and symptoms in children as they cause in adults. Subacute thyroiditis generally makes a child less sick than acute thyroiditis. Subacute thyroiditis affects the whole gland, whereas acute thyroiditis may swell only part of the gland. If acute thyroiditis occurs several times, a malformation may exist in the thyroid that will probably require surgery.

Finding Nodules and Cancer in Children

Although a functioning nodule or a cystic nodule (see Chapter 7) is rarely cancer in an adult, this isn't true in children. Children rarely get thyroid nodules, but when they do, the nodules indicate cancer more frequently than they do in adults. The incidence of nodules in children by examination is about 1 percent. But young adults who are autopsied have an incidence of 13 percent, and older adults are found to have nodules 50 percent of the time, so the true incidence in children may be higher. The signs that make a nodule particularly suspicious for cancer are the same as in adults: rapid growth, painlessness, firmness and fixation, and nodes felt in the neck.

A number of risk factors exist for nodules in children, which include

- ✔ Female sex
- ✔ Family history of thyroid disease
- ✔ Previous thyroid disease
- ✔ Onset of puberty

A very important clue that a child's nodule may be cancerous is past exposure to irradiation. Exposure leads to nodules and cancer in multiple places in the thyroid. (The leading type of thyroid cancer in both children and adults is *papillary* — the type of cancer most closely associated with irradiation exposure.) Exposure to X-rays isn't limited to people living in the area around a nuclear power plant. In the United States, in the not-so-distant past, doctors used X-rays to treat acne and enlarged thymus glands (which lie near the thyroid). Children with Hodgkin's disease also receive X-ray treatment, which may result in cancer later.

Children with a history of exposure to irradiation need to be followed regularly with thyroid function tests and thyroid ultrasound studies. Make sure your child's doctor does these tests every six months to a year.

A doctor does a fine needle biopsy of the nodule if she suspects cancer; the false negative result is only about 4 percent. Doctors should perform the biopsy under ultrasound guidance because the tumors in children tend to be smaller than adult tumors. Solid nodules are cancerous much more often than cystic nodules.

In children, thyroid cancer presents itself as a painless mass about 90 percent of the time. Of all diagnosed thyroid cancer cases in children, 25 percent already have lymph nodes in the neck that can be felt. A thyroid mass that's hard or a thyroid that's fixed and doesn't move with swallowing is more suggestive of thyroid cancer. Thyroid function tests (free T4 and TSH) are usually normal.

Thyroid cancer is the most common malignancy of the endocrine glands in children. Thyroid cancer is the papillary form (see Chapter 8) in 75 percent of cases. The rest are follicular and medullary cancers. Children tend to have more cancer spread in the neck and into the lungs at the time of diagnosis than adults do, but this doesn't make their prognosis worse. The cancer can be managed just like adult cancer with a total thyroidectomy (see Chapter 13), preserving the parathyroid glands and the recurrent laryngeal nerves. Radioactive ablation of the remaining thyroid tissue follows the thyroidectomy. Doctors place the patient on thyroid hormone to replace the thyroid hormone and to suppress growth of new thyroid tissue.

Doctors monitor children with thyroid cancer with thyroglobulin blood tests; this test should read close to 0 shortly after surgery. Doctors do the blood tests every six months to a year. If the level of thyroglobulin rises, a whole body scan is done, looking for tissue that takes up iodine. Doctors can do the scan using the new recombinant TSH (see Chapter 8), so the patient doesn't have to stop taking thyroid hormone to perform this study. If doctors find all the iodine in the neck, local surgery may be enough to eliminate the additional thyroid cancer tissue. If the tissue is spread around the body, a large dose of radioactive iodine destroys it.

Chapter 19

Thyroid Disease and the Elderly

*B*efore we start talking thyroids, let's get our definitions straight. Who is "elderly"? The answer to this question becomes more and more important to me as I get older. For the sake of the information in this chapter, let's accept the definition used in most studies, namely, a person age 65 or older.

Thyroid disease often afflicts elderly people. The trouble with thyroid disease in the elderly, and the reason that I devote an entire chapter to it, is that doctors so often miss it. Doctors miss it for two key reasons. First, when elderly people go to a doctor, hospital, or nursing home, the illness or condition that prompts them to seek care is, naturally, the doctor's primary focus. Second, symptoms of thyroid disease often mirror symptoms of other conditions, so even if the doctor looks for other conditions in the patient, the doctor can easily misdiagnose thyroid disease in an elderly patient.

When doctors are taught about disease, they learn a set of signs and symptoms that are characteristic of the disease. Elderly patients with thyroid disease may have none of the symptoms typical of the disease, or their symptoms may be almost opposite of what doctors expect. The only way doctors are going to discover thyroid disease in many elderly patients is with screening — obtaining thyroid function tests from a person who appears to be healthy.

Screening for thyroid disease in the elderly has its own problems. The main problem is that screening picks up a lot of *subclinical disease* — a situation where one blood test isn't normal but another is, and the patient has no symptoms of the disease. Tremendous controversy exists concerning what to do with subclinical thyroid disease. As a community, doctors haven't yet made any final decisions about whether to treat subclinical thyroid disease, wait for symptoms to develop, or wait for both thyroid blood tests to become abnormal. In this chapter, I share my own biases as I discuss the various diseases.

Thyroid Changes in the Elderly Due to Aging and Nonthyroidal Disease

The blood levels of thyroid hormones differ in the elderly compared to younger individuals. Also, chronic illness, common in the elderly, causes changes in thyroid hormone levels that need to be understood so they will not be thought to be thyroid disease and treated.

Normal aging changes

There are normal changes in thyroid function in the elderly that should not be confused with disease of the thyroid. Among the more important are the following:

- The baseline TSH levels in older people are higher.
- Baseline free T4 and free T3 levels are lower.
- Production of T3 from the thyroid and from removal of iodine from T4 is diminished.
- Uptake of iodine by the thyroid is diminished.

However, the size of the thyroid correlates more with body weight and less with aging.

Changes due to chronic illness or drugs

Thyroid function tests also change in response to nonthyroidal chronic illness and a poor nutritional state, neither very uncommon in the elderly. Drugs (see Chapter 10) may alter thyroid tests as well. The changes, which need to be understood so the person isn't treated as though he has a thyroid condition, include the following:

- A fall in free T3
- A fall in serum TSH
- Later on, a fall in free T4

Knowing whether thyroid disease is present is difficult when doctors find the preceding changes. But if free T3 falls, TSH should rise unless failure of the pituitary to make TSH (secondary hypothyroidism) occurs. If the patient overcomes the chronic illness, these changes return to normal.

When these changes in thyroid hormone levels are found, whether they're the body's way of adjusting to aging or illness in a way that helps the body or are part of the disease and need to be reversed with thyroid hormone isn't clear. Giving patients with these changes thyroid hormone doesn't seem to make a difference.

Real Thyroid Disease in the Elderly

To determine how many elderly people thyroid disease affects, we need yet another definition. How do we define "thyroid disease"? Is having an abnormal TSH level sufficient to make a diagnosis, or must the free T4 level be abnormal as well? (See Chapter 4 for information about these tests.) This is difficult to answer in the elderly, because they often have so many symptoms; many of these symptoms are symptoms of other conditions as well as thyroid disease.

Looking at current definitions of thyroid disease

Some doctors consider an abnormal TSH to be insufficient evidence of thyroid disease; they use the term *subclinical* to describe the situation where the TSH is abnormal but the free T4 is normal. They advocate against treating a patient with subclinical thyroid disease. Yet many studies show that treatment reduces or eliminates many of the symptoms. On the other hand, treating an elderly person, particularly with thyroid hormone, for hypothyroidism may not be entirely benign and helpful, as I discuss later in this chapter in the section on hypothyroidism in the elderly.

The most recent clinical studies in 2005 indicate that subclinical hypothyroidism is associated with damage to the heart and that treatment prevents that damage. Studies from two different groups published in the *Archives of Internal Medicine* in November 2005 showed that heart failure and heart attacks occurred more often in patients with subclinical hypothyroidism than in normal people. Thyroid specialists may reconsider their refusal to treat subclinical hypothyroidism as a result of these findings.

In one study from the United Kingdom, published in the *Archives of Internal Medicine* in January 2001, doctors tested all patients age 65 or older for thyroid disease when they entered the hospital. Out of 280 patients (leaving out those who already were known to have thyroid disease), 9 had hypothyroidism, and 5 had hyperthyroidism. Doctors had previously suspected none of these 14 cases. An additional 21 patients had subclinical hypothyroidism (high TSH, normal free T4), and 12 had subclinical hyperthyroidism (low TSH, normal free T4). The authors stated that overall, nearly 40 percent of the elderly people not thought to have thyroid disease had some evidence of it. Should all these people receive some treatment?

Writing in rebuttal to this study, other authors suggested that many of the people with subclinical disease actually have temporary abnormalities caused by other diseases.

In another study of elderly people who weren't hospitalized, researchers discovered unsuspected hyperthyroidism in 1 percent and unsuspected hypothyroidism in 2 percent of participants. So 3 of 100 elderly people are walking around with clinical thyroid disease. That may not seem like a lot, but in the population of the United States, it means that almost one million elderly people are walking around with undetected and highly treatable thyroid disease. (That number doesn't even account for the age group 35 to 65, which contains many more cases of undiagnosed thyroid disease.)

Large population studies have shown that 10 percent of women over age 65 have elevated TSH levels. Most of them don't have symptoms of thyroid disease.

I find it interesting that no argument exists about screening babies for thyroid disease (when the occurrence of abnormal tests is 1 in 3,750), yet the debate continues about screening the elderly (when doctors may find 3 in 100 cases of clinical thyroid disease).

My own bias is that everyone should be screened for thyroid disease beginning at age 35 and every five years thereafter. Doctors easily perform screening with a TSH test. If this test is abnormal, then the doctor does a free T4 test. If both tests are abnormal, the patient is treated for thyroid disease. If only the TSH is abnormal, taking a careful history and doing a physical examination is reasonable. Then the doctor decides on treatment based on that evaluation. Doctors can take other factors into consideration when making the decision whether to treat; later in the chapter, I discuss these factors in relation to specific diseases.

Trying thyroid hormone for subclinical patients

Doctors find that more than 10 percent of elderly women and 3 percent of elderly men have abnormally high TSH when tested. Among elderly patients with subclinical thyroid disease whose TSH level is less than 10, only half show some clinical improvement after receiving thyroxine (T4 hormone replacement). Such patients should probably not receive treatment if they complain of anginal heart pain. Every patient whose TSH level is over 20 improves with treatment.

An important study, whose results indicate that doctors should treat subclinical hypothyroidism in the elderly, was published in *Clinical Endocrinology* in 2000. It was a study of 1,843 people ages 55 and over. Researchers evaluated all patients for the presence of hypothyroidism and followed the patients for as short a time as just two years. Of those individuals in the study who had an elevated TSH but a normal free T4, the risk of dementia and Alzheimer's disease was three times greater than the risk of those with normal TSH and free T4. The lower the free T4 (though still in the normal range), the higher the incidence of dementia and Alzheimer's. Those individuals who had positive antiperoxidase antibodies also had a higher incidence of dementia. The authors' conclusion was, "This is the first prospective study to suggest that subclinical hypothyroidism in the elderly increases the risk of dementia and Alzheimer's disease."

Another factor that influences treatment decisions is that an elderly patient who has subclinical hypothyroidism along with another autoimmune disorder — such as type 1 diabetes, pernicious anemia, rheumatoid arthritis, or premature graying of the hair — is likely to eventually become clinically hypothyroid. In addition, certain other disorders, such as high blood pressure and nonpernicious anemia, may be associated with hypothyroidism and may reverse with thyroid hormone treatment. The anemia and high blood pressure, in turn, may be damaging to the heart, the brain, and the kidneys.

Make sure your doctor tests you for hypothyroidism if you have recent onset of high blood pressure or anemia.

If you have subclinical thyroid disease and your doctor starts you on thyroid-hormone replacement, there are several reasons why you may want to continue that treatment. If you test positive for thyroid autoantibodies and you have a high TSH, chances are very good that you'll develop clinical hypothyroidism in the future. Also, your cholesterol level may benefit from the thyroid hormone; a measurement of cholesterol before and after taking the pills may show that it has been lowered significantly. The thyroid hormone also often lowers a chemical in the blood called *homocysteine,* which can contribute to heart disease.

Sources of Confusion in Diagnosis

The natural consequences of aging, the many complicating diseases found in the elderly, and medications can all confuse a diagnosis of thyroid disease. Aging and other diseases can cause symptoms that may be identical to those found in thyroid disease. Medications cause changes in laboratory tests that confuse the diagnosis (see Chapter 10).

Other chronic illnesses, conditions, and diseases

Nonthyroidal chronic illness and certain diseases common in the elderly also cause changes in thyroid hormone levels that doctors need to understand so they won't mistake them for thyroid disease. The more common conditions and diseases that confuse thyroid testing are

- Poor nutrition
- Poorly controlled diabetes mellitus
- Liver disease
- Heart failure

Severe illness causes a temporary fall in T4 that doctors may misdiagnose as hypothyroidism.

Medications

Drugs the elderly often take that can alter thyroid function tests include the following:

- **Epilepsy drugs:** Epilepsy drugs such as carbamazine and diphenylhydantoin cause the rapid breakdown of thyroid hormones by the liver, which lowers thyroid hormone levels in the blood.

- **Aspirin:** Aspirin decreases the binding of thyroid hormones to thyroidbinding globulin, thereby lowering the total (but not the free) T4.

- **Arthritis drugs:** Arthritis drugs such as prednisone decrease thyroxinebinding globulin levels.

- **Drugs for abnormal heart rhythm:** These drugs, particularly amiodarone, can cause both hypothyroidism and hyperthyroidism.

- **Heparin:** Heparin, used for anticoagulation, can cause a temporary rise in T4 by displacing it from binding proteins.

For a complete discussion on medications and their effect on the thyroid, please see Chapter 10.

Discovering Hypothyroidism in the Elderly

Victor Brooklyn is a 68-year-old man who has been feeling a bit fatigued lately. He has put on a few pounds, and he feels cold when others seem comfortable. He also notices that he is more constipated than before. Victor thinks that all these changes are the natural effects of aging. He had been constipated for years, but it has recently become a serious problem, and this is what brings him to his doctor. The doctor observes that Victor's pulse is slow and that he has lost some of his eyelashes. He tells Victor that he believes this may be hypothyroidism and sends him for thyroid function tests.

The TSH level comes back high at 9, but the free T4 is within the normal range. Because his doctor is unsure of what to do, he sends Victor to Dr. Rubin. Dr. Rubin tells Victor that he appears to have subclinical hypothyroidism, although he thinks that his thyroid is causing the symptoms that Victor describes. He puts Victor on thyroid-hormone replacement pills.

After two weeks, Victor notices that his bowel movements improve. He is less tired and less cold. He returns to Dr. Rubin for repeat thyroid function tests. The TSH is now 6, so Dr. Rubin increases the dose of thyroid hormone. A month later, the TSH test is down in the normal range, and Victor states that he is now just his mildly constipated self.

Deciphering signs and symptoms

Doctors so easily miss the diagnosis of hypothyroidism in the elderly that I have to admit I've missed it myself on occasion (very rare occasions, of course). The principal reason is that so many of the changes our bodies experience as we grow older are typical findings in hypothyroidism. Some of the most important are the following:

- ✔ Slowing of mental function
- ✔ Slowing of physical function
- ✔ Tendency to have a lower body temperature
- ✔ Intolerance of cold

  ✔ Constipation

  ✔ Hardening of the arteries

  ✔ Elevation of blood fats (especially cholesterol)

  ✔ Weight gain

  ✔ Elevation of blood pressure

  ✔ Anemia

  ✔ Muscle cramps

  ✔ Dry skin

All the above changes are common effects of aging but are also signs and symptoms of hypothyroidism.

On the other hand, some signs found in the elderly tend to point away from a diagnosis of hypothyroidism, making an accurate diagnosis even less likely. For example, the elderly get Parkinson's disease, which results in tremors, or they simply develop senile tremors. Many elderly people lose weight because of poor nutrition; they may also be nervous. These symptoms may point to an overactive thyroid, but they definitely don't neatly fit into the list of symptoms of hypothyroidism.

Many elderly people with hypothyroidism don't have goiters. Just as in younger patients, the most common reasons for hypothyroidism in the elderly are chronic thyroiditis and previous removal of the thyroid for cancer or hyperthyroidism (see Chapter 5).

Getting laboratory confirmation

The only way to know for sure that an elderly person doesn't have hypothyroidism is to obtain thyroid function tests. If hypothyroidism is present, the free T4 should be low, and the TSH should be high (see Chapter 5). Often the TSH is high, but the free T4 is normal — the situation known as *subclinical hypothyroidism*. The only way to determine whether hypothyroidism is having an effect on the patient is to give a trial of thyroid hormone. I am very much in favor of doing this, although, as I explain in the next section, the patient may not feel much different on medication.

Taking treatment slowly

As far as treatment is concerned, it has been thought that it's most important that the doctor go slowly. The doctor should start the patient with a very low dose of thyroxine (for example, 25 micrograms), increasing it every four to six weeks until the TSH is at the upper limit of normal. You don't want excessive treatment, because it can possibly worsen heart pain and increase shortness of breath, palpitations, and rapid heartbeats, as well as nervousness and heat intolerance. Even the first exposure to a small dose of thyroxine may bring on anginal chest pain. An excessive dose causes osteoporosis, a thinning of the bones. These problems may be more theoretical than real. No careful study has shown that older people have more trouble with thyroid hormone than younger ones.

The major problem doctors have when treating elderly patients with hypothyroidism may be one of adherence — ensuring that a patient is taking his or her medication. If you have a parent who must take medication, putting the pills into a case with daily slots may help. Ultimately, only someone standing beside the patient, observing him or her taking the drug, can be sure.

The dose of thyroid that provides normal thyroid function in these elderly patients is usually lower than that of younger patients.

Testing thyroid function on a regular basis is important to ensure that the TSH and free-T4 levels remain normal. Testing every six months should be adequate.

The elderly with hypothyroidism are especially at risk of developing myxedema coma (see Chapter 5). With all their other diseases, myxedema coma is particularly dangerous for this age group.

Hyperthyroidism in the Elderly

Toby Dummy is the 76-year-old aunt of Stacy and Karen Dummy. Her husband has noticed that she seems depressed lately. Although she used to love to cook, she seems to have lost interest. She sits on her couch most of the day, not doing much of anything. She has gained several pounds and seems fatigued most of the time. Toby's doctor suggests that perhaps she is hypothyroid. He obtains thyroid function tests. To his surprise, the free T4 is elevated, and the TSH is suppressed, suggesting a diagnosis of hyperthyroidism. He sends Toby to see Dr. Rubin.

Dr. Rubin, whose practice is filled with members of the Dummy family by this time, examines Toby and finds that she doesn't have a goiter. However, her pulse is somewhat fast. He makes a diagnosis of *apathetic hyperthyroidism* and explains to Toby's husband that this type of hyperthyroidism isn't uncommon in the elderly population. He starts Toby on the antithyroid drug methimazole. After six weeks, Toby's thyroid function tests are normal. Dr. Rubin stops the methimazole and gives Toby radioactive iodine several days later.

Toby is feeling so much better that she invites Dr. Rubin and his wife, Enid, to a delicious dinner in a lovely dining room recently remodeled by Toby's husband.

Sorting through confusing signs and symptoms

Hyperthyroidism is less common than hypothyroidism, but it's still a significant problem among the elderly. As with hypothyroidism, doctors can easily confuse the symptoms of an overactive thyroid with the normal signs of aging. The following characteristics are among the similarities between normal aging and hyperthyroidism:

- Shaking of the hands and fingers
- Weight loss
- Irregular heart rhythms
- Increased threat of congestive heart failure
- Intolerance to heat
- Profuse sweating
- Fatigue and weakness

At the same time, the elderly may have signs that aren't consistent with hyperthyroidism at all. They may appear entirely apathetic, sitting very quietly, acting depressed, and showing fatigue and weight gain. This is the picture of apathetic hyperthyroidism that Toby Dummy illustrates.

Many elderly patients with hyperthyroidism don't have goiters.

Sometimes the first sign of hyperthyroidism is the finding of *atrial fibrillation,* an irregular heartbeat. (If you're diagnosed with atrial fibrillation, you may need to take an anticoagulant to prevent *pulmonary emboli,* blood clots that form in the irregularly beating heart and flow to the lungs, cutting off blood flow when they become stuck. After your heart rhythm is restored to normal, you can stop taking the anticoagulant.)

If your heart rhythm suddenly becomes very irregular, and your doctor tells you that it's atrial fibrillation, ask him or her to order thyroid function tests.

Loss of bone is another important consequence of hyperthyroidism. The elderly, particularly women who already have much diminished bone, can't afford to lose more bone. One study published in the *Journal of Clinical Investigation* in 2000 showed that elderly people with hyperthyroidism had significant reduction in bone density when compared with elderly people without hyperthyroidism. After hyperthyroid patients were successfully treated, their bone mineral density showed improvement within six months.

Other studies show a definite increase in bone fracture risk in people with hyperthyroidism.

Graves' disease is the most common cause of hyperthyroidism in the elderly, just as it is in younger people (see Chapter 6). However, two causes of hyperthyroidism are more common at this age than earlier in life: a toxic nodule, a nodule that produces too much thyroid hormone, and iodine-induced hyperthyroidism, hyperthyroidism that occurs in a person who had previously been deficient in iodine and suddenly takes a large amount of it. Less frequently, thyroiditis may provoke hyperthyroidism temporarily (see Chapter 11).

Securing a diagnosis

Thyroid function tests remain the key method for making a diagnosis of hyperthyroidism in the elderly. If hyperthyroidism is present, the free T4 should be high, and the TSH should be suppressed. Occasionally, the T4 is normal, but the free T3 is elevated, a condition called *T3 thyrotoxicosis* (see Chapter 6). This condition is especially common if a hyperactive nodule is the source of the hyperthyroidism.

When confusion exists about the cause of hyperthyroidism, a thyroid uptake and scan can help to clarify the situation. It shows a high uptake if the hyperthyroidism is due to Graves' disease but a low uptake if autoimmune (chronic) thyroiditis is the cause. Generally this study isn't necessary.

Just as a subclinical form of hypothyroidism exists, a subclinical form of hyperthyroidism exists that doctors find more often in the elderly than younger patients. However, it is a much less common problem. A normal free T4 but a low level of TSH defines subclinical hyperthyroidism. These patients don't have the florid symptoms that patients with high free-T4 levels show, which is why it's called *subclinical.* And just as subclinical hypothyroidism is associated with heart disease that improves with treatment, subclinical hyperthyroidism is also associated with heart disease that improves with treatment. Elderly patients with subclinical hyperthyroidism who don't receive treatment have a higher rate of death from heart disease than those who do receive treatment.

The use of the word *subclinical* is unfortunate. Subclinical patients have a disease, whether hypothyroidism or hyperthyroidism, and need treatment. Doctors have to be more careful in their selection and application of treatment and of all their patients' other medical conditions, but doctors do their elderly patients no favor by ignoring their thyroid condition.

Treating hyperthyroidism in the elderly

The treatment of choice for hyperthyroidism in the elderly is *radioactive iodine* (RAI). A single treatment brings the disease under control in four to six weeks. RAI avoids the problems associated with taking the daily antithyroid pills. However, many people who take RAI develop hypothyroidism and need to be on a daily thyroid hormone pill for the rest of their lives.

The problem with antithyroid drugs in the elderly is one of adherence to daily drugs for at least a year. However, antithyroid drugs are a very acceptable alternative to RAI. Elderly people are actually more sensitive to them than younger people and have a higher remission rate. This may be the treatment of choice in an older individual with few or no complicating diseases who is alert and can be depended on to take her medicine.

Another problem with antithyroid drugs is that agranulocytosis, the loss of white blood cell production, is more common in elderly people treated with antithyroid drugs than younger people. White blood cells protect the body from infection. Using methimazole at a dose of less than 30 milligrams can avoid agranulocytosis. Most elderly patients never need that much to treat their hyperthyroidism.

A beta blocker such as propranolol is also useful in controlling symptoms of hyperthyroidism (such as tremor, nervousness, sweating, and rapid heart rate).

If a doctor gives RAI to a person with a hyperactive thyroid, a sudden release of thyroid hormones may occur as the thyroid tissues break down. This may be dangerous for an elderly person, who could have a sudden worsening of heart failure and a very rapid heart rate, as well as much worse chest pain. To avoid this complication, doctors give antithyroid drugs for six weeks before administering the RAI. When the patient has normal thyroid function on the drugs, the risk of a sudden release of thyroid hormones is eliminated.

Most heart symptoms associated with hyperthyroidism disappear after successful treatment. However, sometimes the atrial fibrillation doesn't reverse. The reason is that the elderly have other damage to the heart, usually from hardening of the arteries, or arteriosclerosis. Reversing the hyperthyroidism doesn't correct arteriosclerosis.

The elderly person with hyperthyroidism is also a more likely candidate to develop thyroid storm (see Chapter 6). It occurs when the hyperthyroidism isn't treated or treated inadequately and the patient develops a complicating illness like pneumonia or suffers some kind of trauma or needs surgery. Even the taking of radioactive iodine to treat the hyperthyroidism in the first place may cause thyroid storm because of the sudden release of so much thyroid hormone. This is a medical emergency. Unfortunately, elderly people with multiple medical problems who develop thyroid storm have a high death rate.

Thyroid Nodules in the Elderly

Nodules are very common in the elderly, but doctors find thyroid cancer less often in elderly people than in younger people. Doctors can study the nodules with a radioactive iodine scan to see whether they're active and with an ultrasound to see whether they're filled with fluid *(cystic)*. Both of these characteristics point the diagnosis to a benign nodule rather than a cancer. Thyroid function tests can show whether the nodule is hyperfunctioning and needs treatment.

People who have had neck irradiation even 50 years ago are still at risk for developing thyroid cancer. Thyroid specialists are seeing less and less thyroid cancer associated with neck irradiation as the population that was irradiated before 1950 is dying out. Neck radiation is more dangerous to people who have been irradiated before age 15, which makes them 70 years of age or older at this time.

Most of the cancers in the elderly (80 percent) are papillary thyroid cancers (see Chapter 8), especially if patients have a history of irradiation to the neck. The next group is follicular cancer, which is more dangerous in the elderly than in younger patients. Follicular cancer spreads to bone and can cause fractures in an older person who already has much loss of bone.

An even less common kind of thyroid cancer in the elderly is medullary thyroid cancer. It has a worse prognosis in the elderly and is often detected at a late stage, especially because most medullary thyroid cancers are sporadic, occurring only in the one individual and not their relatives (familial medullary thyroid cancer). Doctors don't test the sporadic cases early as they do familial cases.

Rarely (1 or 2 in 100 tumors) does an elderly person have anaplastic thyroid cancer. It has a terrible prognosis, and most patients are dead within a year. This is a cancer that almost never appears before the age of 60. Neither surgery nor radiation therapy nor chemotherapy has much use in this cancer.

As doctors do more ultrasound of the neck, they find more small masses in the thyroid. The masses can be biopsied under ultrasound control and may be cancer. Should doctors treat these small tumors in elderly patients the same way as they treat them in younger patients? The current consensus is that they should, especially if the patient belongs to the growing group of healthy elderly.

In the final analysis, a fine needle aspiration biopsy remains the best single test to rule out cancer in a nodule. If this test is positive for cancer, surgery is the treatment of choice, with follow-up similar to any thyroid cancer patient (see Chapter 8). Obviously, surgery is more risky in this patient population. Use of radioactive iodine to ablate remaining thyroid tissue is also a problem because many of these tumors don't take up the radioactive iodine.

Doctors consider patients who can't take up RAI for treatment with chemotherapy. These patients tolerate chemotherapy very poorly, so doctors don't often give it to them.

Chapter 20

Diet, Exercise, and Your Thyroid

This chapter answers important questions you may have about how best to maintain your thyroid health and offers further evidence of the starring role that the thyroid gland plays in your body. Remember that your thyroid gland functions at its best if it finds itself in a healthy body whose tissues are fed by the right nutrients and whose muscles and bones are strengthened by an appropriate level of exercise. For this reason, I give you some basic ideas about diet and exercise here. For a more complete guide to diet, see my book *Diabetes Cookbook For Dummies,* which contains dietary suggestions not just for people with diabetes, but for all people who want to eat healthy food. To learn more about exercise in your lifestyle, see *Diabetes For Dummies,* which presents an exercise program for everyone who wants to feel good in their body. Wiley publishes both these titles.

Guaranteeing Your Best Nutrition

Two friends run into each other, and the first friend asks how the second one feels. The second friend answers, "Lousy — I've got arthritis and a bad back. I'm always tense, and I have insomnia. Miserable. I'm miserable." "And what kind of work are you doing?" the first friend asks. "The same thing — I'm still selling health foods."

This story is good for a chuckle, but the truth is that what you eat (and drink and smoke) has more influence on your health than all the diseases in a medical textbook. In the United States, we spend more than $100 billion on health each year. (That goes a long way toward explaining all the healthy doctors in this country.) The U.S. government is aware of these health costs and knows that its citizens function best when they eat right and exercise. For this reason, the government has long published a list of dietary recommendations, the *Dietary Guidelines for Americans.*

The *Dietary Guidelines for Americans,* updated every five years, is a great place for you to start to turn your body into a suitable "container" for a healthy thyroid gland. You can check them out at www.healthierus.gov/dietaryguidelines. The 2005 version of the guidelines is divided into ten chapters that cover issues such as weight management, physical activity, healthful eating habits, and food safety. Basically they concern your level of fitness, a healthy diet, your alcohol intake, and the safe consumption of food. The following section gets more specific about these recommendations.

Maintaining a healthy weight

If you go online and check out a message board about thyroid disease, you'll probably find that lots of people have lots of questions about how the thyroid affects weight gain and loss. This section helps set the record straight.

A very simple calculation allows you to determine your ideal weight; the calculation differs slightly for men and women:

- ✔ **Men:** Calculate your height in inches. Give yourself 106 pounds for the first 60 inches (5 feet) of height and 6 pounds for each inch above 60. For example, a 5'6" man should weigh 106 plus 6 times 6, or 142 pounds. This is his ideal weight. However, there really is a weight range that is appropriate for each height, because each of us has a different body shape.

  To calculate the range, take 10 percent of the number you calculate as your ideal weight, and add that number to and subtract it from the ideal weight number. For example, the man who is 5'6" would determine that 10 percent of 142 is 14 pounds. He'd add 14 to 142 and subtract 14 from 142 to get his weight range. The range for a 5'6" man is 128 to 156 pounds.

- ✔ **Women:** Calculate your height in inches and give yourself 100 pounds for the first 60 inches (5 feet) and then 5 pounds for each inch over 60. A 5'4" woman has an ideal weight of 120 pounds. Using the same technique I describe for men, the 5'4" woman would calculate that her proper weight range is 108 to 132 pounds.

Now that you know how much you should weigh, do you have to achieve that goal? The answer is no. Are you shocked?

The simple fact is that I, your kindly and wise doctor, want you to achieve a weight at which you'll have no risk of disease. If that weight is 10 or 15 pounds above the top of your "ideal" weight range, I'm telling you that's okay. If you gain much more than that, chances are you'll suffer some medical consequence, but even that isn't certain. If you want to look like a fashion model, that's up to you.

Using the Food Guide Pyramid to make your food choices

In 2005, the government reorganized its Food Guide Pyramid and individualized it. This means that each person has his or her own specific pyramid. Instead of horizontal divisions, the divisions are now vertical, with each one having a thickness that corresponds to the amount of that food group that you should be eating. Your amount depends on your age, sex, and level of physical activity. If you go to www.mypyramid.gov/pyramid/index.html, you can plug in a few numbers and get specific recommendations for your personalized Food Guide Pyramid, along with a host of additional nutrition information.

The old recommendations for servings are gone from this Pyramid. They were confusing. People can relate to amounts like ounces and cups much more easily. The new pyramid consists of the following food groups, which I present below in the recommended order of consumption, more to less:

- **Grains:** The health benefits of grains include reduction in heart disease, constipation, diabetes, and cancer. They also help with weight management. The government wants you to eat plenty of grains, which they help you to calculate, the amount depending on your calorie needs. You should be eating whole grains, grains that contain the whole grain kernel, such as whole-wheat flour, bulgur (cracked wheat), oatmeal, whole cornmeal, and brown rice. The government wants you to eat less refined grain, such as white flour, white bread, and white rice.

- **Vegetables:** You should be eating more dark green vegetables, more orange vegetables, and more dry beans and peas. The health benefits of vegetables are reductions in strokes, diabetes, weight, and loss of bone. The amount you need to consume varies from 1 cup to 3 cups a day based on your age, sex, and level of activity.

- **Fruits:** You need to eat a variety of different fruits, and the amount varies from 1 to 2 cups a day. They can be fresh, canned, frozen, or dried. Fruits benefit you by reducing heart disease, diabetes, high blood pressure, and cancer.

- **Milk and dairy products:** This group includes dairy and cheese. You get the benefit of larger bone mass and reduction of osteoporosis from this group. Consume 2 to 3 cups of milk or something else from this group each day.

- **Proteins:** Meat and beans fit the bill here. The instruction is to "go lean on protein," and you should eat no more than 2 to 6 ½ ounces of protein daily. Proteins give you vitamins, iron, magnesium, and zinc. They are also the building blocks for bones, muscles, cartilage, skin, and blood. Fish, nuts, and seeds, which provide fat in a better form (unsaturated fat), are preferred to beef, which contains more saturated fat and cholesterol, the fats that lead to arteriosclerosis. Beans are also a good source of protein.

Counting calories

The guidelines I explain in the previous section offer a range of ounces of each food group rather than a fixed number of ounces. The reason for this is that your intake of the various food groups depends on your ideal weight. Also, because no two people are exactly alike in their metabolism and in their activity level, a daily calorie level for two people of the same height and weight is different, particularly if they're male and female. But you can get a general idea of how many calories you should be consuming to maintain your ideal weight, and then make adjustments if you find that you need fewer or more calories.

I talk about "ideal weight" just to give you a reference from which to calculate your daily caloric needs. What I want you to achieve is a healthy weight.

Here's a relatively simple formula to use to figure out how many calories you need. Start with the figure for your ideal weight (see the previous section, "Maintaining a healthy weight"). Multiply that number by ten. If you should weigh 140 pounds, for example, your calculation comes to 1,400 kilocalories, which is your basal calorie need. Now you add more depending on your activity level. A person who doesn't exercise much at all increases the basal calorie number by 10 percent to arrive at a daily kilocalorie level of 1,540. A person who does moderate exercise, for example a daily walk for 25 minutes, adds 20 percent to that total to arrive at 1,680 kilocalories. The very active person, who digs ditches all day, for example, needs 40 percent more or even higher to arrive at a daily need of 1,960 kilocalories or greater.

The government has made it easy for you to figure out how much to eat on a daily basis. Go to the Web site www.mypyramid.gov/mypyramid/index.aspx and put in your age, sex, and level of physical activity. For example, I put in a male age 50 who does about 1 hour of physical activity a day. The chart told me that I should eat 8 ounces of grains, 3 cups of vegetables, 2 cups of fruit, 3 cups of milk, and 6½ ounces of protein and beans daily. It told me to aim for four whole grains a day, a variety of vegetables throughout the week, 7 teaspoons of oils a day, and to limit my sugar and fat kilocalories to 360. Then came the caveat, "This calorie level is only an estimate of your needs. Monitor your body weight to see if you need to adjust your calorie intake."

To give you an idea of the difference that age makes, the chart instructs a male age 10 who does the same amount of physical activity to eat 6 ounces of grains, 2½ cups of vegetables, 1½ cups of fruits, 3 cups of milk, and 5 ounces of protein and beans. The chart instructs this boy to eat 6 teaspoons of oil and only 195 kilocalories of additional food from sweets and fats.

If you adhere to these guidelines, you are well on your way to hitting the target of a healthy weight. The next sections fine-tune this information by discussing individual nutrients and why you ought to choose a variety of grains, fruits, and vegetables.

Selecting a variety of foods

Choosing among the many foods that make up each group has many benefits. Most important, when you eat a variety of foods, you ensure that you get all the nutrients your body (including your thyroid) needs. In particular, some foods contain certain vitamins and minerals that aren't present in other foods. Only a variety of foods gives you all the vitamins and minerals that you need. In addition, your meals are more interesting when you eat a variety of foods rather than the same meal again and again.

Keep in mind that despite their differences in color and appearance, most fruits and vegetables share about the same energy sources as other members of their group (see the following "Energy sources" section). The different colors and appearances indicate that they differ in their vitamins and minerals.

Energy sources

The energy that we use to move our bodies comes from one of three sources:

✔ **Protein:** Protein is necessary to build muscles and the organs of the body. Proteins also make up certain hormones. The backbone of the thyroid hormone is an amino acid, one of the several amino acids that combine to make up protein.

You get your protein when you eat animal foods, such as meat, fish, poultry, and milk. These are sources of complete protein. Each of these foods contains all the amino acids that the human body needs to manufacture its own protein, including certain amino acids that the human body can't manufacture called *essential amino acids.* Plants, especially beans and peas, also contain protein, but a single source of vegetable protein doesn't have all the essential amino acids in one food source. Therefore, vegetarians must eat a variety of protein sources.

✔ **Carbohydrates:** Carbohydrates are mainly found in the bread, cereal, rice, and pasta food group, as well as in fruits and some vegetables. When carbohydrates are broken down in the intestine, they're absorbed into the body as sugars, which give you the immediate energy you need to move your muscles. Your body can also store them in your muscles and your liver to provide energy if you need it later on.

✔ **Fats:** Your body needs fats in very small quantities to provide the backbone for certain essential hormones, such as estrogen and testosterone. Fats also store energy in the fat tissues of your body, but when they're present in excessive amounts, they can accumulate in places where they do damage, especially the arteries of the heart. The worst offenders are the *saturated fats,* the kind that are solid at room temperature. Butter and the fat attached to a steak are examples. The calories in this type of fat should make up no more than 10 percent of your total calories. Most of the fats of vegetable origin (like canola oil and olive oil) are *unsaturated fats,* although they're still a source of concentrated calories.

Vegetable fats that are saturated are coconut and palm oils, so use them sparingly. Check out the "Choosing your fats properly" section later in the chapter for more information on this important subject.

Vitamins

Although you only need vitamins in tiny amounts, they're essential for a healthy body. They change the stored energy in the energy sources into energy that the body can use. Your body uses them in many of the chemical reactions that take place in your cells. You need to eat a number of vitamins, because your body can't make them. The various vitamins, their function, and their sources in food include

- ✔ **Vitamin A,** used for vision and growth of bone and teeth, is found in liver, carrots, and spinach.

- ✔ **Vitamin B1,** used for digestion and nervous system function, comes from whole-grain cereals, peas, and nuts.

- ✔ **Vitamin B2,** which helps to release energy and maintain the skin and eyes, comes from liver, milk, eggs, and leafy vegetables.

- ✔ **Vitamin B3,** used for maintenance of the skin and nerves, comes from chicken, salmon, and peanuts.

- ✔ **Vitamin B6** is necessary to make red blood cells and to release energy from the energy sources. It comes from meat, fish, poultry, and peanuts.

- ✔ **Vitamin B12** is essential for the nervous system and red blood cells. It's found in all foods coming from animals, including meat and milk; a person who eats nothing but vegetables won't get this vitamin.

- ✔ **Vitamin C** helps with healing and prevention of infections and is found in citrus fruits, strawberries, and broccoli.

- ✔ **Vitamin D** is necessary for the proper use of calcium and comes in milk, fish, and the yolk of eggs. Fortunately, this is a vitamin that the body can make when the skin is exposed to sunlight.

- ✔ **Vitamin E** has many functions, including prevention of cholesterol buildup and production of red blood cells and muscles. You get it in vegetable oils, peas, and nuts.

- ✔ **Vitamin K** is essential for clotting of the blood so that you don't continue to bleed when you're cut. It comes from broccoli and leafy vegetables.

- ✔ **Folic acid** is another vitamin needed to produce red blood cells and protein. It's found in leafy vegetables, oranges, and peanuts.

Minerals

The minerals aren't *organic* — they aren't of animal or vegetable origin. They come from the earth and are taken up by vegetables, which animals then eat. Minerals consist of the major minerals, which are present in relatively large amounts in the body, and trace elements that are essential but present in only tiny amounts.

The major minerals consist of the following:

- ✔ **Calcium** for strong bones and teeth, for blood clotting, and for muscle function is found in dairy products, almonds, broccoli, and other green vegetables.
- ✔ **Magnesium** for nerve and muscle function is found in milk, seafood, bananas, and green leafy vegetables.
- ✔ **Phosphorus** for the bones and teeth comes from milk, hamburger, and cheese.

The trace elements include the following:

- ✔ **Chromium,** for using carbohydrates properly, is found in organ meats, mushrooms, and broccoli.
- ✔ **Iodine,** the key mineral for the production of thyroid hormones, is found in seafood and iodized salt and bread.
- ✔ **Iron,** for red blood cell hemoglobin, comes from meat, poultry, fish, and raisins.
- ✔ **Selenium,** also used in enzymes that affect thyroid hormones, is found in seafood and whole grains.
- ✔ **Zinc,** needed in the production of insulin, is found in red meat, shellfish, and eggs.

Now you know what these nutrients are, what they do, and where you find them. No discussion of proper nutrition can leave out a discussion of fats, so keep reading.

Choosing your fats properly

You want to limit your fat intake to no more than 30 percent of your total daily calories while limiting your intake of saturated fat to no more than one third of that amount. Eating your calories according to the Food Guide Pyramid keeps you within those limitations if you choose your fats wisely. Select foods that contain unsaturated fat, like vegetable oils (not coconut or palm oils).

You can keep your fats down by looking for low-fat foods, which are plentiful in the supermarkets these days. Just remember not to substitute foods rich in carbohydrates. Food labels can tell you what you need to know about the energy sources in the food as well as the amounts of the vitamins and minerals.

Measuring your cholesterol

The fat that most people think about is cholesterol. You should know your level of cholesterol. Ask your doctor to check your cholesterol level if you don't know it yet. The recommendation is that your total cholesterol should be less than 200. However, a particle in your blood called *high density lipoprotein* (HDL) carries cholesterol away from the arteries back to the liver, where it's broken down. That's why HDL is commonly referred to as "good" cholesterol. You can do a simple calculation to see if your level of cholesterol is dangerous. If you divide the total cholesterol by the HDL cholesterol and the result is less than 4.5, you're at lower risk to have a heart attack. The higher that number, the greater your risk.

You can do something to raise your HDL. The best way is exercise. The more you do (within reason), the higher your HDL and the lower your risk of a heart attack.

High cholesterol and hypothyroidism

High cholesterol is also a well-known effect of hypothyroidism. Moreover, high cholesterol isn't only associated with coronary artery disease and heart attacks, but with peripheral vascular disease (leading to blocked blood flow to the arms and legs) and cerebral artery disease, which can lead to strokes.

The number of people with high cholesterol is far greater than the number of people who have hypothyroidism. Most abnormalities in cholesterol are due to excessive fat in the diet and lack of exercise.

Many cases of undiagnosed hypothyroidism may result in high cholesterol. Studies show that more than 10 percent of people with high cholesterol (levels over 200) have hypothyroidism. Most people with high cholesterol have never been tested for hypothyroidism, and most people don't know that hypothyroidism and high cholesterol have a connection in the first place.

When a patient with high cholesterol receives a diagnosis of hypothyroidism, the treatment is, of course, thyroid hormone. The results can be pretty dramatic, with a major improvement in the fats in the blood. (This result may not be true for people with *subclinical hypothyroidism,* who have an elevated TSH level but a normal free T4.) Reduction in cholesterol by as much as 30 to 40 percent may follow the use of thyroid hormone in a person with hypothyroidism.

The explanation for the increase in cholesterol in hypothyroidism is that the metabolism (or breakdown) of cholesterol declines with hypothyroidism just as the metabolism of everything else in the body declines. However, the production of cholesterol remains the same, leading to a rise in the blood cholesterol.

If your cholesterol is elevated above 200, ask your doctor to check your thyroid function.

Moderating your sugar intake

The U.S. government guidelines recommend choosing beverages and foods to moderate your intake of sugars. Many reasons support this recommendation:

✓ Sugary foods promote tooth decay.

✓ Sugary foods often contain few essential nutrients and replace those foods that have these nutrients.

✓ Sugary foods are the source of many calories. People often eat them in an effort to avoid fatty foods but still end up with too many calories.

You can avoid these problems by keeping your portions of sugary foods like pies, cakes, candies, and cookies small. Substituting fruit for these sugary desserts reduces sugar intake, provides a certain amount of sweetness for your sweet tooth, and provides you with other important nutrients all at once.

The biggest offender when it comes to eating lots of sugar with no nutrition is a bottle of soda. Unless it's diet soda, prepared with noncaloric sweeteners, the typical bottle of soda gives you a huge amount of sugar and nothing else. Twelve ounces of soda has between 100 and 200 unhealthy kilocalories of sugar. Drink one a day for 15 days, and you gain a pound. Even the flavored fruit sodas have this problem. Do yourself a favor and switch to water with lemon or lime or the diet sodas that have no sugar. Be sure to read the label to find out what you're drinking.

Choosing and preparing foods with less salt

The guideline regarding salt intake is meant to protect you from developing high blood pressure. The recommended amount of salt is a teaspoon, or 6 grams, daily. Most people eat twice as much as that or more. One problem is that food manufacturers typically add a lot of salt to their foods. Avoid this by choosing low-salt foods as well as less processed foods and more whole fruits and vegetables.

Another problem is that people are so used to picking up the salt shaker and heavily spraying their food with salt. The result is food that tastes like salt and not much else. Try your food without salt for a change. At first it may taste bland, but then you begin to notice the subtle flavors of the food coming through. When you do, you may never want to go back to eating so much salt again.

Most recipes, especially in older cookbooks, recommend more salt than is necessary for proper preparation of the food. Try reducing the salt in the recipe by half. The food will probably cook just as well, and the taste may even be superior. If you don't tell your family that you're reducing the salt, they'll probably never know.

In the United States and many other countries, iodized salt is the major source of iodine. That teaspoon of salt a day contains twice as much iodine as you are required to eat each day, so you can reduce your salt intake to a half teaspoon and still be assured of getting enough. If you eat one piece of bread, it contains just about your daily requirement of iodine. You don't need to eat excess salt to assure yourself of getting enough iodine.

Drinking alcohol in moderation

Men who consume more than two drinks of alcohol a day or more than ten in a week and women who consume more than one drink a day or five a week should work to reduce those amounts. Like cigarettes, alcohol can damage your body in many ways. It raises your blood pressure, causes liver destruction, and promotes certain cancers. It provides no nutrition and often causes you to eat less of the foods you need for good nutrition. Severe alcoholism results in damage to the nervous system, vitamin deficiency diseases, anemia, and skin damage.

Alcohol also destroys families. When one or more members of a family are alcoholics, the incidence of divorce, accidents, suicide, loss of employment, and disease within that family is much greater than in families that don't have an alcoholic member. Alcoholism can also lead to impotency, making sexual relations impossible.

Keep in mind that alcohol in moderation (as specified by the numbers I've provided) can raise the level of HDL, or "good cholesterol," in your body. Alcohol can also be a pleasant part of a meal and a key element in certain social scenes. Clearly, alcohol isn't going to go away, but you must control its use.

Keeping foods safe to eat

To protect yourself from the chemicals that are sprayed on foods as they're grown and the chemicals present in the soil that fruits and vegetables are grown in, wash all fruits and vegetables before eating them. (Obviously, this doesn't eliminate chemicals inside the food.)

Proper refrigeration of foods that can spoil is essential. You must keep raw meat, fish, and poultry in the refrigerator before cooking them thoroughly.

Keep your hands clean when you handle these foods. And make sure that you clean cutting boards and knives well after you use them for cutting raw meats. The use of a mild bleach solution to cleanse cutting boards is also recommended.

After you cook food, if you want to save it for a later time, keep it in the refrigerator. Leaving it at room temperature allows bacteria to grow that may be present when you eat the food again, even if you reheat it.

For more information on food safety, visit `www.foodsafety.gov`. Clicking on the "Consumer Advice" link is a great place to start for information on food handling, product-specific advice, and information targeted to various groups of people.

Making good food choices

You can easily choose to eat foods that contribute to better health and weight control over those that lead to illness and obesity. You just need to know how to substitute one for the other. In Table 20-1, I show you the wiser choices that you can make every day. By making these choices, you notice a little loss of taste but a definite improvement in your health and your ability to lose weight.

Table 20-1	Choosing Healthier Foods	
Food Group	*Better Choice*	*Worse Choice*
Breads	Whole-grain breads, whole-grain and bran cereals, rice, pasta	Refined-flour breads and cakes, croissants, cookies, pastries
Vegetables	Dark green, leafy vegetables; yellow-orange vegetables; cabbage; broccoli	Avocados, vegetables in butter or cream sauce
Fruits	Citrus fruits, berries, apples, pears	Coconut, fruit pies, or pastries
Dairy	Low-fat cheese, low-fat or nonfat milk, sherbet	Whole milk, butter, sweet cream, ice cream, cream cheese, hard cheeses
Meats	Lean meats, chicken, fresh fish, cooked dry beans and peas, egg whites	Fatty meats, lunch meats, tuna in oil, egg yolks (or whole eggs), sausages

Clarifying the Thyroid-Weight Connection

Certain misconceptions exist about how your thyroid reacts to weight loss and how your weight reacts to a change in your thyroid function. In this section, I hope to dispel these misconceptions by showing you how your thyroid and your weight really interact.

Does my metabolism slow when I lose weight?

People who lose weight on a diet often regain the weight after a time. If you've had this experience, maybe you've heard that the reason you can't keep the weight off is that your thyroid and metabolism slow down after you lose some pounds, so the weight comes back on more easily. This reasoning implies that your body establishes a "set-point" weight and tries to maintain it by changing your thyroid function and your metabolism whenever you move away from that weight. The idea is that if you lose weight, your metabolic rate falls because your thyroid function declines. Researchers have studied this idea to determine its validity.

In a study in the *American Journal of Clinical Nutrition* in November 2000, researchers tested thyroid function and metabolic rates for 24 overweight women in the process of losing weight. When they were actively losing weight, the women's resting metabolic rates and free T3 hormone levels declined. But after they reached their ideal weight, their free T3 levels and resting metabolic rate were normal as well. This study contradicts the idea of a "set-point" weight.

If you're having trouble keeping off the weight you lose and your thyroid is functioning normally, this study shows that you can't blame your thyroid. You may want to take a closer look at your exercise and eating habits instead.

If I'm treated for hyperthyroidism, am I doomed to gain weight?

Many people who receive treatment for hyperthyroidism with radioactive iodine complain that they can't lose weight after they become hypothyroid and are placed on thyroid-hormone replacement. If this describes your situation, you should consider a number of possible explanations:

- You may not be taking enough thyroid hormones to replace your deficit. Checking that your thyroid-stimulating hormone (TSH) is in the normal range and ideally less than 2.5 is important.

- You may need to take T3 hormone replacement as well as T4, even if your TSH is normal (see Chapter 4).

- You may be eating some food that interferes with thyroid hormone absorption, such as soy protein, around the time you take the thyroid hormone.

Then again, maybe none of the above explain your weight gain.

A study in the *Journal of the American College of Nutrition* in 1999 attempted to address this issue. The authors studied ten people who received radioactive iodine for hyperthyroidism. The researchers looked at the participants' total food energy intake; their T4, T3, and TSH levels; and their height and weight at the time of treatment and at one, two, three, six, and twelve months afterward. The participants' thyroid hormone levels declined in the first months of treatment but increased later. Even when thyroid hormone levels increased, the participants continued to gain weight. Interestingly, the average weight of the participants before the development of hyperthyroidism was about 170 pounds; at the time of treatment, 148 pounds; and after a year, about 168 pounds. Their final average weight was actually *lower* than their average weight before hyperthyroidism developed. The study concluded that weight gain after treatment of hyperthyroidism was initially due to a fall in the metabolic rate that accompanied the drop in thyroid hormone but later was due to food intake or lifestyle choices.

Another study in the *Journal of Clinical Endocrinology and Metabolism* in 1998 showed where the weight gain occurs in the body when you receive treatment for hyperthyroidism. The researchers showed that most of the weight gain in the first three months occurred as fat in the waist area and in muscle tissue, whereas weight gain later on was in the fat under the skin. This study shows very clearly that the weight loss that occurred before treatment for hyperthyroidism was loss of lean tissue, the muscle mass — further proof that using excess thyroid hormone for weight loss leads to loss of muscle.

Many people treated for hyperthyroidism gain more weight than they want to after treatment. In most cases, this occurs either because their thyroid hormone levels aren't in the range they should be or because they don't alter their eating and exercise habits after treatment. If you're in this situation, keep in mind that you probably increased your food intake and decreased your activity level when your body was hyperthyroid. You need to make lifestyle adjustments after treatment in order to bring your body back to its healthy weight.

The thyroid and celiac disease

Celiac disease is an autoimmune disease of the small intestine that results in poor absorption of fat, protein, carbohydrates, iron, and vitamins A, D, and K. The consequences of celiac disease are diarrhea, *osteomalacia* (poorly mineralized bone), signs of vitamin deficiency, and anemia. Studies show that as high as 21 percent of patients with celiac disease also have autoimmune hypothyroidism, and 3 percent of people with thyroid disease have celiac disease.

The treatment for celiac disease is to remove gluten from the patient's diet. Gluten is present in wheat, barley, oats, rye, and as a filler in many prepared foods and medications. When gluten is removed from the diet, not only does the celiac disease disappear, but the patient's thyroid disease is cured as well.

A study in the *American Journal of Gastroenterology* in March 2001 found that out of 241 patients with celiac disease, 31 (13 percent) also had hypothyroidism. Of the 31, 29 had subclinical hypothyroidism with an elevation in TSH but a normal T4. When they received treatment for a year by avoiding gluten in their diet and the celiac disease was cured, the thyroid abnormalities disappeared in all of them as well.

Thyroid disease is so commonly associated with celiac disease that everyone with celiac disease should be tested for thyroid disease. If present, both the celiac disease and the thyroid disorder may respond to gluten withdrawal.

Getting Enough Iodine in a Vegetarian Diet

Because iodine is a key element of thyroid hormones, iodine is a necessary part of your daily diet.

Vegetarians avoid eating the key foods that contain iodine, such as fish, seafood, eggs, meat, and milk. You must have sufficient iodine in your diet to have good thyroid health. A study of vegetarians in the *British Journal of Medicine* in December 1998 found that 63 percent of the females and 36 percent of the males had inadequate iodine intake.

If you follow a vegetarian diet, you may want to take iodized salt or iodine supplements. If you have any doubt about whether you're getting enough iodine, ask your doctor to check your iodine level (with a urine test). A teaspoon of salt a day or a piece or two of bread takes care of your iodine needs as a vegetarian.

Exercising for Your Thyroid

If you're being successfully treated for a thyroid condition and tests show that you have normal thyroid function, you can exercise as much as you want. (Just be sure to listen to your body and slow down if you feel like you're overextending yourself.) You should be doing aerobic exercise, which forces your heart to beat faster, to keep your heart healthy and your body fat under control. You should also be doing strength training to retain and build muscle.

The amount of exercise that you do determines its effect on your body. If you do 30 minutes of aerobic exercise daily, you achieve aerobic fitness. If you do 60 minutes of aerobic exercise daily, you're able to maintain weight loss. If you do 90 minutes of aerobic exercise daily, you lose weight.

A study in the November 2005 issue of the *Archives of Internal Medicine* looked at the long-term effects of exercise at different levels of intensity for different durations. The study divided 500 people into four exercise groups: a moderate, intensity-low frequency group; a moderate, intensity-high frequency group; a hard, intensity-low frequency group; and a hard, intensity-high frequency group. The heart rate during exercise determined the intensity of the exercise. Low frequency was three to four days per week, while high frequency was five to seven days per week. All groups showed significant improvement in cardiorespiratory fitness by six months and maintained that fitness over two years. However, only the group that combined hard exercise with high frequency showed improvement in blood fats.

Avoiding iodine before thyroid studies

The results of thyroid uptake studies are more valuable if the subjects avoid foods that contain iodine for a time before the test. The purpose of most such studies is to determine the size and shape of the thyroid and whether a given abnormality of the thyroid takes up iodine.

If your doctor is testing you for hyperthyroidism, you don't have to avoid iodine. In fact, avoiding iodine may confuse the diagnosis, because you're looking for abnormally high uptake of the iodine, and you don't want to artificially enhance the test results by following a low-iodine diet.

If you're having a thyroid scan done for reasons other than hyperthyroidism, follow a low-iodine diet for several days:

- ✔ Use only noniodized salt.
- ✔ Avoid milk or milk products.
- ✔ Avoid commercial vitamin preparations unless they definitely don't contain iodine.
- ✔ Steer clear of eggs.
- ✔ Don't eat seafood, fish, shellfish, seaweed, or kelp.
- ✔ Avoid cured or corned foods.
- ✔ Don't use bread products made with iodine dough conditioners.
- ✔ Avoid foods that contain Red Dye #3, chocolate, molasses, or soy.

If you have a thyroid condition that hasn't yet been treated, you need to be aware of some special considerations regarding exercise. In this section, I discuss these situations and talk about how to use exercise to maximize your health in general.

If you are older than 35 and starting an exercise program, especially a vigorous one, talk to your doctor first.

Recognizing the natural consequences of aging

Don't confuse the natural effects of aging with the consequences of having thyroid disease. As you get older, your ability to do aerobic exercise decreases, as does your strength. If you go to the gym for the first time in years and find that you can't last as long on the treadmill as you used to, chances are that your thyroid isn't the culprit.

Your ability to take in oxygen is a measure of your physical condition. Your oxygen uptake peaks around age 25, and after that, it steadily declines no matter what you do to prevent it. Your strength also seems to peak around the same time, but it remains more or less the same until around age 40, when it starts to decline steadily. We all lose about 25 percent of our maximum strength by age 65. We also lose flexibility with aging — our tendons, ligaments, and joint capsules become stiffer.

You've certainly heard the old saying, "You will only be young once." Take my word for it: It's true.

At any age, you can maximize your strength, your stamina, and your flexibility by doing plenty of exercise. By plenty, I mean at least 30 minutes, four or more times per week, preferably every day.

Working out with hypothyroidism

When you have an underactive thyroid, the fatigue that accompanies this condition limits your ability to exercise. After you begin taking the proper replacement dose of thyroid hormone, you should be able to exercise normally. But if you still can't exercise because of fatigue, consider the two common reasons:

- ✔ You may not be receiving sufficient thyroid hormone, so your TSH is between 0.5 and 2.5. If your symptoms linger even after taking the hormone replacement, don't settle for a TSH of 3 or higher.

- ✔ You may need to take T3 hormone in addition to T4 to fully replace your missing thyroid function.

Hypothyroidism does affect the functioning of your heart, which can become apparent during exercise. If you're receiving treatment with thyroid hormone, your heart function should return to normal (assuming that you don't have any other heart conditions).

Heart function during exercise may actually be a greater issue for patients with *subclinical hypothyroidism* (where your TSH is elevated, but your free T4 is normal), because these patients aren't necessarily treated with thyroid hormone. (See Chapter 19 for a detailed discussion of the debate over treatment.) Subclinical hypothyroidism is associated with mild abnormalities in the heart, which aren't measurable when you're resting but are detectable when you exercise. The normal heart's adaptation to effort is diminished in subclinical hypothyroidism. Subclinical hypothyroidism also results in a rise in the form of cholesterol that leads to heart attacks and a fall in the form that's protective against heart attacks. Some thyroid specialists believe that these subtle changes are reason enough to treat subclinical hypothyroidism with thyroid hormone.

The muscles of a person with subclinical hypothyroidism show abnormal energy metabolism that leads to early fatigue, which thyroid hormone also corrects. Subclinical hypothyroidism also impairs the ability of blood vessels to open up to allow more blood flow, which is further evidence of the need for treatment, particularly before the condition worsens.

Exercising with hyperthyroidism

If you're hyperthyroid, your heart rate and the amount of blood pumped per heartbeat are both elevated when you're resting, but they don't respond to exercise in a normal fashion. After you achieve normal thyroid function through treatment, these abnormalities disappear.

Careful study of the hearts of hyperthyroid patients shows that their resting heart rates are abnormally high, as are the frequent occurrences of abnormal heart rhythms. Abnormal thickening of the heart muscle increases the size of the heart.

With exercise, the hyperthyroid heart can't increase its workload the way that a normal heart can. The result is that the hyperthyroid person can't exercise as long as she used to, and her peak level of exercise is reduced. This is true even in subclinical hyperthyroidism, where the TSH is suppressed below the normal range, but the free T4 remains normal. When a person takes the beta blocker propranolol to slow the heart, the patient feels an improvement in exercise capacity.

An elderly person with hyperthyroidism must be especially careful with exercise, because she has an increased risk of heart failure and may experience abnormal heart rhythms (which may not improve even when the hyperthyroidism is brought under control). Chest pain can get worse as hyperthyroidism continues.

Not only heart muscle but also skeletal (arm, leg, and trunk) muscles are abnormal in hyperthyroidism. Hyperthyroid skeletal muscle requires more energy to perform the same amount of work as healthy muscle. As a result, it can be fatigued much earlier.

Meeting your minimal exercise needs

While you're recovering from hypothyroidism or hyperthyroidism, you may not be able to do much exercise and certainly not the amount necessary for good health. After you're cured, however, you want to get up to speed. You want to do two types of exercise, which I describe in the following sections.

Aerobic exercise

Aerobic exercise is used to improve heart and lung function and raise the healthy cholesterol. Any exercise that gets the heart beating faster for a sustained period is aerobic exercise. Doctors used to recommend a formula for determining the ideal heart rate during exercise: Subtract your age from 220, and your ideal heart rate is 60 to 75 percent of that number. Now we know that many people can sustain aerobic exercise at higher heart rates. Perhaps the best way to know whether you're meeting your exercise goals is to rank the exercise as follows: very, very light; very light; fairly light; somewhat hard; very hard; and very, very hard. If you stay at the level of *somewhat hard* while you get into shape, you're doing the right amount of aerobic exercise.

You should sustain aerobic exercise for 20 to 30 minutes every day. By doing this, despite the normal loss of exercise capacity with aging, you're maximizing what you have and adding significant time to your life.

 One way of insuring that you get enough exercise is to get yourself a pedometer, a little device you wear on your belt that counts your steps. If you count your daily steps for a week, you likely find that you average around 3,000 to 4,000 a day. Your ultimate goal is to average 10,000 steps a day, and you can achieve this rapidly or more slowly. Setting some athletic event in the future as your reason for building up your walking ability is often a good idea. That gives you a goal to work toward and permits you to compare your time over the years to see how fit you're becoming (or not).

Anaerobic exercise

Don't forget to do muscle strengthening anaerobic exercises as well. Anaerobic exercise strengthens muscles and increases stamina. Using light weights of 10 to 15 pounds, three times a week, you want to do at least three or four different exercises to work your arms and legs and strengthen your back. I recommend the following exercises for strengthening your muscles:

- Bicep curls
- Shoulder presses

✔ Lateral raises

✔ Bent-over rowing

✔ Good mornings

✔ Flys

✔ Pullovers

You can find the details for performing these exercises in my book *Diabetes For Dummies,* 2nd Edition as well as in *Weight Training For Dummies* (both published by Wiley, Inc.). You should do each exercise 15 times and repeat the whole set twice. Doing this every few days greatly increases your strength.

Uncovering a New Hormone: Connecting Leptin to Weight Loss and the Thyroid

Leptin is a relatively new hormone that has an important role in normal thyroid function. First described in 1994, *leptin* is a hormone made by fat cells that's a major regulator of body weight. As your body fat goes up, the leptin in your body increases.

When a person fasts, he or she has a fall in T3 and TSH. A fall in leptin may be responsible for this, which could explain a decline in weight loss that occurs over time in a fasting individual. In the future, the use of leptin during a diet may promote increased weight loss. This section explains the brief history of our knowledge of leptin and what we know so far about its relationship with thyroid hormone.

Learning the functions of leptin

Researchers conducted the first studies of this hormone on a strain of obese rats, which they found to have a genetic mutation that resulted in failure of leptin production. Administering leptin to these mice resulted in weight loss — the mice reduced their food intake and had increased energy. The same thing was found when leptin was given to normal-weight mice — they lost fat mass. Researchers then discovered leptin in human beings, which was hailed as the obesity gene. Unfortunately, injections of leptin in human beings didn't lead to substantial weight loss.

Obesity isn't the result of a genetic mutation in the leptin gene. However, several families have been found to have a mutation of the leptin gene that leads to severe obesity at a young age. This gene is a recessive trait, meaning that family members who have only one abnormal leptin gene instead of two don't show the disease. When people with the disease take leptin, they experience significant weight loss and the reversal of metabolic abnormalities.

Further studies showed that leptin was doing more than just signaling to the body that it had too much fat. When researchers compared body-fat percentages and leptin levels of women and men, they found that women's leptin levels were as much as two to three times that of men. But even though women typically have more fat mass than men, this result doesn't fully explain the difference. Studies now show that the female sex hormone, estrogen, stimulates leptin production, while the male sex hormone, testosterone, suppresses leptin.

Researchers know that girls go into puberty when they reach a certain weight. Puberty begins when a hormone from the *hypothalamus,* a part of the brain, begins to be released. This hormone is called *gonadotrophin-releasing hormone* (GnRH). The question arose, what was the signal to release GnRH? The presence of leptin proved to be the answer to that question, because it clearly indicates when the fat mass is sufficient for puberty to begin.

Interacting with thyroid hormone

Researchers have now shown that leptin interacts with several other hormones in the body, especially insulin, which appears to have an important place in regulating leptin secretion. Leptin interacts with the adrenal gland and growth hormone as well. Because thyroid hormone increases the metabolic rate, which increases the body temperature, researchers thought that leptin (which also regulates metabolism and body temperature) may interact with thyroid hormone.

Researchers have now shown that leptin helps to regulate the part of the brain that releases *thyrotrophin-releasing hormone* (TRH), and it also regulates the release of thyroid-stimulating hormone. When a person fasts, both the thyroid hormone and leptin concentrations fall. If leptin is given to the fasting individual, the TSH and the T4 hormone return to normal.

On the other hand, researchers have found that thyroid hormone controls leptin production to some extent. In animals without thyroids, leptin is increased, but when thyroid hormone is replaced, leptin is suppressed. So far in humans, researchers haven't shown that thyroid hormone causes either a rise or a fall in leptin concentration.

The understanding of the role of leptin is at an early stage. Much more will be learned in the next few years. Doctors and scientists are just starting to clarify leptin's place in thyroid disease; stay tuned.

Part IV
The Part of Tens

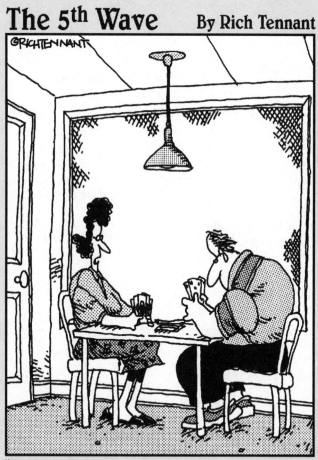

The 5th Wave   By Rich Tennant

"Look—an abnormal thyroid can make you irritable, nervous, and weak in the upper arms. But you can't blame it for the rotten game of gin you're playing."

In this part . . .

As you would expect, a part of your body as important as the thyroid prompts all sorts of myths and
mistaken ideas. Here you find the ones I consider the most
important (and possibly the most damaging if you believe
them). I show you what you can do to make sure that you
maximize your thyroid health in ten easy steps. And
finally, I answer ten representative questions that I've
received from readers since the first edition of this book
was published.

Chapter 21

Ten Myths about Thyroid Health

*T*hanks to the Internet, you have access to incredible amounts of information about your thyroid. Unfortunately, much (perhaps most) of it isn't accurate. Much of what you read online is based on the experiences and opinions of one or a few people who took this or that medicine or herb and got better in two weeks. Maintaining a healthy degree of skepticism is important.

In this chapter, I try to clear up some commonly held myths concerning the thyroid and its diseases.

I'm Hypothyroid, so I Can't Lose Weight

If you have hypothyroidism, or if you've received treatment for a thyroid condition and the cure resulted in your becoming hypothyroid, you may find that you have a hard time losing weight. The myth is that you *can't* lose weight if you have hypothyroidism, even when you receive proper treatment.

A large percentage of people who are receiving successful treatment for hypothyroidism weigh almost the same after treatment as they did before they developed the disease.

I've occasionally seen hypothyroid patients — mostly elderly people — who actually lose weight rather than gain it after they receive replacement thyroid hormone. This occurs when a patient is receiving poor nutrition, which the complacency that can accompany hypothyroidism makes worse, because he or she may not take in enough calories.

Keep in mind that hypothyroidism is associated with fatigue. Many patients with hypothyroidism reduce their physical activity as a result. They may not restore their previous level of activity after they receive proper treatment for their hypothyroidism. Therefore, first look to whether your level of activity is sufficient (I provide suggestions for determining the answer in Chapter 20).

If you struggle to lose the weight that you've gained after becoming hypothyroid, and if your activity level has remained the same, your thyroid treatment may be inadequate (which a TSH test can determine), or you may need to take T3 replacement hormone in addition to T4 (see Chapter 5).

You may also have another autoimmune condition. Because the most common cause of hypothyroidism is autoimmune thyroiditis (see Chapter 5), your doctor should look for diabetes mellitus type 1 or autoimmune adrenal insufficiency (Addison's disease — failure to make the hormone cortisol), among other conditions. A blood glucose test for diabetes or a serum cortisol level for autoimmune adrenal insufficiency easily determines whether you have one of these conditions.

The bottom line is that we all follow the principle of conservation of energy. If we take in too much energy compared to what we need, we gain weight. If we take in too little energy compared to what we need, we lose weight.

Your thyroid health and the Internet

You're not completely on your own when it comes to reading thyroid sites on the Net. If you're lucky enough to find a statement on a Web site indicating that it adheres to the Health on the Net Foundation Code of Conduct (HONcode), you can feel sure that the information is accurate. The Health on the Net Foundation has established a set of principles that any site on the Internet can adhere to. A site that follows the HONcode principles agrees to the following:

Principle 1: Medical advice will be given by qualified professionals (or the site will state that this is not the case).

Principle 2: The information supports, but does not replace, the patient/physician relationship.

Principle 3: Confidentiality of visitors to the site is respected.

Principle 4: Information is supported by references.

Principle 5: Claims about the benefits of specific treatments are supported by references.

Principle 6: Information is provided in the clearest possible manner, with contacts provided for more information — including the Webmaster's e-mail address.

Principle 7: Support for the site is clearly identified (especially commercial support).

Principle 8: If a site is supported by advertising, it's clearly stated, along with the advertising policy. Advertising is clearly differentiated from nonadvertising material.

In addition, at the back of this book in Appendix B and on my Web site (www.drrubin.com), I list sites that I consider authoritative and accurate. Just go to my site, click on "Useful Addresses" on the home page, select "Thyroid Sites" on the next page, and read to your heart's content.

Another truth is that our metabolic rate declines, as does our tendency to move around, as we age. Both changes tend to make weight loss more difficult, but it's still possible.

If you've had hypothyroidism and are on the proper dose of thyroid hormone, you're able to lose weight with sufficient diet and exercise.

I'm Hyperthyroid, so I Can't Gain Weight

The myth that weight loss always accompanies hyperthyroidism is a source of confusion in making an accurate diagnosis. Although the majority of patients do lose weight when they become hyperthyroid, some patients actually gain weight — the elderly, in particular.

A study published in the *Journal of the American Geriatric Society* in 1996 compared 19 classical signs of hyperthyroidism in older patients and younger patients. Researchers found three signs in more than 50 percent of older patients: rapid heartbeat, fatigue, and weight loss. However, some people experienced no weight loss or weight gain. Researchers found seven signs less frequently in older patients than in younger patients. Researchers found only two signs — loss of appetite and an irregular heart rhythm —more often in the older patients. Overall, of the 19 classical clinical signs, older people had only six of them on average, while younger people had 11.

Another study published in *Thyroidology* in 1992 showed very similar results. It also emphasized the importance of checking levels of thyroid hormones and TSH in the elderly population before making a diagnosis of hyperthyroidism.

Weight loss, as well as other symptoms of hyperthyroidism, may not always be present in hyperthyroid patients, especially in the elderly population. The best way to rule out thyroid disease is to get thyroid blood tests every five years, beginning at age 35.

Breastfeeding and Antithyroid Pills Don't Mix

For years, doctors advised women who took antithyroid pills for hyperthyroidism during pregnancy not to breastfeed. The fear was that the medication would enter the baby's circulation through the breast milk and make the baby hypothyroid. Doctors now know this is a myth.

Two important studies have shown that this belief is incorrect. In one study published in the *Journal of Clinical Endocrinology and Metabolism,* researchers gave 88 mothers one of the two major antithyroid drugs, methimazole, for 12 months. Researchers then measured the levels of methimazole in the babies' blood. In addition, they tested the babies for thyroid function, urinary iodine, thyroid autoantibodies, intelligence quotient (IQ), and verbal and functional ability. All of the babies of treated mothers had normal thyroid function. They grew normally, and their IQ, verbal, and functional tests were identical to children who breastfed from mothers without hyperthyroidism. In a second study, researchers gave the other major antithyroid drug, propylthiouricil (PTU), to breastfeeding mothers; some took as much as 750 milligrams of PTU daily. Again the thyroid function tests of the babies were entirely normal, as were the babies' development.

A hyperthyroid mother taking methimazole or propylthiouricil to control her hyperthyroidism may safely breastfeed her new baby.

Brand-Name Thyroid Hormone Pills Are Best

Because the number of people taking thyroid-replacement hormone in the United States and throughout the world is enormous, the amount of money people spend on thyroid-hormone replacement pills is also huge. The company that captures the largest share of the market makes its stockholders very happy.

The myth is that generic preparations of thyroxine (T4 hormone) aren't equal in potency to brand-name thyroxine, aren't standardized over time, and shouldn't be used in the treatment of hypothyroidism.

This myth began, as so many do, with research that was correct at the time but is now outdated. In 1980, an article appeared in the *Journal of the American Medical Association* showing that generic preparations weren't equal to brand-name thyroxine. Sometimes the generic preparations were weaker, and sometimes they were stronger; they weren't uniform from lot to lot. This type of information continued to appear in medical literature as late as 1995.

However, a study completed in 1990 — but didn't appear until 1997 in the *Journal of the American Medical Association* — looked at the problem again. Twenty women who were receiving successful treatment for hypothyroidism were put on four different preparations at the same dosage for six weeks at a time. Blood tests taken during this study showed absolutely no difference in any of the preparations. All the preparations met the Food and Drug Administration criterion for equivalent activity. The conclusion was that the preparations, including two brand names and two generics, were sufficiently equal in their activity, and that no reason supported choosing any one over the others. I'm happy to add that my great thyroid mentor, Dr. Francis Greenspan, among others, performed this study.

Some allege that one of the brand-name companies making thyroid-hormone replacement originally paid for the preceding study, and that when the study didn't show that its product was better, the company suppressed the study's results.

Generic thyroid preparations save you money, and you can use them interchangeably with brand-name thyroxine. Because hypothyroidism may not be a stable condition, you still want to have your doctor check your thyroid function regularly (perhaps yearly).

I Have to Take Thyroid Medication for Life

Doctors tell many patients that once they're on thyroid-hormone replacement, they must take it for life. For many people, this is true. Any treatment that removes or destroys much of the thyroid (such as surgery or radioactive iodine) requires treatment with thyroxine (T4 hormone) for life. However, in certain situations, hypothyroidism is temporary; you may need thyroxine for a time, but you later stop taking it. Sometimes the fact that you no longer need the medication may be obvious, but other times you and your doctor may need to attempt a trial period off thyroid for four to six weeks to see if you still need it.

The following are some of the conditions that require thyroid-hormone replacement for a limited amount of time. I explain each in detail in Chapter 11:

- *Subacute thyroiditis* causes the temporary breakdown of thyroid cells and the release of thyroxine from the thyroid. As this condition improves, your thyroid begins to make and store thyroxine again, and oral thyroxine is no longer necessary.

- *Silent* and *postpartum thyroiditis* also cause temporary loss of thyroxine, which the body restores with time.

- *Acute thyroiditis* occasionally requires temporary treatment with thyroid hormone.

The most common diagnosis that requires thyroid hormone treatment but may later subside so you don't need thyroid hormone pills for life is chronic thyroiditis (see Chapter 5). This condition is the result of antibodies that block TSH from sufficiently stimulating the thyroid to produce enough thyroid hormone. Occasionally, levels of blocking antibodies fall. The only way you know if this happens is by measuring the antibodies (which isn't well standardized) or stopping the thyroid hormone and testing thyroid function four to six weeks later. If your thyroid function remains normal, you may not have to take thyroxine any longer.

Depending on your diagnosis, you may be able to stop thyroid hormone treatment at some point. Checking is well worth it, particularly if you're under 40.

Natural Thyroid Hormones Are Better Than Synthetic Hormones

Scientist extracted the first thyroid hormones used to treat people with low thyroid function from the thyroids of animals and called them *desiccated thyroid* (see Chapter 5). After decades of use, synthetic thyroid hormones made in the laboratory replaced desiccated thyroid. Some holdouts still believe that desiccated thyroid is superior to synthetic thyroxine (T4 hormone) for treating hypothyroidism.

As long ago as 1978, an article appeared in the *American Journal of Medicine* titled "Why does anyone still use desiccated thyroid USP?" The article declared desiccated thyroid an obsolete therapy. The hormone extracted from animals has plenty of problems:

- ✔ Desiccated thyroid can't be standardized from dose to dose, because one animal has a different amount of the thyroid hormones in its thyroid than the next animal.

- ✔ Desiccated thyroid has impurities that may cause immune reactions.

- ✔ The use of desiccated thyroid confuses the thyroid testing. If doctors measure only the total T4 hormone, that result is often low because of the large amount of T3 in the medication. The patient may receive even more thyroid hormone and actually become hyperthyroid.

- ✔ The dose of T4 and T3 that desiccated thyroid supplies doesn't provide the same levels as what the normal thyroid releases.

These problems have had their consequences in the past. Patients have been undertreated or overtreated by different preparations of desiccated thyroid. Doctors have found some patients to be hyperthyroid for a few hours a day due to the large amount of T3 in some desiccated thyroid pills.

One thing to be said for desiccated thyroid is that it does contain some T3, which most synthetic hormone replacements don't have. However, a synthetic preparation of T3 does exist, and it's far superior to the mixture in desiccated thyroid.

Synthetic thyroxine is currently the medication of choice in the treatment of hypothyroidism. In the future, a combination of T4 and T3 in the exact ratio that it leaves the thyroid may replace T4 alone.

Conducting proper medical studies

Scientists who conducted studies using control groups (people who didn't get active medicine or treatment but thought they did) and treatment groups (people who got the active medicine or treatment but weren't certain that they did) have found the myths in this chapter to be just that — myths. In studies using control and treatment groups, even the doctors administering the treatment or medicine don't know who is getting real treatment and who isn't. Only by conducting studies this way can scientists make a fair comparison between groups. This is the famous *double blind placebo–controlled study,* and scientists arrange it in the following manner:

✔ No patient knows what he or she is getting, nor does the doctor, but all patients get something — either real treatment or a placebo.

✔ The benefits for the patient getting the real treatment must be significantly better than those for the patient getting a placebo to prove the treatment's value.

✔ The side effects for each group should be about equal so the patient with the disease isn't having many more side effects than the person serving as a control.

Thyroid Disease Is Contagious

Understanding why this myth has become so entrenched in the minds of the public isn't hard. Most thyroid disease is hereditary; so the likelihood of finding the same disease in two sisters or a mother and her daughter is relatively high, potentially suggesting that their physical closeness to one another causes them to have the same disease. Furthermore, in areas where people don't consume enough iodine, practically everyone has thyroid disease — again seeming to suggest that it may be catching.

Another situation that seems to suggest that thyroid disease is catching is the occurrence of thyroid disease after large-scale radiation exposure. Just about everyone comes down with some illness in this situation. Children, especially, often develop goiters, nodules, and thyroid cancers.

An understanding of the way these diseases develop quickly clarifies the situation:

✔ The hereditary thyroid diseases affect the females of a family, usually sparing the males.

✔ The incidence of thyroid disease rapidly declines in iodine-deficient areas after iodine is supplied to the population.

✔ Children who take iodine pills or avoid exposure to radioactive iodine generally won't get thyroid diseases, while those who don't do.

You can't catch thyroid disease, nor can you give it to someone else in the way that germs pass from person to person.

Iodine Deficiency Is a Medical Problem

Because iodine deficiency (see Chapter 12) causes hypothyroidism, goiter, and cretinism (when severe), you may think that it's a clear-cut disease that should respond to medical treatment with iodine. If this were so, the disease would have disappeared years ago.

As with any major medical problem (like AIDS, breast cancer, and prostate cancer), iodine deficiency is a social, economic, and political problem as much as, or more than, a medical problem.

To begin with, an understanding about the cause of hypothyroidism in iodine-deficient areas is often lacking. The people are poor, work very hard, and have little time for the intricacies of the cause of disease. Their poverty means that they can't afford to pay for nurses to give them medication or inject them with iodized oil. They don't understand that certain foods, like cassava, worsen the problem, so they continue to consume large quantities of them.

Often the local or federal government pumps in lots of money to improve the situation by providing iodine supplementation. But it provides no punishment for those who don't follow the regulations. Manufacturers may fail to put any iodine into their so-called "iodized" salt and claim the subsidies for it anyway. Much of that money disappears after it leaves government control.

Sometimes attempts to solve the problem run up against the realities of salt production. This has been the case in Indonesia, for example, where numerous salt farmers rather than a centralized salt-production facility make salt (as salt is made in China). Consequently, altering salt production to make enough iodized salt was easier and more productive in China than in Indonesia.

When a tremendous need for a substance like iodine exists, the cheats try to profit from people's misery. They charge more for iodized salt and then fail to actually iodize the salt. They also underprice the government's iodized salt so that people buy their salt rather than true iodized salt from the government.

The instability of poor governments also plays a role. For example, when Communist East Germany recognized the problem of iodine deficiency, the government provided iodine and brought the disease under fairly good control. After the reunification of East and West Germany, the combined government neglected the problem, and iodine deficiency began to reappear.

The solution to a clearly medical problem like iodine deficiency may have to involve social, cultural, and economic changes that populations often resist, making a cure exceedingly difficult.

The Higher My Autoantibody Levels, the Worse My Thyroid Disease

This myth derives from a phenomenon that seems obvious: The more you have of something that denotes a disease, the worse that disease must be. For example, if your temperature is 102 degrees Fahrenheit, you're probably sicker than someone whose temperature is only 99 degrees Fahrenheit. When it comes to thyroid autoantibodies, however, this isn't the case.

When doctors measure and compare the levels of autoantibodies with the severity of a patient's thyroid disease, they find no correlation. Some of the sickest patients with hyperthyroidism due to Graves' disease have relatively low levels of autoantibodies, while people with milder cases of Graves' may have high levels.

Adding to the confusion is the fact that the disappearance of thyroid autoantibodies after treatment with antithyroid drugs is a marker for improvement and suggests that the disease won't recur.

Very low levels of autoantibodies are often present in elderly women. But unless those women have abnormal thyroid function tests, the autoantibodies have little importance. Although people with low levels of autoantibodies should be retested occasionally, they don't require treatment unless a thyroid condition develops.

Doctors shouldn't compare autoantibody levels between laboratories. Laboratories practice little consistency in the methods they use in their tests, so a level of a thousand at one laboratory means something very different from a level of a thousand at another laboratory.

Very high thyroid autoantibody levels don't indicate that you have a bad case of autoimmune thyroiditis. They simply confirm the diagnosis if other signs and symptoms exist.

Clinical Symptoms Are More Reliable Than Blood Tests

Thyroid disease can be very confusing. In certain age groups, particularly the elderly, the expected signs and symptoms may not exist. Sometimes doctors find opposite symptoms. For example, some people gain weight as a result of hyperthyroidism.

Many people, including some physicians, believe that clinical signs and symptoms are more accurate than laboratory tests when diagnosing thyroid conditions.

What would a doctor who relies on symptoms do with an elderly woman who is apathetic, doesn't have an enlarged thyroid, and is depressed but has a free T4 level of 3.5 and a TSH of less than 0.3? Her clinical signs and symptoms point to hypothyroidism, but her tests show hyperthyroidism. Relying on symptoms alone, a doctor may give this patient thyroid-hormone replacement. Lots of luck.

I've relied upon thyroid-function tests to diagnose disorders of thyroid function for 33 years. Especially in the last decade, as the TSH test has become more accurate and the free T4 and free T3 have become available, I've felt extremely confident that I have the right diagnosis.

The proof of the pudding is in the eating. When I treat patients with confusing clinical signs according to their lab test results rather than their clinical findings, they invariably get better.

Signs and symptoms of hypothyroidism can be very subtle, just like many other diseases. The signs and symptoms mimic those of diseases like depression, menopause, and aging.

The placebo effect of any drug is another problem. If you give a group of patients a pill that's not supposed to have any effect on the disease in question, a few of them get better. This doesn't mean that the pill is the reason they improve.

A good physician bases his or her treatment on evidence-based medicine. This means that single instances of improvement don't prove that a treatment is correct; they can just as easily mean that the original diagnosis is wrong.

Don't allow a doctor to treat you for a thyroid disease, such as hyperthyroidism or hypothyroidism, unless the thyroid function tests confirm the diagnosis.

Chapter 22

Ten Ways to Maximize Thyroid Health

. . . .

In This Chapter

▶ Keeping an eye out for thyroid disease

▶ Getting enough iodine

▶ Managing hyperthyroidism and cancer

▶ Avoiding drug interactions and radiation

▶ Staying up-to-date

. . . .

*I*f you've been reading this book from beginning to end, we've come a long way together. Now the time has come to put the icing on the cake or perhaps the exclamation point at the end of the sentence. In this chapter, I discuss the steps you can take to ensure your best thyroid function. You may have thought that there was little you could do — that your thyroid, like the Mississippi River, would just keep rolling along. As I show you here, you can do a lot to maximize thyroid health (so much, in fact, that I've included 11 ways to maximize your thyroid health in this edition, instead of just 10).

You can make sure that you have thyroid testing done at the right intervals. You can do some self-examination to determine whether the shape of your thyroid is normal. You can make sure that you're getting the proper nutrients so that your thyroid can make its hormones in sufficient quantities. And perhaps most important of all, you can be knowledgeable about all the new discoveries concerning thyroid health and disease that appear on an almost daily basis.

By doing these things, you're doing all that you can to take care of that little gland that weighs less than an ounce but plays such an important role in your life and your health. And don't forget to take care of all those cells, tissues, and organs that surround that 20-gram gland. It won't be of much use if all the rest of you is falling apart.

Screening at Appropriate Intervals

Many symptoms of hypothyroidism are subtle or are similar to symptoms of aging or menopause (see Chapters 5 and 19). Hyperthyroidism can also be tricky because symptoms may not be prominent (especially in elderly people), and sometimes symptoms appear to point toward an underactive thyroid even though the thyroid is overactive (see Chapter 19).

The most common form of thyroid disease is autoimmune thyroiditis. It probably affects 10 percent of the population of the United States, although only a small fraction of people with this disease actually develop hypothyroidism.

Hypothyroidism often begins when a woman is in her 30s. For this reason, and because of the confusion that can exist between the diagnosis and the signs and symptoms a patient experiences, doctors recommend that you start screening for abnormal thyroid function at age 35 and continue at five-year intervals for the rest of your life. This applies to both sexes. Of course, if tests reveal a thyroid condition, your doctor will perform testing much more frequently.

Your doctor uses a blood test, the TSH (thyroid-stimulating hormone) test, to screen for abnormal thyroid function. Although the normal range is usually given as 0.5 to 5, the true normal range may be narrower, 0.5 to 2.5 (see Chapter 5). If your doctor tells you that your screening test is normal, but you still have symptoms consistent with hypothyroidism, ask the doctor for the exact number of your TSH. If it's above 2.5, ask your doctor to consider giving you a trial of treatment with thyroid-hormone replacement.

Checking Thyroid Function As Your Body Changes

If you're taking thyroid hormone treatment, you're on a fixed dose of medication. However, many physical states, particularly pregnancy (see Chapter 17), create chemical changes in your body that can alter the amount of thyroid hormone that you need to maintain normal function. The same is true as you get older.

Chemical changes that cause you to make more thyroid-binding proteins (see Chapter 4) require you to take an increased dose of thyroid medication. Any condition that increases your estrogen is an example, such as pregnancy and taking oral contraceptive pills. As your body makes more thyroid-binding proteins, more of your dose of thyroid is bound to the proteins and less is available to enter your cells. You must increase your dose of thyroid hormone. Blood tests determine when you again have enough.

Chemical changes that cause you to make less thyroid-binding proteins require a decreased dose of thyroid hormone. If you take androgens (see Chapter 10) or have a disease that causes your body to produce androgens excessively, you may need your dosage of thyroid hormone reduced. Less thyroid-binding protein means less binding of your thyroid dose so more is available to enter cells. If you don't reduce your dose of thyroid hormone in this circumstance, you can become hyperthyroid.

Another situation that occurs in pregnancy is the reduction in autoimmunity (see Chapter 17). If you're being treated for hyperthyroidism with antithyroid pills, you may need a lower dose or none at all until the pregnancy is completed. Then you need treatment again.

During times of major body change such as pregnancy or illness, your need for thyroid hormone or antithyroid medication may change. The only way to be sure you are on the right dose is to have thyroid function tests at regular intervals, usually every three months.

Performing a "Neck Check"

The American Association of Clinical Endocrinologists (AACE), recognizing that many people have thyroid disease that's not diagnosed, proposes that everyone perform the thyroid "neck check." You can find details at their Web site, www.aace.com. Under "Awareness Campaigns," click on "Patient Awareness Campaigns." On the page that comes up, click on "Thyroid Awareness 2005." At the next page, scroll down to "When the Blues Hit" and click on that. The page that comes up has a choice that you can click on called "Neck Check."

You can detect abnormalities in the size and shape of your thyroid gland. If you think you have an enlarged thyroid, seek your doctor's help to determine whether you have any problem.

AACE urges everyone to "think thyroid."

You need to follow five steps to do a neck check. You need a hand-held mirror and a glass of water. The steps are as follows:

1. **Hold the mirror in your hand, focusing on the area of your neck just below the Adam's apple and immediately above the collarbone.** Your thyroid is located in this area of your neck.

2. **While focusing on this area in the mirror, tip your head back.**

3. **Take a drink of water and swallow.**

4. **As you swallow, look at your neck. Check for any bulges or protrusions in this area when you swallow.** *Reminder:* Don't confuse the Adam's

apple with the thyroid gland. The thyroid gland is located farther down on your neck, closer to the collarbone. You may want to repeat this process several times.

5. **If you do see any bulges or protrusions in this area, see your physician.** You may have an enlarged thyroid gland or a thyroid nodule, and your doctor should check to determine whether cancer is present or if you need treatment for thyroid disease.

Getting Enough Iodine to Satisfy Your Thyroid

Though iodine deficiency isn't as vast a problem in the United States, Canada, and Western Europe as in other parts of the world, a few considerations still need addressing.

If you're a vegetarian, you may not eat the foods that are the major sources of iodine in the diet, namely fish, and, to a lesser extent, meat, eggs, and milk. Little iodine is present in fruits and vegetables.

Because high blood pressure is such a concern these days, your doctor may urge you not to add salt to your food because salt raises the blood pressure. However, the American Heart Association's nutritional recommendations are to limit salt intake to less than 6 grams daily, slightly more than a teaspoon. This amount contains plenty of iodine for your diet.

How do you act when you receive contradictory recommendations from health professionals? ("You need sufficient iodine." "Don't eat salt!") You can certainly use a small quantity of salt daily, and this contains enough iodine for your needs because 1 teaspoon of salt contains about 400 micrograms of iodine. Or you can eat a couple slices of bread each day. Each slice of bread contains about 150 micrograms of iodine. The recommended intake of iodine daily is 150 to 200 micrograms.

Stopping Thyroid Medication, If Possible

You're always better off if you let your normal body thyroid physiology work for you than if you try to replace it with an external source of thyroid hormones.

During my many years of medical practice, I've seen numerous people who were taking thyroid hormone who had never been tested with thyroid function tests. They had developed symptoms of fatigue or had gained a few pounds and had been put on medication. Most of these patients, when taken off thyroid hormone, proved to have normal thyroid function on their own. Often, if questioned about whether the thyroid hormone had made a difference, they admitted that they were still fatigued and still had trouble losing weight, even on the medication. These people should never have been placed on thyroid hormone in the first place but should certainly have had a trial off of thyroid hormone replacement over the years.

Another group of patients who have been put on thyroid hormone replacement because of laboratory evidence of low thyroid function may also get off thyroid hormone at some point. These are patients who have hypothyroidism due to chronic thyroiditis (see Chapter 5). Their hypothyroidism is the result of antibodies that block the action of thyroid-stimulating hormone. Up to 25 percent of these patients may be able to come off treatment. The level of these blocking antibodies may possibly fall to the point that the thyroid gland is able to make its own thyroid hormone. Stopping the thyroid hormone after a few years of treatment to see if the thyroid can function on its own is certainly worthwhile.

If you have hypothyroidism due to chronic thyroiditis and have been taking thyroid hormone pills for a few years, ask your doctor if you can stop the thyroid hormone replacement for a month and check your thyroid function tests.

Using Both Types of Thyroid Hormone

The thyroid gland makes two different thyroid hormones: T4, the major component, and T3, considered to be the active form of thyroid hormone but made in much lower amounts by the gland (see Chapter 2).

Because drug manufacturers have had the ability to synthesize it, T4 is the only treatment doctors give when patients need thyroid hormone. Doctors give it so that a patient's TSH level returns to normal, as does the free T4 in the blood. This suggests that most people who receive treatment for hypothyroidism may have a deficiency of T3.

In practical terms, over the years a deficiency of T3 hasn't proven to be a significant problem. However, I've noted in my thyroid practice, as have other specialists, that a few patients continue to complain of symptoms of low thyroid function despite normal laboratory test results. These patients may improve if their doctors add T3 to their treatment.

Measuring this kind of improvement objectively is difficult, because the test results remain in the normal range. This is a case where I've been willing to accept the subjective symptoms of the patient indicating that he or she feels better on the combination therapy compared to T4 alone.

This is still a gray area in medicine. I've seen a handful of patients who didn't feel better regardless of how much T3 I added, even though their thyroid tests were normal. And the latest studies, which I quote in Chapter 5, suggest that additional T3 makes no difference in treatment.

I hope that in the future doctors will have some objective test that will tell them that thyroid function is perfectly normal by a measurement separate from thyroid function tests — for example, a new blood test measuring a chemical that we don't even know about yet or a nonblood test.

If you have symptoms of hypothyroidism and are taking T4 hormone replacement alone, ask your doctor to prescribe a small dose of T3. You may do better on the combination.

Preventing the Regrowth of Thyroid Cancer

If you've had thyroid cancer, you have probably had thyroid surgery followed by irradiation to eliminate the remaining thyroid tissue. Now you want to prevent any regrowth of thyroid cancer. You prevent regrowth by taking sufficient thyroid hormone to suppress the production of thyroid-stimulating hormone. The goal is for your TSH level to drop below the normal range. The lower level of the normal range is about 0.5, so you want a reading of 0.3 or below to be sure your thyroid isn't being stimulated.

But how low is too low? If a reading of 0.3 is good, would a reading of 0.1 be better? A study published in *Thyroid* in 1999 addressed this issue. The researchers had two groups of cancer patients: One group's TSH levels were suppressed to below 0.1; the other group's TSH levels were kept between 0.4 and 0.1. The study found that residual thyroid tissue was no more suppressed when the TSH was less than 0.1 than when it was between 0.4 and 0.1. The researchers concluded that thyroid cancer patients should receive suppressive doses of T4, but that greater suppression is no better than lesser degrees of suppression.

Excessive suppression of thyroid hormone runs the risk of causing osteoporosis, heart problems, and loss of muscle tissue. The advantage of taking the least suppressive dose of thyroid hormone possible is that you have less risk of developing osteoporosis or rapid heartbeats, particularly if you're middle aged or older.

Using the Same Thyroid Preparation

The American Association of Clinical Endocrinologists' campaign for Thyroid Awareness Month in 2005 (Thyroid Awareness Month is January of each year) was "A Healthy Thyroid: You Make the Difference." The focus of this year's theme was that fact that "the body is sensitive to even small changes in thyroid hormone levels," along with "the importance of knowing the brand and dose of your thyroid medication." But you, you genius, already know all about it because you're reading this book.

Although it would be wonderful if a dose of 0.125 mg of Levoxyl, 0.125 mg of Synthroid, and 0.125 mg of levothyroxine were interchangeable, the fact is that they aren't. Despite the best efforts of the Food and Drug Administration, these medications are made slightly differently, and their potency is slightly different. That means if you get on one of these preparations, staying with the same preparation is important to be sure you experience no change in your thyroid function.

What conditions may cause your preparation to change? If you change pharmacies, the new pharmacy will likely use a different source for its medications. The pharmacy you use, even if you don't change, may change its source. If you change health plans, your new health plan may use a different manufacturer. If you buy your drugs from Canada or Mexico, you can bet you're getting a different potency. If you change doctors, the same thing can happen.

Will you realize you're on a new preparation? Probably not, because the changes in your body may be too subtle for you to notice. But the different strength may cause damage to your body, depending on whether it's too much or too little.

How can you prevent this from happening?

- ✔ Check the name of the medication on your new bottle each time you get a refill of your thyroid medication.

- ✔ Ask your pharmacist if he or she is using the same source each time you refill.

- ✔ Try to use the same pharmacy or drug program each time you refill.

- ✔ Avoid discounted sources of thyroid medication. It should be a very inexpensive drug.

If all else fails and you have to change the source of your thyroid medication, get thyroid function tests four to six weeks after you make the change.

Anticipating Drug Interactions

So many drugs interact with thyroid hormones that you must check with your doctor whenever he or she places you on a new medication or takes you off an old medication (see Chapter 10).

Your thyroid function can be affected not only when you start a new medication but also if your doctor takes you off an old medication or changes the dosage significantly.

The way to avoid a problem is to perform (or have your doctor perform) a search for interactions between thyroid hormone and the drugs you'll be taking.

Drugs can affect thyroid function at any level. They can increase or decrease the release of thyrotrophin-releasing hormone, which affects how much thyroid-stimulating hormone (TSH) your body creates. They can increase or decrease the release of thyroid hormone from the thyroid. They can change the ratio of T4 hormone versus T3. They can affect the uptake of thyroid hormone by cells. They can increase or decrease the action of thyroid hormone within the cells.

The major drugs that you should be concerned about are the following, which I discuss in Chapter 10:

- ✔ Lithium
- ✔ Amiodarone
- ✔ Estrogen
- ✔ Steroids
- ✔ Aspirin (in doses greater than 3,000 milligrams)
- ✔ Iron tablets
- ✔ Iodine
- ✔ Propranolol

Chances are that you'll take one or more of these drugs in your lifetime.

Just about every drug affects thyroid function in one way or another. Fortunately, your thyroid gland makes some adjustment to overcome most of the effects. But if you're on a fixed treatment dose of thyroid hormone, your thyroid can't adjust as it would normally. Having your thyroid function tested four to six weeks after you start a new medication or stop an old one is wise.

Protecting Your Thyroid from Radiation

One million or more Americans received neck irradiation for various conditions in the years between 1920 and 1960, and they're at higher risk for thyroid cancer. Close to 10 percent of people who were so treated have developed thyroid cancer to date.

If you received irradiation to your neck area as a child because of enlarged tonsils, acne, an enlarged thymus, or some other condition, you're at increased risk for thyroid cancer and should inform your doctor.

If you've had any kind of radiation treatment to your head, chest, or neck in the past, you should perform the "neck check" I describe earlier in the "Performing a 'Neck Check'" section of this chapter. If you feel something unusual in shape or size, see your doctor. If you don't, see your doctor anyway, because changes may be very subtle, and the incidence of thyroid cancer is definitely higher if you've been irradiated. The exception here is that radiation treatment for hyperthyroidism doesn't increase your risk of cancer.

A thyroid scan or a thyroid ultrasound (see Chapter 4) should find any significant abnormality that exists. If one is found, the usual next step is a fine needle biopsy of the thyroid.

What about follow-up if nothing is found? Having an examination of your thyroid on at least an annual basis is probably a good idea if you have a history of thyroid exposure to radiation.

Even those of us who were never exposed to radiation as part of a medical treatment need to be aware of the risks of radiation. That's because as sources of fossil fuel for energy are used up, like it or not, energy companies will probably turn more and more to nuclear energy.

You want to be prepared to avoid taking in a lot of radioactive iodine if a nuclear accident occurs at the power plant near you. Fortunately, the Nuclear Regulatory Commission takes this threat seriously. It has arranged to have stockpiles of iodine available to take in the event of a nuclear accident. By taking a large dose of iodine daily for several days, you block the uptake of iodine into the thyroid.

The other thing you can do to protect yourself is to stay indoors. The radiation can't affect you if you don't come in contact with it.

Exposure of your thyroid to radiation in the past (other than for treatment for hyperthyroidism) definitely increases your risk of thyroid cancer. However, should cancer occur, it's no more dangerous than thyroid cancer not associated with radiation as long as you receive proper treatment.

Keeping Up-to-Date with Thyroid Discoveries

This book is an excellent start in your quest for knowledge about the thyroid gland and how it affects you. Most of the information here will be useful for at least ten years or so. Given the pace of research, however, a book can't keep you completely up-to-date with new findings about thyroid physiology and pathology. You need to seek them out for yourself. Where do you look?

An obvious start is to wait for an updated version of this book, which will generally have all the important information since the last publication. You can also try the Internet.

In Appendix B, you find the Internet sites that I believe are most accurate and reliable with respect to thyroid function and disease. I list the Web sites of large organizations like the American Association of Clinical Endocrinologists, the American Thyroid Association, the American Association of Endocrine Surgeons, and the American Association of Thyroid Surgeons.

You also find smaller sites belonging to individuals and groups who have various thyroid conditions or are advocates for those conditions. You can learn a great deal about the experience of having a particular thyroid disease by reading their comments.

Several government sites provide a ton of free information about the thyroid. Likewise, many institutions of higher learning want to provide information with the hope that you seek out their specialists for your ongoing care.

The various drug companies that make thyroid medications have Web sites that contain information, especially about their products, and often general information about the thyroid as well.

If you speak French, go to the site of the Thyroid Foundation of Canada, where you can find everything you want to know in a French version. This site also has an International Directory of Thyroid-related Organizations. Among the countries the site lists are Denmark, Germany, Italy, Japan, and the Netherlands.

So many different organizations provide the same information about the thyroid that I often wonder why some of them don't pool their resources to provide one major source. I suppose too many egos are involved to take this logical step, but I still think it's a good idea. Perhaps you're thinking, "Why, Dr. Rubin, with all this information available, did you bother to write this book?" My answer is, of course, that this book is unique. No other one out there is quite like it, believe me.

Chapter 23

Ten Questions Readers Have Posed

In This Chapter

▶ Basing the dose of methimazole on the TSH

▶ Treating a teenager with radioactive iodine or tapazole

▶ Taking all the tapazole at one time

▶ Managing hypothyroidism during pregnancy

▶ Considering side effects of long-term thyroid hormone

*T*he number of e-mails that I've received from my readers has been very gratifying. You've thanked me for writing this book with comments like the following:

✔ I just finished reading your *Thyroid For Dummies* book, and I have to tell you, I thoroughly enjoyed reading it!

✔ I want to thank you for your *Thyroid For Dummies* book.

✔ I just want to tell you that your book has been extremely helpful to me.

✔ I read your wonderful book *Thyroid For Dummies* and was so impressed.

✔ I've recently read your book and thoroughly enjoyed it.

At the same time, you've posed a lot of excellent questions that apply not just to you but to many of my readers. The purpose of this chapter is to answer the ten most common questions you've sent me. I'm sorry if I don't answer your particular question here. However, I try to answer all questions that are general in nature by return e-mail, so don't hesitate to write me at `thyroid@drrubin.com`; I promise to reply. If your question applies to enough people, it will probably get into the next edition of this book. I can't answer specific questions about your case, however, without the opportunity to talk to you and examine you myself. To do so would be unethical.

I can't pose your questions better than you do, so this chapter basically replicates your questions. I've tried to omit any information that can identify you, because I consider your privacy extremely important. Thank you again for all your support and interest.

Taken as a whole, your questions have led me to consider a number of interesting issues. I have listed some of the conclusions I've drawn here so you can benefit from the insights that your questions have provoked.

✔ Not all so-called "specialists" know what they're talking about.

✔ You're the one who should make the final decision about your treatment with the help of your doctor.

✔ No doctor has the right to demand that you take a certain treatment.

✔ Even the best treatments change over time, because they too are subject to new research.

✔ We as doctors don't have the answers to all your questions, but we keep trying.

Basing Doses of Methimazole on TSH

On 8/23/05, follow-up lab work indicated normal FT3 and FT4 levels again, but TSH had dropped to 0.19. Endocrinologist increased dosage of methimazole to 20 mg. twice daily, and patient is to return in 6 weeks for follow-up and lab work. I have read conflicting reports that dosing for Graves' should not be based upon the TSH alone, especially when FT3 and FT4 are normal. However, I don't want to be "under-medicated" and have my eyes worsen or go into a thyroid storm either. Do you think my endocrinologist is right on track?

The answer is a definite *no*! Your endocrinologist doesn't seem to be aware that the TSH can remain low for months after the free T4 returns to normal, which doesn't mean you still have active hyperthyroidism. Once the free T4 returns to normal, your doctor should gradually lower your dose of the antithyroid drug to keep the free T4 normal for at least a year. Then your doctor can consider stopping the antithyroid drug, depending on your clinical situation. For example, if the thyroid gland is still large after a year, I would keep the patient on the drug a longer time.

Sometimes, even when taking the lowest dose of an antithyroid drug, your free T4 falls below normal and your TSH rises above normal, indicating you're now hypothyroid. Should you stop the drug at this point? My answer is no, because I believe you need to give your thyroid at least a year of medication to reverse the hyperthyroidism. Instead of stopping the antithyroid drug, I recommend adding thyroid hormone to the antithyroid medication to keep your thyroid function normal.

If your doctor's advise doesn't agree with what you read in this book or some other reliable source, go find another opinion.

Reversing Cold Sensitivity

Two years ago, months before my 40th birthday, I was diagnosed with hypothyroidism. My doctor put me on 50mcg of Synthyroid medication. Within several months, most of my previous symptoms such as low energy, hair fall etc. were reversed and I was feeling pretty good. That is with the exception of my sensitivity to cold and insensitivity to heat. After I started taking Synthyroid, this issue has completely reversed itself to the point of being a real bother to me.

You're saying that, although you had cold sensitivity before taking the Synthroid, you're now sensitive to heat as well. My opinion is that you are probably now getting too much thyroid hormone. People who are hypothyroid are sensitive to cold, but people who are hyperthyroid, whatever the reason, are sensitive to heat, which is one example of many ways the two conditions are the reverse of one another. Table 23-1 shows other examples:

Table 23-1	Comparisons of Signs of Hypothyroidism versus Hyperthyroidism
Hypothyroidism	*Hyperthyroidism*
Gain weight	Lose weight
Slow pulse	Fast pulse
Dry skin	Moist skin
Increased menstrual flow	Decreased menstrual flow
High cholesterol	Low cholesterol
Decreased body temperature	Increased body temperature

I could list many more opposites. But keep in mind that some people don't exhibit the classic signs of hypothyroidism or hyperthyroidism. The elderly, for example, may have hypothyroidism but lose weight because they eat so little.

If you have hypothyroidism or hyperthyroidism, receive treatment, and begin having symptoms opposite to what you had before, your doctor may have overtreated you. Have your thyroid blood tests done to find out.

Treating a Teenager for Hyperthyroidism

We have seen a pediatric endocrinologist who recommended both the meds: PTU (temporarily) and then the radiation treatment. As parents we are leaning towards the RAI treatment and planning on getting it scheduled in a week or two. But we still have questions... Won't her body still be making the antibody for the thyroid? How does this treatment deal with that? How can we get rid of the antibody attack? Does this RAI treatment do that? What about her eyes? – Does the replacement hormone take care of that risk? In general, what is the best treatment for a 16-year-old?

I believe that antithyroid medication is the best treatment for a 16 year old with hyperthyroidism or almost anyone at any age with the condition. As far as I know, radioactive iodine and surgery don't reverse the underlying pathology, the autoimmune reaction. Antithyroid drugs do. Studies of patients who've been on antithyroid drugs for more than ten years demonstrate the drugs' excellent control of hyperthyroidism without side effects. In my own practice, I have patients who, after initial treatment with antithyroid drugs, have gone more than ten years without taking any medication and enjoy normal thyroid function.

If you elect radioactive iodine (or surgery), your 16 year old will likely be hypothyroid for the rest of her life, needing to take a pill every day. In addition, some evidence suggests that the eye disease of hyperthyroidism continues to progress after radioactive iodine or surgery but not after taking antithyroid drugs.

Surgery is probably the best choice for a person with obstruction due to a large thyroid around the esophagus and trachea. Radioactive iodine may be better for a person who can't be depended upon to take antithyroid drugs regularly or has a reaction to the drugs. The same person, however, probably won't take the thyroid pill necessary after radioactive iodine.

Some doctors say that a very large thyroid gland doesn't respond well to antithyroid drugs, but this hasn't been my experience.

My preferred treatment for Graves' disease (hyperthyroidism) is antithyroid medication, for patients of any age and in almost all circumstances.

Taking Methimazole All at Once

I wanted to ask you something. I've been on methimazole 10mg 4x per day (40mg total per day) for 4 weeks. I just went to my doctor who said my levels had dropped by 1/2 and I was doing very well. I do feel 100% better. He now wants me to take all 40mg at once for the next month. I checked with my pharmacist and she said that's not the way it's usually done. You mention this spaced out dosing in your book also. Have you ever heard of this dosing schedule. I asked my doctor and he said that first it's taken spaced out, then it's taken all at once, then the dosage is reduced.

Your doctor is correct. Doctors usually begin prescribing methimazole in divided doses but prescribe a single dosage once the thyroid is under control. As you know, methimazole and the other antithyroid drug, propylthiouricil, take three to six weeks to bring the thyroid under control. Methimazole isn't like penicillin or allergy medications, which begin to work within minutes of taking them. Because a dose of methimazole takes weeks to work, you might as well take your daily dosage all at once. You may even question why we start with multiple daily doses. As Tevya says in *Fiddler on the Roof,* it's tradition.

Taking several pills at one time often helps you remember to take the medication. You can more easily remember to take your pills once instead of multiple times a day.

I usually give more medication to the person who has a higher free T4 and less to the person with a close to normal free T4. But I suspect that the lower dose works just as well in both cases.

Insisting on Radioactive Iodine Treatment

*At my insistence I was placed on PTU and Inderal. (**Author's note:** This is the same as propranolol.) My endocrinologist never even suggested it, they wanted me to do radioactive iodine and I refused, insisting I wanted to try the anti-thyroid drug first. Anyway, I have done great on a block and replace regimen and my endocrinologist is now wanting me to stop the PTU to see if I obtain remission. I am more than willing to do that, however, my endocrinologist has made it clear that if remission is not obtained he is insisting on RAI and stated he "would discharge me as a patient" if I did not agree to the RAI. I feel that I am being bullied into this treatment and I am very concerned as I have some eye involvement. I have called around and thus far all the endo's that I have contacted all have the same mindset . . . RAI or nothing!!!*

You must find some doctors near you who will listen! As I note above, my preferred treatment is antithyroid drugs. If you can't find a doctor who will go along with your wishes, check Chapter 3 and find a doctor according to the ways I suggest. You don't have to take any treatment that you don't want, even if (although it's not the case here) the treatment is life-saving. You may consider a trip to Europe, where all the doctors use antithyroid drugs in preference to radioactive iodine. If you figure out the cost of office visits and medicine in the United States, you may find out you save money.

I've received a large number of e-mails exactly like this one. Doctors tell their patients they have to take radioactive iodine, which is ridiculous and very unsatisfactory. No doctor has the right to tell patients they have to do anything.

You have the final decision about how you want to be treated. If a doctor insists on something you don't want, find another physician.

Treating with Thyroid after Pregnancy

I was diagnosed at around age 6 with a goiter and hypothyroidism due to Hashimoto's. When I was twenty I had a baby and ever since then I don't seem to be able to get my thyroid 'under control'. Does it seem that having a baby can literally make things worse for my condition? My son (my only child) will be ten this year. Over the past few years I have had trouble maintaining a constant TSH. Recently I quit my meds and my TSH shot up to 23. I started back on meds at .150 mg and went back to the doctor. I went down to .125 mg/Levoxyl and my TSH is within range (around 3) but I still have symptoms of hypothyroid. Does adding T3 really help some people with symptoms?

When you have a baby, your body undergoes major changes. One of them is a significant reduction in autoimmunity. If you have chronic thyroiditis (Hashimoto's thyroiditis), you may stop producing as much blocking autoantibody and may not need as much or any thyroid for the duration of the pregnancy. (Similarly, people with hyperthyroidism may stop making stimulating antibodies, decreasing their hyperthyroidism in severity during the pregnancy.) Usually both hypothyroidism and hyperthyroidism come back like before once the pregnancy is over.

If you were last pregnant ten years ago, the pregnancy probably isn't playing a role in your current thyroid function. Antibody levels can rise and fall, and your disease may worsen, requiring more thyroid hormone, or improve, requiring less thyroid hormone, as your antibodies rise and fall. In addition, be careful of changing your type of thyroid from one brand to another; the brands may not be biologically equivalent. Your TSH and free T4 need to be tested six to eight weeks after starting a new brand.

Try never to stop thyroid on your own without consulting your doctor. Thyroid takes weeks to build back up in your body, leaving you hypothyroid as it does. Additionally, as I mention in Chapter 5, a TSH of 3 may not mean you have normal thyroid function, even though a TSH of 3 is within the normal range.

The severity of autoimmune thyroiditis can wax and wane, and different brands of thyroxine have different potencies, so stabilizing your thyroid function may be difficult.

Explaining Joint Problems

*I was wondering if you can tell me (and I have found little research on this) why thyroid troubles can result in tendon troubles and trigger fingers. (**Author's note:** Trigger finger is a catching feeling in a finger due to obstruction of the free movement of the tendon that moves the finger) I have had a huge flare-up of deQuervains Tendinitis, and a few triggerfingers develop, and have found other women with the same problems (or fibromyalgia.)*

In Chapter 5, I discuss the other autoimmune conditions that may accompany autoimmune thyroiditis. Among them are arthritis and other joint conditions. Although the "thyroid troubles" aren't to blame for the tendon troubles and trigger finger, they suggest that you may be prone to other diseases. The main ones besides arthritis are celiac disease, hypoadrenalism, diabetes type 1, and pernicious anemia. Each of these conditions has its own set of symptoms. The fact that you have thyroid troubles along with arthritic problems suggests that you're suffering from another disease as well.

Ideally, you may be able to cure your other troubles by curing your thyroid disease. Unfortunately, other conditions run their own course, so you may suffer from other symptoms even if your thyroid condition becomes normal.

If you have autoimmune thyroiditis (chronic thyroiditis), you have a tendency to suffer from other autoimmune diseases. Although you're still unlikely to experience them, your chances of getting one are greater than someone who doesn't have autoimmune thyroiditis.

Taking Antithyroid Drugs Long Term

My husband bought Thyroid For Dummies so that we could learn more about my hyperthyroidism. I was stunned to read that no rule says that antithyroid pills cannot be given for more than a year, because I was led to believe otherwise. I was told that I could only take methimazole for 1 1/2 to 2 years after which I would have to take radioactive iodine if my thyroid did not go into remission. About 3 months after ending methimazole, tests showed I was again hyperthyroid and I was advised to take radioactive iodine.

As I've noted previously, no reason exists not to take antithyroid drugs for as long as you need them. About 50 percent of the patients who take antithyroid drugs go into remission. If you don't fall into this lucky group, you can still go back on the antithyroid drugs for another trial. Many of my patients have gone into remission after a year on antithyroid drugs, but some have required two or even three years. I eventually try to take all of them off of methimazole, because I don't like to use drugs as a general rule. But if a patient has a recurrence and is willing to continue to try drugs, I don't hesitate to put her on antithyroid drugs again.

However, some people are allergic to antithyroid medication, while others experience a fall in white blood cell count when taking the drug, which reverses when they stop taking it. In such cases, I first try the other common antithyroid drug. If that too is a problem, I go on to radioactive iodine.

Patients have been on antithyroid drugs for 10 years and longer with no harmful effect. I am frankly at a loss to explain the reluctance of many endocrinologists to use these drugs for as long as it takes to accomplish a remission.

Antithyroid drugs are safe and effective. They may be a better form of treatment than radioactive iodine and surgery, except in certain circumstances I describe here and in Chapter 6. No reason exists for not using them for years if necessary.

Reversing Chronic Thyroiditis

I am a 41-year-old practicing surgeon. I obtained your book which stated up to 25 percent of the chronic thyroiditis patients have reversal. I stopped taking the meds on my own and I feel pretty darn good after only 7 days. Of course, I will check my TSH in 5 weeks from now to see if the disease is in remission. I am now bench pressing 365 lbs which I have not done since 1982, this is only after 7 days. I asked the internist and the endocrinologist can the chronic thyroiditis go away and they both said never. I showed them your book and they are now reviewing all their patients with Hashimoto's. Myself as well as the other physicians are wondering 3 things: 1) Do anabolic steroids trigger Hashimoto's? 2) After reversal how long does it take before the body is normalized (arthralgias, weakness, etc.)? and 3) What is the chance of the Hashimoto's returning?

I don't recommend stopping your antithyroid drugs to improve your weight lifting. I think it's a coincidence that you're stronger seven days after stopping your medication, because the effect of antithyroid drugs lasts four to six weeks or longer. As for your questions, as far as I know, anabolic steroids don't trigger Hashimoto's, and I found nothing in the thyroid literature that suggests this could happen. Chronic thyroiditis (Hashimoto's) is an autoimmune disease passed down in the family. Anabolic steroids do reduce the blood levels of thyroid-binding globulins, but thyroid function remains normal.

As chronic thyroiditis reverses, a gradual reduction in the levels of blocking autoantibodies occurs, which may take years. A gradual reduction in the need for thyroid hormone may accompany the reduction in the blocking autoantibodies, although this may be very subtle. Your other symptoms may be due to another autoimmune disease that doesn't reverse, explaining why your symptoms may continue.

If the autoantibodies have fallen, they probably won't return, so the lucky 25 percent who have reversal of the Hashimoto's are probably free from the disease from now on.

Chronic thyroiditis goes into remission in about 25 percent of patients. After you've been on thyroid for several years, I recommend discussing with your doctor the possibility of coming off the thyroid medication for four to six weeks to test for a return of normal thyroid function.

Changing Thyroid Dosage

I'm a 20+ year hypothyroid patient, and I enjoyed reading your book. Most of my questions concern dosage changes over time — for example, over the 20+ years of treatment, my optimal dosage of thyroid hormone has significantly decreased (from .2mcg to .125mcg). This drop in dosage took place quickly — over a two to three year period. I have never come across any literature thoroughly explaining why this decreased tolerance occurred in such a sort time period. Another dosage question I have is whether dosage varies depending upon patient's weight — do heavier patients require a higher dosage than thin patients of the same height? Does a heavy patient who looses substantial weight normally remain at the same dosage?

Your questions are excellent. You say that your thyroid dosage declined over a two- to three-year period. Your decline in dosage was probably due to what I described in the previous question, a fall-off in your thyroid autoantibodies. No one knows how slowly or quickly a fall-off in thyroid autoantibodies can take place, so your situation may not be unusual. It suggests that you may eventually be able to come off the thyroid completely. You should discuss this with your doctor.

The next question is whether the dosage varies according to the patient's weight. Because patients with more blocking antibodies need more thyroid than those with fewer antibodies, weight is one consideration that determines the amount of thyroid needed. However, all things being equal, lean body mass, which is the size of the muscles and bones regardless of how much fat a person has, determines how much thyroid a person needs. In a study from the *Journal of Clinical Endocrinology and Metabolism* from March 2005, doctors evaluated patients with thyroid cancer who had all their thyroid removed to see how much thyroid patients needed to bring their TSH down to a certain value. The best correlation was with the lean body mass, which means that a heavy person who loses substantial weight remains at the same dosage because the fat loss doesn't change the lean body mass.

Your muscle and bone mass determines how much thyroid you have to take, not the amount of fat in your body. A tall person who is thin probably needs more thyroid than a small person who is fat, because the tall person has much more lean body mass.

Part V
Appendixes

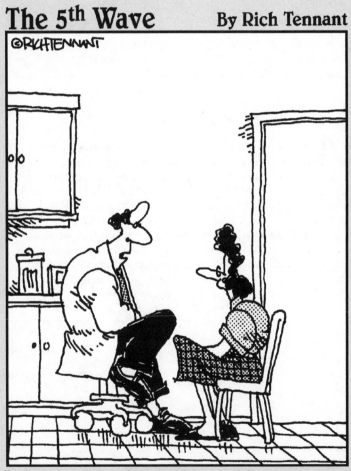

"Yes, perspiration and a rapid pulse could indicate a hyperthyroid. But the fact that these symptoms occur only when the pool boy is working in the yard next door does raise some questions."

In this part . . .

Appendix A is a glossary of the terms you encounter as you read and hear about the thyroid gland, its function, and its diseases. All the strange words you meet for the first time in the text of the book are listed here and defined. Appendix B shows you where to look for more information as well as the latest research findings on the thyroid. There is a huge amount of research focusing on every aspect of normal thyroid function and abnormal thyroid conditions. This book gives you a good working knowledge of the subject, but there is always more to know, and these Web sites are where to find it.

Appendix A

A Glossary of Key Terms

Acute thyroiditis: A bacterial infection of the thyroid.

Allele: One of two or more genes that determine which enzyme will be made or which body characteristic will prevail.

Antigen: A foreign protein that prompts the production of antibodies to destroy it.

Autoimmune thyroiditis: Inflammation of the thyroid associated with the production of antibodies against thyroid tissue.

Beta blocking agent: One of a group of drugs given to block some of the adverse effects of excess thyroid hormone.

Chorionic gonadotrophin: A hormone made by the placenta, which shares some properties with thyroid-stimulating hormone.

Chromosome: One of 23 pairs in the nucleus of every human cell that carry all the genes that determine the characteristics of the body.

Chronic thyroiditis: Another name for *autoimmune thyroiditis*.

Cretinism: A syndrome affecting children; its most outstanding feature is mental retardation that results from a lack of iodine during pregnancy.

Cyst: A saclike structure containing fluid.

Cytomel: A brand name for T3 medication.

Dominant gene: The gene that determines which particular enzyme or body characteristic will be expressed when two different genes are present.

Ectopic thyroid: Thyroid tissue found in an abnormal site, such as the base of the tongue.

Exopthalmus: Eye disease associated with Graves' disease.

Fine needle aspiration biopsy (FNAB): The process of putting a tiny needle into tissue, in this case the thyroid, for the purpose of determining the nature of that tissue. This process is particularly helpful for identifying thyroid cancer.

Free thyroxine (FT4): The tiny fraction of the T4 hormone that isn't bound to protein and is therefore available to enter cells.

Free thyroxine index (FTI): An obsolete test once used for determining thyroid function. The product of multiplying the total T4 by the T3 resin uptake.

Free triiodothyronine (FT3): The tiny fraction of the T3 hormone that isn't bound to protein and is therefore available to enter cells.

Gestational transient thyrotoxicosis: A brief period of hyperthyroidism during pregnancy that results from the large production of human chorionic gonadotrophin (which acts as a thyroid stimulator).

Goiter: An enlarged thyroid gland.

Graves' disease: An autoimmune condition that combines hyperthyroidism, eye disease, and skin disease.

Hashimoto's thyroiditis: Another name for autoimmune or chronic thyroiditis.

Heterozygous: Possessing two different genes for an enzyme or trait.

Homozygous: Possessing two of the same gene for an enzyme or trait.

Hyperthyroidism: A hyperactive state caused by the excessive production or taking of thyroid hormone.

Hypothyroidism: A hypoactive state produced by the diminished production or intake of thyroid hormone.

Isthmus of the thyroid: The thyroid tissue that connects both lobes of the thyroid.

Leptin: A hormone produced by fat cells that signals the brain that the intake of calories is excessive.

Levothroid: A brand name for synthetic thyroxine (T4).

Levoxyl: A brand name for synthetic thyroxine (T4).

Liothyronine: A generic name for T3 medication.

Liotrix: The generic name for the combination of T3 and T4 medication.

Medullary thyroid cancer: A cancer in the thyroid associated with cells called *parafollicular,* or *C-cells,* which make a hormone called *calcitonin.*

Multinodular goiter: An enlargement of the thyroid associated with many nodules, or outgrowths.

Multiple endocrine neoplasia: Hereditary production of tumors in several endocrine glands — one of the tumors may be a medullary thyroid cancer.

Mutation: An unexpected change in the enzyme or body characteristic produced by an alteration in a particular gene.

Myxedema: Another name for hypothyroidism.

Myxemeda coma: A severe form of hypothyroidism usually found in elderly people usually brought on by a complicating factor, such as infection or trauma, which may result in coma and death.

Postpartum thyroiditis: Inflammation of the thyroid after a pregnancy that is associated with thyroid autoantibodies and may go through stages of hyperthyroidism, normal thyroid function, and hypothyroidism. It may resolve or end in hypothyroidism.

Pyramidal lobe of the thyroid: An accessory lobe rising from the isthmus of the thyroid.

Recessive gene: A gene that will determine an enzyme or body characteristic only when it's present on both chromosomes. (Otherwise, the dominant gene prevails.)

Resin T3 uptake: A test of thyroid function (now obsolete) that provides an assessment of the amount of T4 bound to protein compared to the free T4.

Riedel's thyroiditis: A rare form of thyroid inflammation that is often associated with thyroid antibodies. It results in fibrosis of thyroid tissue, and sometimes parathyroid tissue, with tight adherence to the trachea.

Silent thyroiditis: A form of thyroiditis that's identical to postpartum thyroiditis but can occur at any time of life.

Subacute thyroiditis: A viral inflammation of the thyroid that's associated with pain in the thyroid.

Subclinical hypothyroidism: An elevation of the TSH, with a normal free-T4 level and minimal to no symptoms of hypothyroidism.

Synthroid: A brand name for synthetic thyroxine (T4).

Thiocyanate: A chemical found in some foods that may interfere with thyroid function.

Thyroglobulin: Material in the follicle of the thyroid in which thyroid hormones are stored.

Thyroid agenesis: Failure to produce a thyroid gland.

Thyroid autoantibodies: Proteins that react against the thyroid, sometimes to suppress or destroy it and sometimes to stimulate it.

Thyroid dysgenesis: Failure of the thyroid to grow or move into its proper place in the neck, attached to the trachea below the Adam's apple.

Thyroid hypoplasia: Production of a thyroid gland that's inadequate for the needs of the body.

Thyroid scan and uptake: Use of radioactive iodine to outline the thyroid, determine if tissue is actively producing thyroid hormone, and determine the level of activity of the gland.

Thyroid-stimulating hormone (TSH): A hormone from the pituitary gland that stimulates the thyroid to produce more thyroid hormone.

Thyroid storm: A very severe form of hyperthyroidism with high fever and severe sickness — a medical emergency.

Thyroid ultrasound: Use of sound waves to outline the thyroid and determine if growths are solid or cystic.

Thyrolar: Brand name for combined synthetic T3 and T4 medication.

Thyrotrophin-releasing hormone (TRH): A hormone from the hypothalamus in the brain that stimulates the production and release of thyroid hormone through thyroid-stimulating hormone (TSH).

Thyroxine (T4): The major thyroid hormone.

Thyroxine-binding protein: Several proteins that bind the T3 and T4 hormones, making them unavailable to enter cells.

Total thyroxine: The sum of the thyroxine bound and unbound to thyroid-binding proteins.

Transient congenital hypothyroidism: Temporary hypothyroidism in newborns that often results from prematurity.

Triiodothyronine (T3): The active form of thyroid hormone.

Unithroid: Brand name for synthetic thyroxine (T4).

Vitiligo: Patchy loss of skin pigment sometimes occurring in autoimmune diseases.

Appendix B

Sources of More Information

The Web sites I describe in this appendix offer a vast array of information on thyroid disease, thyroid research, specialists in the field of thyroid health and disease, and companies that make thyroid products. If you can't find what you're looking for here, it probably doesn't exist. Many of the sites point to other links that provide still more information. You can access all these sites from my Web page: www.drrubin.com. On the left-hand side of the page, under "Related Websites," select "Thyroid," and you can click on all the addresses that follow.

You can generally depend on the information in these sites (although some of them may point you toward other sites where the information is less reliable). But no matter what you read online, never make changes in your thyroid care without consulting your physician.

American Association of Clinical Endocrinologists
www.aace.com

This organization was founded in 1992 to serve as the voice of clinical endocrinologists, those actually seeing patients. The site provides practice guidelines, a calendar of important events in endocrinology, and a place both to find an endocrinologist and for endocrinologists to find a position.

American Association of Endocrine Surgeons
http://endocrinesurgery.org

This organization is dedicated to the advancement of endocrine surgery, and the site is a place to find a thyroid surgeon.

If you live outside the United States, go to the site of the **International Association of Endocrine Surgeons** (www.iaes-endocrine-surgeons.com) and select your home area.

American Thyroid Association
www.thyroid.org

This organization was founded in 1923 to promote research in thyroid disease, to spread new knowledge of thyroid disease, and to guide public policy on issues related to thyroid disease. On this important site, you find patient information and guidelines for physicians.

Asia and Oceania Thyroid Association
www.aota.or.kr

This organization was founded to promote thyroid research and education throughout Asia and Oceania.

Endocrine Society
www.endo-society.org

This organization, founded in 1916, is a leading source for research and information on all branches of *endocrinology,* the study of the glands that produce hormones.

European Thyroid Association
www.eurothyroid.com

This organization of European thyroid specialists promotes research and education about thyroid disease.

Latin American Thyroid Society
www.lats.org

This site is dedicated to thyroid research and knowledge in Latin America.

The Mayo Clinic
www.mayoclinic.com

This site is an excellent source of patient information on major thyroid conditions.

Medline Plus Thyroid Diseases
www.nlm.nih.gov/medlineplus/thyroiddiseases.html

This service of the National Library of Medicine provides information about thyroid disease management and research.

Merck Thyrolink
www.thyrolink.com/servlet/PB/menu/1247710/index.html

This service of Merck Pharmaceutical Company offers patient information in English, German, and French.

National Graves' Disease Foundation
www.ngdf.org

This support group, now more than ten years old, is dedicated exclusively to Graves' patients.

Online Mendelian Inheritance in Man
www.ncbi.nlm.nih.gov/entrez/query.fcgi?db=OMIM

This site is a huge database of diseases that are inherited by getting a single gene. If you search by "thyroid," you find all the currently known thyroid disorders in this database.

Synthroid Information Network
www.synthroid.com

This site was founded by Abbott Laboratories, the makers of Synthroid (a form of thyroxine hormone replacement), to provide information concerning their drug.

Thyroid Disease Manager
www.thyroidmanager.org

This is an excellent source for authoritative information on all aspects of thyroid disease. It may be a little technical, but check it out. It's constantly updated and revised.

Thyroid Federation International
www.thyroid-fed.org

This organization was founded in 1995 to deal with the problems of thyroid disease on a global basis. It's mainly involved in helping people start a thyroid patient organization in their country or locale.

Index

• *E* •

• R •

Notes

Notes

Notes

JSINESS, CAREERS & PERSONAL FINANCE

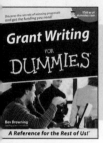

0-7645-5307-0

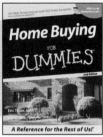

0-7645-5331-3 *†

Also available:
- ✓ Accounting For Dummies †
  0-7645-5314-3
- ✓ Business Plans Kit For Dummies †
  0-7645-5365-8
- ✓ Cover Letters For Dummies
  0-7645-5224-4
- ✓ Frugal Living For Dummies
  0-7645-5403-4
- ✓ Leadership For Dummies
  0-7645-5176-0
- ✓ Managing For Dummies
  0-7645-1771-6

- ✓ Marketing For Dummies
  0-7645-5600-2
- ✓ Personal Finance For Dummies *
  0-7645-2590-5
- ✓ Project Management For Dummies
  0-7645-5283-X
- ✓ Resumes For Dummies †
  0-7645-5471-9
- ✓ Selling For Dummies
  0-7645-5363-1
- ✓ Small Business Kit For Dummies *†
  0-7645-5093-4

OME & BUSINESS COMPUTER BASICS

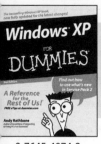

0-7645-4074-2

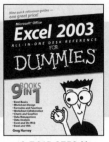

0-7645-3758-X

Also available:
- ✓ ACT! 6 For Dummies
  0-7645-2645-6
- ✓ iLife '04 All-in-One Desk Reference
  For Dummies
  0-7645-7347-0
- ✓ iPAQ For Dummies
  0-7645-6769-1
- ✓ Mac OS X Panther Timesaving
  Techniques For Dummies
  0-7645-5812-9
- ✓ Macs For Dummies
  0-7645-5656-8

- ✓ Microsoft Money 2004 For Dummies
  0-7645-4195-1
- ✓ Office 2003 All-in-One Desk Reference
  For Dummies
  0-7645-3883-7
- ✓ Outlook 2003 For Dummies
  0-7645-3759-8
- ✓ PCs For Dummies
  0-7645-4074-2
- ✓ TiVo For Dummies
  0-7645-6923-6
- ✓ Upgrading and Fixing PCs For Dummies
  0-7645-1665-5
- ✓ Windows XP Timesaving Techniques
  For Dummies
  0-7645-3748-2

OD, HOME, GARDEN, HOBBIES, MUSIC & PETS

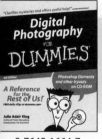

0-7645-5295-3

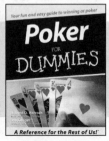

0-7645-5232-5

Also available:
- ✓ Bass Guitar For Dummies
  0-7645-2487-9
- ✓ Diabetes Cookbook For Dummies
  0-7645-5230-9
- ✓ Gardening For Dummies *
  0-7645-5130-2
- ✓ Guitar For Dummies
  0-7645-5106-X
- ✓ Holiday Decorating For Dummies
  0-7645-2570-0
- ✓ Home Improvement All-in-One
  For Dummies
  0-7645-5680-0

- ✓ Knitting For Dummies
  0-7645-5395-X
- ✓ Piano For Dummies
  0-7645-5105-1
- ✓ Puppies For Dummies
  0-7645-5255-4
- ✓ Scrapbooking For Dummies
  0-7645-7208-3
- ✓ Senior Dogs For Dummies
  0-7645-5818-8
- ✓ Singing For Dummies
  0-7645-2475-5
- ✓ 30-Minute Meals For Dummies
  0-7645-2589-1

NTERNET & DIGITAL MEDIA

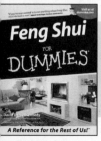

0-7645-1664-7

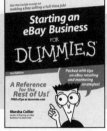

0-7645-6924-4

Also available:
- ✓ 2005 Online Shopping Directory
  For Dummies
  0-7645-7495-7
- ✓ CD & DVD Recording For Dummies
  0-7645-5956-7
- ✓ eBay For Dummies
  0-7645-5654-1
- ✓ Fighting Spam For Dummies
  0-7645-5965-6
- ✓ Genealogy Online For Dummies
  0-7645-5964-8
- ✓ Google For Dummies
  0-7645-4420-9

- ✓ Home Recording For Musicians
  For Dummies
  0-7645-1634-5
- ✓ The Internet For Dummies
  0-7645-4173-0
- ✓ iPod & iTunes For Dummies
  0-7645-7772-7
- ✓ Preventing Identity Theft For Dummies
  0-7645-7336-5
- ✓ Pro Tools All-in-One Desk Reference
  For Dummies
  0-7645-5714-9
- ✓ Roxio Easy Media Creator For Dummies
  0-7645-7131-1

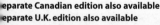

eparate Canadian edition also available
eparate U.K. edition also available

ilable wherever books are sold. For more information or to order direct: U.S. customers visit www.dummies.com or call 1-877-762-2974.
. customers visit www.wileyeurope.com or call 0800 243407. Canadian customers visit www.wiley.ca or call 1-800-567-4797.

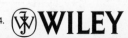

SPORTS, FITNESS, PARENTING, RELIGION & SPIRITUALITY

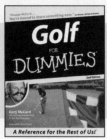
0-7645-5146-9

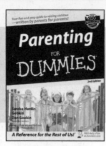
0-7645-5418-2

Also available:

- Adoption For Dummies
  0-7645-5488-3
- Basketball For Dummies
  0-7645-5248-1
- The Bible For Dummies
  0-7645-5296-1
- Buddhism For Dummies
  0-7645-5359-3
- Catholicism For Dummies
  0-7645-5391-7
- Hockey For Dummies
  0-7645-5228-7

- Judaism For Dummies
  0-7645-5299-6
- Martial Arts For Dummies
  0-7645-5358-5
- Pilates For Dummies
  0-7645-5397-6
- Religion For Dummies
  0-7645-5264-3
- Teaching Kids to Read For Dummies
  0-7645-4043-2
- Weight Training For Dummies
  0-7645-5168-X
- Yoga For Dummies
  0-7645-5117-5

TRAVEL

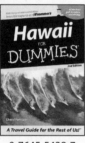
0-7645-5438-7

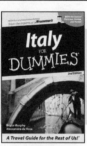
0-7645-5453-0

Also available:

- Alaska For Dummies
  0-7645-1761-9
- Arizona For Dummies
  0-7645-6938-4
- Cancún and the Yucatán For Dummies
  0-7645-2437-2
- Cruise Vacations For Dummies
  0-7645-6941-4
- Europe For Dummies
  0-7645-5456-5
- Ireland For Dummies
  0-7645-5455-7

- Las Vegas For Dummies
  0-7645-5448-4
- London For Dummies
  0-7645-4277-X
- New York City For Dummies
  0-7645-6945-7
- Paris For Dummies
  0-7645-5494-8
- RV Vacations For Dummies
  0-7645-5443-3
- Walt Disney World & Orlando For Dummies
  0-7645-6943-0

GRAPHICS, DESIGN & WEB DEVELOPMENT

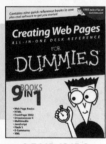
0-7645-4345-8

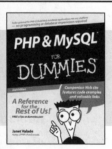
0-7645-5589-8

Also available:

- Adobe Acrobat 6 PDF For Dummies
  0-7645-3760-1
- Building a Web Site For Dummies
  0-7645-7144-3
- Dreamweaver MX 2004 For Dummies
  0-7645-4342-3
- FrontPage 2003 For Dummies
  0-7645-3882-9
- HTML 4 For Dummies
  0-7645-1995-6
- Illustrator cs For Dummies
  0-7645-4084-X

- Macromedia Flash MX 2004 For Dummies
  0-7645-4358-X
- Photoshop 7 All-in-One Desk Reference For Dummies
  0-7645-1667-1
- Photoshop cs Timesaving Techniques For Dummies
  0-7645-6782-9
- PHP 5 For Dummies
  0-7645-4166-8
- PowerPoint 2003 For Dummies
  0-7645-3908-6
- QuarkXPress 6 For Dummies
  0-7645-2593-X

NETWORKING, SECURITY, PROGRAMMING & DATABASES

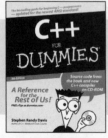
0-7645-6852-3

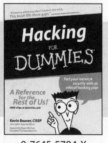
0-7645-5784-X

Also available:

- A+ Certification For Dummies
  0-7645-4187-0
- Access 2003 All-in-One Desk Reference For Dummies
  0-7645-3988-4
- Beginning Programming For Dummies
  0-7645-4997-9
- C For Dummies
  0-7645-7068-4
- Firewalls For Dummies
  0-7645-4048-3
- Home Networking For Dummies
  0-7645-42796

- Network Security For Dummies
  0-7645-1679-5
- Networking For Dummies
  0-7645-1677-9
- TCP/IP For Dummies
  0-7645-1760-0
- VBA For Dummies
  0-7645-3989-2
- Wireless All In-One Desk Reference For Dummies
  0-7645-7496-5
- Wireless Home Networking For Dummies
  0-7645-3910-8

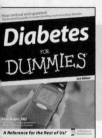

0-7645-6820-5 *†

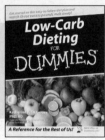

0-7645-2566-2

Also available:

- Alzheimer's For Dummies
  0-7645-3899-3
- Asthma For Dummies
  0-7645-4233-8
- Controlling Cholesterol For Dummies
  0-7645-5440-9
- Depression For Dummies
  0-7645-3900-0
- Dieting For Dummies
  0-7645-4149-8
- Fertility For Dummies
  0-7645-2549-2

- Fibromyalgia For Dummies
  0-7645-5441-7
- Improving Your Memory For Dummies
  0-7645-5435-2
- Pregnancy For Dummies †
  0-7645-4483-7
- Quitting Smoking For Dummies
  0-7645-2629-4
- Relationships For Dummies
  0-7645-5384-4
- Thyroid For Dummies
  0-7645-5385-2

UCATION, HISTORY, REFERENCE & TEST PREPARATION

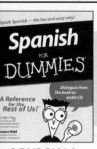

0-7645-5194-9

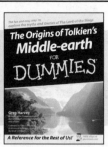

0-7645-4186-2

Also available:

- Algebra For Dummies
  0-7645-5325-9
- British History For Dummies
  0-7645-7021-8
- Calculus For Dummies
  0-7645-2498-4
- English Grammar For Dummies
  0-7645-5322-4
- Forensics For Dummies
  0-7645-5580-4
- The GMAT For Dummies
  0-7645-5251-1
- Inglés Para Dummies
  0-7645-5427-1

- Italian For Dummies
  0-7645-5196-5
- Latin For Dummies
  0-7645-5431-X
- Lewis & Clark For Dummies
  0-7645-2545-X
- Research Papers For Dummies
  0-7645-5426-3
- The SAT I For Dummies
  0-7645-7193-1
- Science Fair Projects For Dummies
  0-7645-5460-3
- U.S. History For Dummies
  0-7645-5249-X

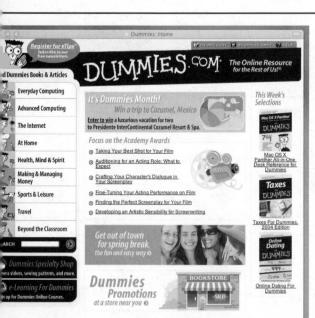

Get smart @ dummies.com®

- **Find a full list of Dummies titles**
- **Look into loads of FREE on-site articles**
- **Sign up for FREE eTips e-mailed to you weekly**
- **See what other products carry the Dummies name**
- **Shop directly from the Dummies bookstore**
- **Enter to win new prizes every month!**

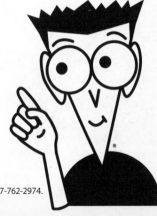

parate Canadian edition also available
parate U.K. edition also available

lable wherever books are sold. For more information or to order direct: U.S. customers visit www.dummies.com or call 1-877-762-2974.
customers visit www.wileyeurope.com or call 0800 243407. Canadian customers visit www.wiley.ca or call 1-800-567-4797.

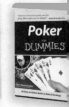
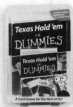
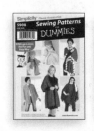
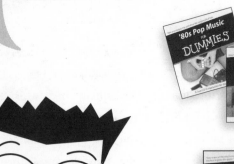
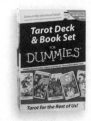
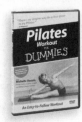
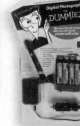
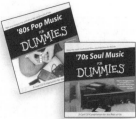
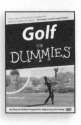
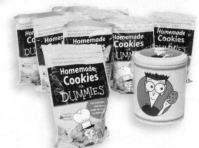
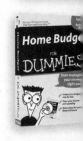